Ultrasound

MEDICAL APPLICATIONS, BIOLOGICAL EFFECTS, AND HAZARD POTENTIAL

Ultrasound

MEDICAL APPLICATIONS, BIOLOGICAL EFFECTS, AND HAZARD POTENTIAL

Edited by

M. H. Repacholi

Royal Adelaide Hospital
Adelaide, South Australia

M. Grandolfo

Superior Institute of Health
Rome, Italy

and

A. Rindi

National Institute of Nuclear Physics
Frascati, Italy

Plenum Press • New York and London

Library of Congress Cataloging in Publication Data

International School of Radiation Damage and Protection (6th:1985: Erice, Sicily)
  Ultrasound: medical applications, biological effects, and hazard potential.

  "Proceedings of the Sixth Course of the International School of Radiation Damage
and Protection on Advances in Biological Effects and Dosimetry of Ultrasound, held
September 6–15, 1985, at the Ettore Majorana Center for Scientific Culture, Erice,
Sicily, Italy"—T.p. verso.
  Bibliography: p.
  Includes index.
  1. Ultrasonic waves—Physiological effect—Congresses. 2. Ultrasonic waves—
Toxicology—Congresses. 3. Ultrasonics in medicine—Congresses. I. Repacholi,
Michael H. II. Grandolfo, Martino. III. Rindi, Alessandro. IV. Title.
QP82.2.U37I55 1985   616.07'543   86-22705
ISBN-13: 978-1-4612-9013-1   e-ISBN-13: 978-1-4613-1811-8
DOI: 10.1007/ 978-1-4613-1811-8

Proceedings of the sixth course of the International School of Radiation Damage
and Protection, on Advances in Biological Effects and Dosimetry of Ultrasound, held
September 6–15, 1985, at the Ettore Majorana Center for Scientific Culture,
Erice, Sicily, Italy

© 1987 Plenum Press, New York
Softcover reprint of the hardcover 1st edition 1987
A Division of Plenum Publishing Corporation
233 Spring Street, New York, N.Y. 10013

To
BETTY-JO, GABRIELLA, and ROSELLA

PREFACE

This volume contains the lectures presented at the International School of Radiation Damage and Protection at the "Ettore Majorana" Centre for Scientific Culture in Erice, Italy, September 6-15, 1985. The sixth course of the School, entitled "Advances in Applications, Biological Effects, and Dosimetry of Ultrasound," provided an in-depth review of all facets of ultrasound interactions and their biological effects on living systems, allowing an assessment of the hazard potential of the various applications of ultrasound. Particular reference was made to possible health risks associated with medical ultrasound exposure since this use is by far the most prevalent.

Since the initial application of ultrasound to submarine detection, medical diagnostic and therapeutic applications have become predominant over the past 20 years. The question of safety of this physical agent is an extremely important one. In many industrialized countries most pregnant women receive at least one diagnostic ultrasound examination before the birth of the child. Thus, potential hazards to the fetus are of prime concern. This problem has been aggravated by the fact that the medical diagnostic applications of ultrasound have far outpaced research efforts on biological effects. A further compounding factor of concern to clinicians and scientists has been the use of higher and higher intensities by the manufacturers of ultrasound equipment, particularly higher peak pulse intensities.

Low average intensities combined with higher peak pulse intensities increase the possibility that biological effects in vivo could occur via a nonthermal mechanism. The search for cavitational and nonthermal, noncavitational interaction mechanisms in vivo is a particularly difficult one since adequate research techniques to identify these mechanisms and effects have yet to be established.

The papers in this book were organized to give descriptions of the characteristics of ultrasonic fields, detection principles, interaction mechanisms, and biological effects ranging from in vitro cell systems to human studies. Ultrasound standards and safety guidelines are summarized. Particular attention was given to the many diagnostic and therapeutic applications of ultrasound, to provide an appreciation of the present and future uses of medical ultrasound and the intensities they employ.

This text is addressed to workers in the field of medical ultrasound, both clinical and technical support personnel, and to scientists in universities, research organizations, and government institutions. Students will also find that this text provides a comprehensive overview of the bioeffects research field.

Michael H. Repacholi
Martino Grandolfo
Alessandro Rindi

April, 1986

ACKNOWLEDGEMENTS

    We are indebted to the: Italian Association of Radiation Protection, Italian Ministry of Education, Italian Ministry of Scientific and Technological Research, Istituto Superiore di Sanità, Sicilian Regional Government and Siemens Medical System for sponsoring the Course.
    We acknowledge with appreciation the cooperation and contributions of: Michelina Guarna and staff of the Royal Adelaide Hospital, South Australia, Mrs.Franca Grisanti and Mr.Giacomo Monteleone of the Istituto Superiore di Sanità, Rome, Italy, and Dr.Alberto Gabriele and Miss Pinola Savalli of the E.Majorana Center in Erice, Italy.

CONTENTS

HISTORICAL OVERVIEW

Wesley L. Nyborg

Physics Department
University of Vermont
Burlington, Vermont 05405   USA

In this lecture my aim is to trace the development of some basic ideas and applications relating to biological effects of ultrasound, and of methods for characterizing exposure. Only a part of the subject can be treated here. Excellent sources for further reading include books by El'piner (1964), Dunn and O'Brien (1976) and Wells (1977), and also a review paper by Fry (1979).

THE PERIOD 1927 - 1930

Systematic studies of physical, chemical and biological changes produced by ultrasound began with the aid of technologies and devices which were developed early in the 1900's: vacuum tube electronics pioneered by Lee de Forest, and piezoelectric transducers based on principles discovered by Pierre Curie. An early publication is by Wood and Loomis (1927); they used equipment based on the circuit shown in Fig. 1. Using a two kilowatt oscillator, a bank of oil condensers, and a number of large coils, voltages up to 50,000 were applied to the quartz transducer, which rested on a sheet of lead at the bottom of a dish containing transformer oil. By using quartz discs of different thicknessess, ultrasound was generated in the oil bath at frequencies from 100 to 700 kHz. The ultrasound was communicated to various objects of interest by bringing these into contact with the oil.

Wood and Loomis created considerable scientific excitement by the findings reported in their 1927 paper, which they termed "a preliminary survey of what appears to be a wide field for investigation." Among the phenomena they reported are:
Radiation pressure.
When exerted against the free surface of the oil a mound appeared, with height as much as 7 cm, the "summit erupting oil drops like a minature volcano." When exerted against a glass disk (Fig. 2) the force was sufficient to "support a weight of 150 grams."

1

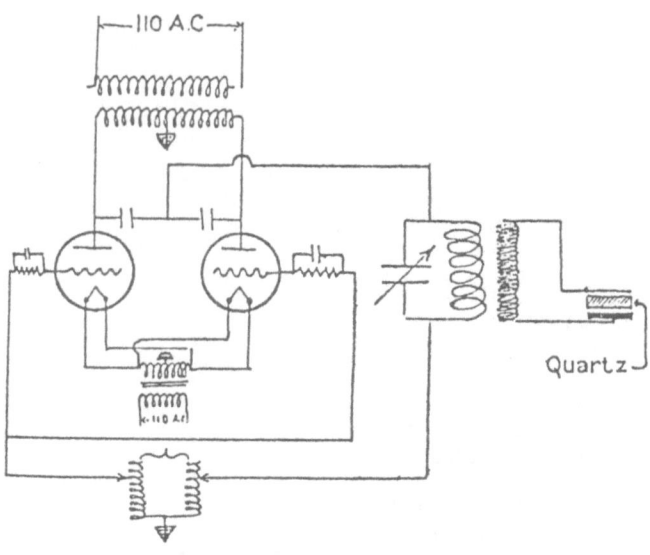

Fig. 1. Oscillator used by Wood and Loomis (1927).

Emulsification
   When two non-miscible liquids such as oil and
   water were simultaneously subjected to ultrasound
   (in a beaker lowered into the oil bath) a colloidal
   suspension was formed.
Atomization
   When a beaker containing benzol was lowered into the
   oil, the beaker filled "rapidly with a cloud of
   white smoke, a benzol fog, the surface of which
   was in tumultuous motion."
Flocculation
   Under some conditions ultrasound caused small particles in suspension to rush together, forming clusters.
Biological effects
   Filaments of spirogyra in suspension were torn to
   pieces and the cells ruptured. Also red cells in
   saline were rapidly destroyed. Paramecia "were
   rendered immobile by a short treatment to vibration
   of moderate intensity, subsequently recovering, but
   were killed by a longer exposure, many of them being
   torn open." Small fish and frogs were killed by an
   exposure of one or two minutes while mice were not
   killed, but temporarily immobilized, after an exposure of 20 minutes. The cause of death was not
   determined but heating was considered possible.

   The Wood-Loomis work was quickly followed by one involving collaboration between Harvey and Loomis (1928). They
devised an arrangement whereby biological cells could be observed under a high-power microscope while being subjected to
ultrasound. This was done by mounting a quartz disk on the
microscope stage, with suitable provision for applying a
driving voltage at the required frequency (400 kHz). Their
observations included the following:

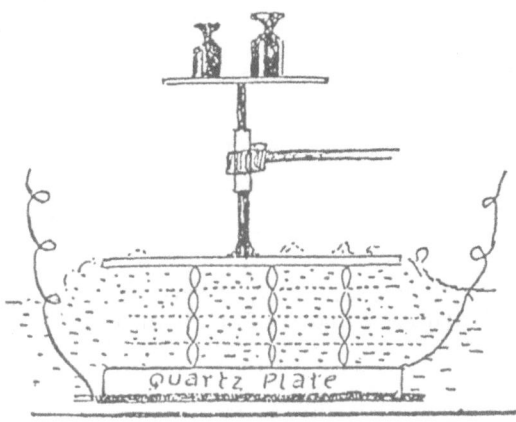

quartz plate

Fig. 2. Arrangement used by Wood and Loomis (1927) to
demonstrate radiation pressure.

Rotation of oil droplets
When an emulsion of oil was viewed a particular
droplet was singled out for observation. It could
be "made to rotate rapidly in either direction at
speeds that could be accurately controlled by
varying slightly the frequency of the oscillating
circuit."
Intracellular stirring
In a leaf of Elodea the protoplasm was observed to
rotate at a speed which increased as the voltage to
the quartz increased. Related intracellular motion
was observed in Nitella and moss cells. The authors
concluded that the "stirring of the cell contents is
one of the most characteristic effects of ultrasonics ".

While Wood, Loomis and Harvey were proceeding with their
investigations in the Eastern United States (Loomis Laboratories in New York, and Princeton University in New Jersey)
Schmitt and co-workers were taking up ultrasound studies in
the West (University of California at Berkeley). Schmitt
(1929) used the arrangement in Fig. 3 for applying ultrasound
locally to individual amoeba and marine eggs while observing
results through a microscope. Ultrasound could be transmitted
from the quartz source to a pyrex tube which had been bent and
drawn down to accommodate a quartz microneedle; the latter
could be manipulated into contact with an individual cell and
set into ultrasonic vibration. The needle vibration was complicated, being partly transverse and partly longitudinal, but
interesting findings were made for two kinds of cells:
Amoebae
Vibration of the needle internal to an amoeba
caused rotation of the granules, whose speed could
be controlled by adjusting the equipment. Even
violent churning of the protoplasm did not immediately hinder amoeboid movement although the protoplasm became coagulated, and death occurred, after a
lengthy period of severe treatment.

3

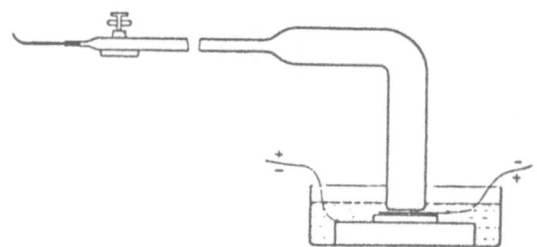

Fig. 3. Arrangement used by Schmitt (1929) for local-
         ized application of ultrasound.

Marine eggs
    When the needle was inserted into the cytoplasm and
    caused to vibrate, the neighboring protoplasmic
    granules rotated about the needle; also the
    nucleolus (which was remote from the needle) moved
    about within the nucleus, following an elliptical
    orbit.

    Preliminary studies of chemical changes produced by
ultrasound were carried out by Richards and Loomis (1927),
using the same apparatus as that used by Wood and Loomis (Fig.
1).   Among their findings were the following:
    Degassing
        A flask of water previously saturated with air be-
        came filled with bubbles of gas when radiated with
        ultrasound. At the same time the temperature of the
        water increased and its solubility therefore de-
        creased. However, the amount of gas released was
        measured and found to be several times greater than
        the amount expected on the basis of reduced solu-
        bility.

    It was demonstrated by Schmitt, Johnson and Olson (1929)
that some chemical reactions, which occur in liquids, can be
accelerated considerably by ultrasound. They also presented
evidence for the importance of "cavitation", defined here as
activity of gas bubbles, such as those produced by the degassing process described by Richards and Loomis. In doing this
they followed a method which has since been often used by
other investigators:
    Inhibition of cavitation by applied superpressure.
        In experiments where ultrasound was applied to a
        reaction (e.g., the production of iodine from potas-
        sium iodide) in a closed vessel, increased pressure
        was supplied from an oxygen tank. The reaction
        rate increased with increasing pressure up to a
        certain value (several atmospheres), then decreased.
        The ultrasound generated no reaction product at all
        when the super pressure exceeded a critical value,
        equal to about 5 atm.

    Johnson (1929) applied the method just described to ex-
periments in which ultrasound was applied to aqueous suspensions of unicellular organisms, and red blood cells. At
atmospheric pressure "vigorous cavitation of air bubbles was
observed, and 30 seconds of radiation sufficed completely to
disintegrate the organisms." When superpressure up to 4 atm

4

was applied the "effervescence of bubbles of visible size was entirely prevented" and the cells were practically unaffected by the ultrasound. Another method for dealing with gases was also found to be successful:

Inhibition of cavitation by degassing

Exposures were carried out on suspensions of red blood cells from which gases had been removed by evacuation. There was then no appreciable hemolysis. However, when the suspension was resaturated with gas and again exposed to ultrasound considerable hemolysis occurred.

Harvey (1930) reviewed the findings on biological effects of ultrasound, and concluded that these (including the "whirling of protoplasm" and related intracellular disturbances to which he gave much importance) are "simply the expression in cells of more general physical and chemical phenomena in liquid media." He classed these phenomena as follows:

"(1) Heating of media which absorb the waves.
(2) Movement of particles into nodes of standing wave patterns, and radiation pressure.
(3) Flocculation (or movement into large aggregates) of particles above a critical size.
(4) Dispersion at liquid-gas, liquid-liquid and liquid-solid surfaces.
(5) Expulsion of gases or vapors from solution (cavitation)... .
(6) Compression and expansion of media through which sound waves pass... .
(7) Acceleration of chemical reactions."

It can be surmised from the preceding discussion that the period 1927-1930 was one of excitement, in which several groups of investigators set out to explore possibilities for ultrasound, a new field of study. While much has been learned in the half-century that has elapsed since that period, important ideas were put forward then which are still accepted. Also, some of the phenomena which intrigued the early workers are still not fully understood, and continue to present challenges to research workers.

DEVELOPMENT OF IDEAS ON CAVITATION

An example of a topic which was recognized as critical from the beginning and which is still a lively one, is that of the role of gas. Considerable insight came from the physical theory developed by Minnaert (1933), who showed that spherical bubbles of gas in water will execute breathing oscillations in response to a time-varying pressure field. The mathematical analysis used by Minnaert was analogous to that used by physicists to solve problems involving vibrating masses and springs. For the gas bubble the "spring" comes from elasticity of the gas and the "mass" represents inertia presented by the surrounding liquid. He considered relative volume changes in the bubble to be small so that linear conditions prevail. On this basis he showed that the bubble-oscillator is characterized by a resonance frequency, analogous to that for a mass-spring system. Neglecting effects of surface tension (which become important for bubbles in the micron and sub-micron range).

Minnaert's expression for the resonance frequency (f_{res}) is:

$$f_{res} = \frac{(3\gamma P_0/\rho)^{\frac{1}{2}}}{2\pi R_0} \qquad (1)$$

Here γ is the ratio of specific heats for the gas (1.4 for air), P_0 is the prevailing hydrostatic pressure, ρ is the liquid density and R_0 is the equilibrium radius of the bubble. Thus an air bubble of radius 10 μm in water at standard atmospheric pressure has a resonance frequency of 325 kHz. After Minnaert's publication, much attention was given to the dynamics of gas bubbles in acoustic fields, partly because of their effectiveness as scatterers of underwater sound. The expression in Eq. 1 was confirmed experimentally at frequencies up to 100 kHz and beyond. Also, theory for acoustic energy losses associated with vibrating bubbles was developed. An excellent review of knowledge on linear oscillations of spherical gas bubbles was published by Devin (1959).

The theory of Minnaert and successors help considerably in understanding some of the observations reported in the 1927-1930 period. For example, by recognizing that the momentary force on a bubble in a sound field is proportional both to its volume and to the gradient of pressure in the surrounding liquid, interesting conclusions were reached about time-averaged forces and motions. The following conclusions, arrived at from theory, have been confirmed experimentally:

  i) Bubbles smaller than resonance size move toward each other and, in water, coalesce to form large bubbles. This probably explains, in part, the degassing process, reported by Richards and Loomis (1927) and the "expulsion" of gases noted by Harvey (1930). In solutions where the bubbles become coated with organic material they may be prevented from coalescing but will form bubble clusters (foam). This clustering is a form of the "flocculation" noted by Harvey (1930).

  ii) In standing-wave fields where there are maxima and minima of the pressure amplitude, bubbles smaller than resonance size move to the pressure maxima. At a pressure maximum the collected bubbles may coalesce to form larger ones until bubble diameters approach the resonance value. As this occurs the bubbles vibrate with increasing amplitude. Thus the greatest activity occurs at pressure maxima.

On the other hand, bubbles larger than resonance size go to pressure minima, where they are relatively inactive.

Other phenomena, such as acceleration of chemical reactions, which were found in the 1927-1930 investigations to be associated with "cavitation", could not be accounted for by linear theory. Satisfactory explanations came after development of nonlinear equations of motion by Plesset (1949), Noltingk and Neppiras (1950) and Neppiras and Noltingk (1951). Using computational methods the latter investigators found solutions to the nonlinear equation, giving the response of a spherical gas bubble in water to an ambient sound field. Plots of bubble radius versus time showed the possibility of dramatic occurrences. A typical example showed the bubble expanding during an acoustic cycle to a radius somewhat more than twice its original size, then collapsing at an accelerating rate, reaching speeds comparable to the speed of sound in water. During collapse the predicted internal pressure and temperature become very large; however, this highly compressed state lasts only a short time, after which the spherical-bubble theory predicts reexpansion of the bubble. Temperatures up to thousands of degrees Kelvin are predicted when the bubble is most compressed, and it is reasonable to suppose that these momentary high temperatures lead to the observed acceleration of chemical reactions. While details of the theory have not been confirmed experimentally, its main features have received wide acceptance.

Much has been learned about cavitation and its biophysical significance since the early studies. A review covering the literature up to about 1975 was prepared by Coakley and Nyborg (1978). Important advances have occurred since that time, which are discussed in the lecture by Professor Carstensen.

RADIATION FORCE, ACOUSTIC STREAMING AND RELATED TOPICS

The arrangement used by Wood and Loomis (Fig. 2) was the forerunner of important methods for measuring the acoustic output characteristics of ultrasonic devices. For example, in one method an ultrasonic beam passes through water and impinges on a sheet of material which absorbs essentially all of the acoustic energy. A force is then exerted on the sheet equal to the total acoustic power divided by the velocity of sound in water. Thus a total power of 1 mW leads to a force of 68 g, which can be measured with a sensitive balance if care is taken to avoid disturbances. (Rooney, 1973). Another method depends on measuring the radiation force exerted on a small steel sphere; this force is proportional to the intensity at the location of the sphere, and thus provides a means of measuring local intensity. (Dunn and Fry, 1972). The use of radiation force methods in characterizing ultrasound fields is discussed further by Dr. Giese.

Mathematically, the theory of radiation force is a topic in nonlinear acoustics, treated as a second-order approximation (one step beyond linear theory). Examples of second-order phenomena were treated by Raleigh (1945) in his classic treatise, first published in 1877. Another second-order phenomenon is "radiation torque", a time-averaged torque exerted on objects in a sound field, causing them to rotate. Still another is "acoustic streaming" a steady circulatory or eddying motion set up by sound in a fluid.

Knowledge of second-order acoustics helps considerably in reaching an understanding of some of the findings reported in the 1927-1930 period.

Thus the movement of particles into positions in standing wave patterns, mentioned by Harvey (1930), is according to theory for radiation forces on small particles. The rotation of oil drops noted by Harvey and Loomis (1928) and the rotations of intracellular granules reported by Schmitt (1929) are apparently caused by radiation torque. Examples of small-scale acoustic streaming are seen in the intracellular stirring and whirling movements reported by Harvey and Loomis (1928) and by Schmitt (1929).

Ultrasonically induced intracellular stirring was studied by Dyer (1972) in an interesting way. He applied ultrasound locally to the boundary of moss protonema while cell division was occurring, thus setting the incipient cross wall into steady rotation. After this treatment he found that cell division proceeded in a number of instances, but that the daughter cells and their progeny were abnormal, the abnormality persisting throughout a series of cultures.

Investigations of biophysical applications of second-order phenomena continue to the present time. Some aspects of the subject are treated in reviews by Nyborg (1978, 1982). The topic is treated further by Dr. ter Haar in one of her lectures.

HEATING; PHYSICAL THERAPY

In the list given by Harvey (1930) of physical and chemical phenomena associated with ultrasound, the first item is "heating of media which absorb the waves." The heating process was recognized very early as a means of characterizing the acoustic output of a device. If the ultrasound beam from the device is passed into a medium where it is completely absorbed, the total heat generated (expressed in appropriate units) per unit time is just equal to the total acoustic power. Thus calorimetric measurements lead to a determination of output power; this general approach, suitably refined, is the basis of standard methods in use today.

That ultrasound produces heating in tissues was soon recognized as useful for applications to physical therapy (Pohlman et al., 1939). Contemporary usage has been reviewed by Lehmann et al. (1978), by Lehman (1982), by Stewart, et al. (1982), and by Dyson (1985). Dyson shows that in some applications the mechanism for therapeutic action of ultrasound is nonthermal. The present status of knowledge on therapeutic applications is discussed in a lecture by Dr. ter Haar.

FOCUSED ULTRASOUND

Perhaps the first biological use of focused ultrasound was by Lynn et al. (1942). These authors used the method of Gruetzmacher (1935) who showed that focusing could be achieved by using as source a quartz crystal which had been ground to a concave shape. The arrangement used by Lynn and co-workers is shown in Fig. 4. They applied the ultrasound in short bursts to blocks of paraffin and beef liver (through a water path), showing that localized regions of altered medium occurred "instantaneously" near the focus. Applications of focused ultrasound to the brain of cats, dogs and monkeys (Lynn and Putman, 1944) led to the formation of lesions in the brain, but were accompanied by injury to the skin and soft tissues overlying the brain.

Starting in the late 1940's an intensive effort was launched at the University of Illinois by W. J. Fry and co-workers to use focused ultrasound as a tool for investigating the central nervous system. In exposing the brain a part of the skull cap was removed, to avoid problems experienced by

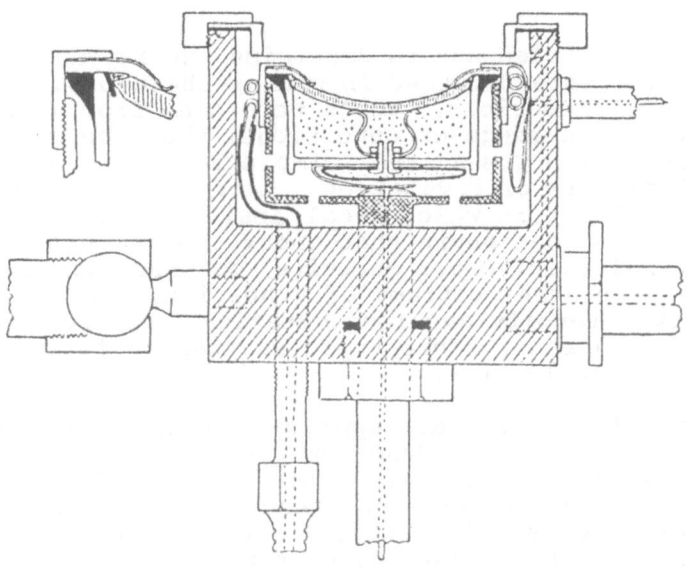

Fig. 4. Focused ultrasound generator used by Lynn et
        al. (1942)

Lynn and Putnam (1944), and to improve acoustic coupling. As
described in a review by W. J. Fry (1958), the desired localization was accomplished by using four separate focusing
transducers (Fig. 5). These were adjusted so that their foci
were coincident and so that their pressure fields were in
phase at the common focus.

     Techniques employing miniature thermocouples were devel-
oped for characterizing the focused fields. Systematic

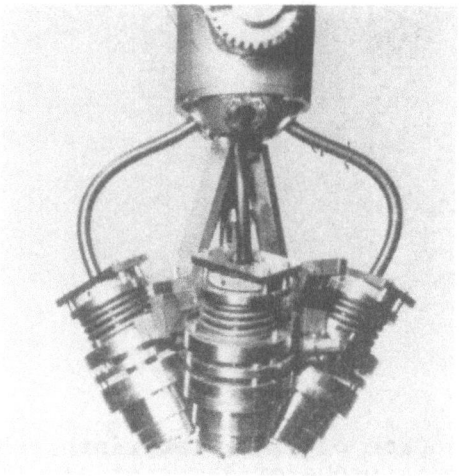

Fig. 5. Multibeam focusing arrangement. From W. J. Fry
        (1958) with permission of the publisher.

studies were carried out to determine the intensity levels at which lesions were produced in brain; these proved to be accurately reproducible. Tests were done from which it was concluded, for a range of conditions, that the mechanism for lesion production was neither simple temperature elevation nor any familiar form of cavitation. Later work, by the Illinois group and others, in which focal lesions were produced in various organs, has shown that under special conditions (high-intensity pulses of short duration) destructive cavitation occurs; at the other extreme of conditions (pulses of relatively low intensity and long duration) the mechanism has been found to be thermal. This topic is treated further by Dr. Williams in his lecture.

In the last few years applications have been made of the fact that focused ultrasound can create heat in a designated small region remote from the source. Lele (1985) has described techniques for treating cancer with controlled hyperthermia created by using steered beams of focused ultrasound. He will be discussing the topic of ultrasonic hyperthermia in one of his lectures.

ULTRASONIC TREATMENT OF MENIERE'S DISEASE

Meniere's disease is a disorder of the middle ear which results in attacks of vertigo and, if untreated, often leads to complete loss of hearing. In 1952 Arslan began applications of ultrasound to this disease; he later published a review of his findings (Arslan, 1965). In 1960 James and co-workers developed an improved method for applying 3 MHz ultrasound to bone over the semicircular canal together with effective water cooling. (Fig. 6). Gratifying results were obtained (James, 1963). Ultrasonic methods for treating Meniere's disease are now in routine use, though developments have taken place in the procedures used, and although the mechanisms of action are still not established. (Wells, 1977).

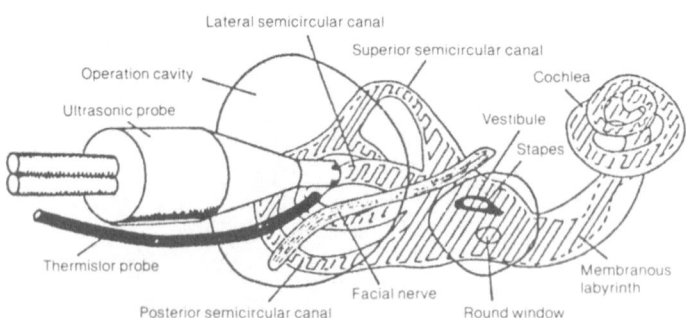

Fig. 6. Diagram of right labyrinth, showing the ultrasonic probe of James et al. (1963) in position for irradiating the lateral semicircular canal. From Wells (1977) with permission of the author and publisher.

REFERENCE

Arslan, M. and Sala, O., 1965, Chapter 11. Action of ultrasound on the internal ear, in "Ultrasonic Energy," E. Kelly, ed., University of Illinois Press, Urbana.

Coakley, W. T. and Nyborg, W. L., 1978, Chapter II. Cavitation; dynamics of gas bubbles; applications, in "Ultrasound: Its Applications in Medicine and Biology," F. J. Fry, ed., Elsevier Scientific Publishing Co., Amsterdam.

Devin, C., Jr., 1959, Survey of thermal, radiation, and viscous damping of pulsating air bubbles in water, J. Acoust. Soc. Am., 31:1654.

Dunn, F. and Fry, F. J., 1972, Ultrasonic field measurement using the suspended ball radiometer and thermocouple probe, in "Interaction of Ultrasound and Biological Tissues," J. R. Reid and M. R. Sikov, eds., DHEW Publication (FDA) 73-8008, Food and Drug Adminstration, Rockville, MD.

Dunn, F. and O'Brien, W. D., 1976, "Ultrasonic Biophysics," Dowden, Hutchinson and Ross, Inc., Stroudsburg, Pennsylvania, USA.

Dyer, H. J., 1972, Structural effects of ultrasound on the cell, in "Interaction of Ultrasound and Biological Tissues", J. R. Reid and M. R. Sikov, eds, DHEW Publication (FDA) 738008, Food and Drug Adminstration, Rockville, MD.

Dyson, M., 1985, Chapter 11. Therapeutic applications of ultrasound, in "Biological Effects of Ultrasound," W. L. Nyborg and M. C. Ziskin, eds., Churchill Livingstone, New York.

El'piner, I. E., 1964, "Ultrasound; Physical, Chemical and Biological Effects", Consultants Bureau, New York.

Fry, F. J., 1979, Biological effects of ultrasound--a review, Proc. IEEE, 67:604.

Fry, W. J., 1958, Intense ultrasound investigations of the central nervous sytem, in "Advances in Biological and Medical Physics", C. A. Tobias and J. H. Lawrence, eds., Academic Press Inc., New York.

Gruetzmacher, J., 1935, Piezoelektrischer kristall mit ultraschallkonvergenz, Ztschr. f. physik, 96:342.

Harvey, E. N., 1930, Biological aspects of ultrasonic waves, a general survey, Biol. Bull. 59:306.

Harvey, E. N. and Loomis, A. L., 1928, High frequency sound waves of small intensity and their biological effects, Nature, 121:622.

James, J. A., 1963, New developments in the ultrasonic therapy of Meniere's disease, Ann. R. Coll. Surg. Engl. 33:226.

Johnson, C. H., 1929, The lethal effects of ultrasonic radiation, Jour. Physiol., 67:356.

Lehman, J. F., 1982, "Therapeutic Heat and Cold," 3rd Edition, Williams and Wilkins, Baltimore.

Lehmann, J. F., Warren C. G. and Guy, A. W., 1978, Chapter X. Therapy with continuous wave ultrasound, in "Ultrasound: Its Applications in Medicine and Biology", F. J. Fry, ed., Elsevier Scientific Publishing Co., Amsterdam.

Lele, P. P., 1985, Chapter 12. Local hyperthermia by ultrasound for cancer therapy, in "Biological Effects of Ultrasound", W. L. Nyborg and M. C. Ziskin, eds., Churchill Livingstone, New York.

Lynn, J. G. and Putnam, T. J., 1944, Histology of cerebral lesions produced by focused ultrasound, Amer. J. Path. 20, 637.

Lynn, J. G., Zwemer, R. L., Chick, A. J. and Miller, A. E.,
    1942, A new method for the generation and use of focused
    ultrasound in experimental biology, J. Gen. Physiol.,
    26:179.
Minnaert, M., 1933, On musical air-bubbles and the sound of
    running water, Phil. Mag. (Series 7), 16:235.
Neppiras, E. A. and Noltingk, B. E., 1951, Cavitation produced
    by ultrasonics: theoretical conditions for the onset of
    cavitation, Proc. Phys. Soc. B (London), 64B:1032.
Noltingk, B. E. and Neppiras, E. A., 1950, Cavitation produced
    by ultrasonics, Proc. Phys. Soc. B (London), 63B:674.
Nyborg, W. L., 1978, Chapter 1. Physical principles of ultra-
    sound, in "Ultrasound: Its Application in Medicine and
    Biology", F. J. Fry, ed., Elsevier Scientific Publishing
    Co., Amsterdam.
Nyborg, W. L., 1982, Chapter 2. Biophysical mechanisms of
    ultrasound, in "Essentials of Medical Ultrasound," M. H.
    Repacholi and D. A. Benwell, eds., The Humana Press,
    Inc., Clifton, NJ 07015.
Plesset, M. S., 1949, The dynamics of cavitation bubbles, J.
    Appl. Mech., 16:277.
Pohlman, R., Richter, R., and Parow, E., 1939, Uber die
    Ausbreitung und Absorption des Ultraschalls in Menschlic-
    hen gewebe und seine therapeutisch Wirkung an ischias
    und Plerusneuralgia, Deutsch. Med. Wischr., 65:251.
Rayleigh, J. W. S., 1945, "The Theory of Sound," Dover Publi-
    cation, Inc., New York.
Richards, W. T. and Loomis, A. L., 1927, The chemical effects
    of high frequency sound waves. I. A preliminary survey,
    J. Am. Chem. Soc., 49:3086.
Rooney, J. A., 1973, Determination of acoustic power outputs
    the microwatt-milliwatt range, Ultrasound in Med. &
    Biol., 1:13.
Schmitt, F. O., 1929, Ultrasonic micromanipulation, Protoplas-
    ma, 7:332.
Schmitt, F. O., Johnson, C. H. and Olson, A. R., 1929, Oxida-
    tions promoted by ultrasonic radiation, J. Am. Chem.
    Soc., 51:370.
Stewart, H. F., Repacholi, M. H. and Benwell, D. A., 1982,
    Chapter 6. Ultrasound therapy, in "Essentials of Medi-
    cal Ultrasound", M. H. Repacholi and D. A. Benwell, eds.,
    The Humana Press Inc., Clifton, NJ 07015.
Wells, P.N.T., 1977, "Biomedical Ultrasonics", Academic Press,
    London.
Wood, R. W. and Loomis, A. L., 1927, The physical and biologi-
    cal effects of high-frequency sound-waves of great inten-
    sity, Phil. Mag. (Series 7), 4:417.

FUNDAMENTALS OF ACOUSTIC WAVE THEORY

Martino Grandolfo and Paolo Vecchia

Physics Laboratory, Istituto Superiore di Sanità

00161 Rome, Italy

SOUND WAVES

Ultrasound radiation, which is included among Non-Ionizing Radiation (NIR) with electromagnetic radiations such as radiofrequency,microwaves, visible light etc., differs from these because of its mechanical nature. Sound waves are produced as a result of disturbances taking place in a material medium: these disturbances cause the particles from which the medium is formed to be set into vibration. The vibration of particles is an essential characteristic of acoustic propagation and, for this reason, it is impossible for sound to travel through a vacuum.

Sound propagates in waves, or disturbances whose amplitude varies with space and time according to the wave equation. For a displacement u of a particle this equation takes, in the simplest case (one dimension), the following form:

$$\frac{d^2 u}{dx^2} = \frac{1}{c} \frac{d^2 u}{dt^2} \qquad (1)$$

It could be shown that eq.(1) is satisfied by a whole class of solutions, namely by any function having an argument x+ct or x-ct, i.e.:

$$f(x+ct) \qquad \text{or} \qquad f(x-ct) \qquad (2)$$

or any linear combination of such functions. The parameter c represents the propagation speed of the wave. $f(x_0, t_0)$, the function at a given point x_0 and time t_0, takes the same value at a later time $t_0 + \Delta t$ in a point $x_0 + \Delta x$, where $\Delta x = \pm c \Delta t$ (the sign depending on the propagation direction).

Of all possible solutions of a form given in (2), periodic functions have special importance from a practical point of view. Consideration is limited to sinusoidal functions without any loss of generality because any periodic function can be expressed as a suitable combination of sinusoidal functions, through an analytical technique known as Fourier analysis.

Consider the following special solution of eq.(1):

$$u(x,t) = u_o \sin k(x-ct) \qquad\qquad (3)$$

representing a harmonic oscillation of amplitude u_0 ; k is called wave number, and $\lambda = 2\pi/k$ is the wavelength. It is possible to obtain directly from eq.(3) the well known expressions relating to the oscillation period T and frequency f:

$$T = \lambda/c \qquad\qquad f = c/\lambda \qquad\qquad (4)$$

Thus a sinusoidal wave is fully characterized by three independent parameters: propagation speed, frequency and amplitude. In the following paragraphs is more detail on the meaning of each of these quantities for sound waves.

CHARACTERISTICS OF SOUND

The transmission of sound consists of an ordered and periodical movement of the molecules of a medium, which may be solid, liquid, or gas. As a consequence of an external perturbation, a number of molecules oscillate in phase, thus transmitting their kinetic energy to neighboring molecules. In this way, energy is transferred from one molecule to another, with no associated transfer of matter. The direction of energy propagation may be parallel or perpendicular to the direction of oscillation of the particles; the corresponding waves are termed longitudinal and transverse, respectively.

Transverse waves are especially important in solids, but other waves such as shear waves, torsion waves, flexural (or Lamb) waves, surface Rayleigh waves, and Love waves also exist. Among these, only shear waves, also called rotational waves, are of interest in ultrasonics. Transverse waves travel only through solids, because liquids and gases do not support shear stresses under normal conditions.

Longitudinal waves on the contrary can pass through all types of media and are more important with regard to interactions with biological systems. In longitudinal waves, the collective motion of particles creates alternate regions of compression and rarefaction, i.e. a periodical pressure variation. This variation has the same propagation speed and frequency of oscillations of particles. The sound wave can therefore be described in terms of the pressure p:

$$p(x,t) = p_0 \sin k(x-t) \qquad\qquad (5)$$

Eq.(5) does not give the absolute value of pressure at a given point; it gives the time varying pressure term responsible for the sound, to which the imperturbed pressure should always be added in order to obtain the total pressure value. The following paragraphs address this varying term, which is called acoustic pressure.

It is important to point out that eq.(5) represents a special case of vibration, namely a wave propagating in one direction from a source (assumed to be a point). In practice, a sound wave is emitted from an extended source radiating energy in all directions, and the distribution pattern may be quite complex.

In principle, the problem of an extended source of finite dimensions could be solved by considering it as the sum of a large number of point sources, each emitting waves in all directions with the same intensity.

Such waves, radiating isotropically in space, are called spherical waves and are mathematically described by an equation similar to eq.(5), but in three dimensions:

$$\frac{\partial^2 p}{\partial x^2} + \frac{\partial^2 p}{\partial y^2} + \frac{\partial^2 p}{\partial z^2} = \frac{1}{c^2} \frac{\partial^2 p}{\partial t^2} \qquad (6)$$

For the symmetry, any solution of eq.(6) will be given by a function taking the same value in all points at the same distance from the source. If r is the radius of the surface of a sphere which is the locus of these points, the sinusoidal solution is:

$$p(r,t) = p_0 \sin k(r-ct) \qquad (7)$$

The direction of the radius r changes from point to point on the spherical surface. For large distances from the source (compared to the sound beam wavelength), the propagation axes may be considered to be parallel for all waves within a given region. This corresponds to replacing a portion of spherical surface with a plane and to approximating molecular vibrations with parallel oscillations, called plane waves. In practice, the plane wave approximation is applicable when the distance between wavefront and source is much greater than the wavelength.

Summing the contributions from point sources is simple in principle, but in practice the overlapping of a virtually infinite number of spherical waves may give rise to enormous mathematical difficulties. How to manage the problem of sources of finite dimensions will discussed later in more detail. However, if the distance of the wavefront from the source is large enough, the latter may be considered a point.

Let us now consider in more detail the parameters which characterize a sound wave, namely its propagation speed, frequency and amplitude.

a. Propagation speed

The propagation speed of sound in a medium depends on the physical properties of the medium itself. For longitudinal waves, the following relations:

$$c = \sqrt{\gamma p / \rho} \qquad\qquad c = \sqrt{1/\beta\rho} \qquad (8)$$

express the propagation speed in gases and in liquids, respectively, where $\gamma = C_p/C_v$ is the ratio of specific heats at constant pressure and volume, β is the liquid compressibility, and ρ is the density of the medium.

In solids, the sound speed is:

$$c = \sqrt{\frac{E}{\rho} \frac{1-\nu}{(1+\nu)(1-2\nu)}} \qquad\qquad c = \sqrt{G/\rho} \qquad (9)$$

for longitudinal and transverse waves, respectively. Here, E is the Young's modulus for the medium, G is the rigidity modulus, and ν is the Poisson's ratio, i.e. the ratio of the transverse contracting strain to the elongation strain (typical values range from 0.2 to 0.5). In a solid rod with cross-sectional dimensions considerably smaller than the wavelength the transverse strain may be neglected, and the first of eqs.(9) reduces to:

$$c = \sqrt{E/\rho} \qquad (10)$$

Because both the density and the elastic moduli vary with the tempe-

15

rature, the sound speed will also vary, generally increasing with increasing temperature.

The speed of sound in solids is higher than in liquids, and very much higher than in gases. Table 1 gives the approximate values of the acoustic speed of some commonly used materials.

Table 1. Approximate values of the acoustic speed (m/s) of some materials at room temperature and standard pressure

Material	Longitudinal waves	Transverse waves
Aluminium	6400	3100
Steel	6000	2900
Copper	4700	2300
Water	1400	--
Hydrogen	1300	--
Air	330	--

It is also seen in the table that, in solids, transverse waves travel at about half the speed of longitudinal waves. These differences in sound speed give rise to noticeable effects at interfaces between different media, such as air and biological tissue.

b. Frequency

Sound waves are divided into infrasound (frequency ranging between 0 and 16-20 Hz), audible sound (from 16-20 Hz to 16-20 kHz) and ultrasound (above 16-20 kHz). The limits are not clearly defined because of the variability in response of the human ear. This distinction is more important from the physiological point of view than the physical description, and this is the reason why one speaks of sound in general rather than of ultrasound in particular.

In optics, light radiation of a single frequency corresponds to a pure colour (called monochromatic); in the same way, a perfectly sinusoidal acoustic wave corresponds to a pure tone. Whereas many sources of monochromatic light do exist, the same is not true for acoustic sources. Sound emitted from a real source results from the overlapping of many vibrations of different frequency, amplitude and duration. To quantitatively describe sound is therefore an extremely complicated task, which can be solved in an approximate way by averaging the different physical quantities over finite intervals of time, space, or frequency.

For practical reasons the whole spectrum of acoustic frequencies is divided into frequency bands. If f_1 and f_2 are the lower and upper limit of each band, the partition into proportional bands occurs where the ratio f_2/f_1 is the same for each band. Limiting frequencies are in a geometric, rather than arithmetic, progression. This criterion allows one to cover an extremely wide frequency range with a limited number of bands and, what is most important, corresponds to the physiological response of the human ear.

According to the geometric progression of frequencies, a centre frequency is defined for each band, as the geometric mean of the limiting frequencies, i.e.:

$$f_0 = (f_1 f_2)^{1/2} \qquad (11)$$

An octave is defined as an interval corresponding to the doubling of frequency. An octave band incorporates those frequencies between f_1 and f_2 where $f_2 = 2f_1$. In a similar manner, a third octave band is characterized by $f_2 = 2^{1/3} f_1$; in general, a n-th octave band is such that $f_2 = 2^{1/n} f_1$. It follows from the above definition that the centre frequency is 1/2n-th octave above f_1 and below f_2:

$$f_2 = 2^{1/2n} f_0 \qquad\qquad f_0 = 2^{1/2n} f_1 \qquad (12)$$

Eqs.(12) show that any proportional frequency band is completely defined by its centre frequency and by n.

c. Amplitude

As mentioned above, a sound wave is described by an equation giving the acoustic pressure as a function of space coordinates and time, so that the distribution of any complex sound is described in terms of a time-varying pressure field. Sound amplitude, or its root mean square, could therefore be measured in pascal. For reasons related to the physiological response of the human ear, sound amplitude is usually expressed through a quantity varying as the logarithm of acoustic pressure. This quantity, defined as:

$$L_p = 10 \log \frac{p^2}{p_{ref}^2} = 20 \log \frac{p}{p_{ref}} \qquad (13)$$

is termed sound pressure level (SPL) and is measured in decibels (dB).

In eq.(13) p is the acoustic pressure, whereas p_{ref} is a reference pressure which must be specified when dealing with absolute levels; the value generally chosen is $20 \, \mu Pa$. However, differences between SPLs are independent of the reference pressure, since:

$$L_{p_2} - L_{p_1} = 10 \log \frac{p_2^2}{p_1^2} \qquad (14)$$

Eq.(14) shows that equal differences between SPLs correspond to equal ratios between sound pressures. For example, a 20 dB difference between two levels corresponds to a ratio of 10 between rms pressures.

ACOUSTIC ENERGY

The propagation of a sound wave corresponds to an energy transfer without a transfer of matter. This can be deduced from the wave equation (5). It is an expression of the energy conservation principle, and may be regarded as the equivalent in acoustics to Poynting's theorem of electromagnetic radiation. If w is the acoustic energy density, i.e. the energy per unit volume, eq.(5) may be expressed as:

$$\frac{\partial w}{\partial t} + \vec{\nabla} \cdot \vec{I} = 0 \qquad (15)$$

where $\vec{I} = p\vec{v}$, and $\vec{v}$ is the velocity of particles.

The vector $\vec{I}$ represents the energy flow per unit time through the unit surface perpendicular to the propagation direction, and is termed acoustic energy flux or, more frequently, acoustic intensity. This quantity is of fundamental importance in acoustics. Using the analogy of other branches of physics, we can define a field as an intermediary in interactions between physical systems (whose properties are functions of the space coordinates and time). The "acoustic field" (or "ultrasonic field", in the case of ultrasound) can be expressed in terms of acoustic intensity.

From the fundamental equations of fluid dynamics, it can be shown that the energy density w is made of two terms:

$$w = \frac{1}{2} \left(\rho\, v^2 + \frac{p^2}{\rho c} \right) \tag{16}$$

the first of which is called the acoustic kinetic energy, the second the acoustic potential energy.

The interpretation of eq.(15) as an energy conservation law is more immediate if it is integrated over a finite volume. If W is the total acoustic energy enclosed in the volume, we obtain:

$$\frac{dW}{dt} = \frac{d}{dt} \int_v w\, dV = - \int_s \vec{I} \cdot \vec{n}\, dS = - \Phi_s (\vec{I}) \tag{17}$$

This shows that the variation of W per unit time equals the flux of vector $\vec{I}$ through the external surface ($\vec{n}$ is the unit vector outgoing perpendicularly from the surface element dS).

Eq.(15) may be interpreted in terms of another important physical quantity, namely the acoustic power, which is defined as the energy variation per unit time:

$$\mathscr{P} = dW/dt \tag{18}$$

If a volume V encloses a sound source, then the acoustic energy flux through the limiting surface gives the instantaneous power of the source.

Eqs.(15) and (16) become simpler and more meaningful in the case of plane waves. Here the velocity v of particles is related to the sound propagation speed c by the expression:

$$v = p / \rho c \tag{19}$$

and one obtains:

$$\frac{1}{2} \rho v^2 = \frac{1}{2} \frac{p^2}{\rho c^2} = \frac{1}{2} w \qquad\qquad I = cw \tag{20}$$

The first of eqs.(20) states that in a plane wave the kinetic and potential energy are the same, the second that the acoustic energy travels with speed c along the propagation direction.

Units for the acoustic power and intensity are respectively the watt (W) and the watt per square meter (W/m^2). A sound intensity level L_I and a sound power level L_W are also defined, respectively, as:

$$L_I = 10 \log \frac{I}{I_{ref}} \qquad\qquad L_W = 10 \log \frac{W}{W_{ref}} \tag{21}$$

Commonly used reference values are 1 picowatt (1 pW = 10^{-12} W) and 1 picowatt per square meter, respectively.

CONTINUOUS AND PULSED WAVES

An ideal wave, defined by eq.(7), is characterized by a single frequency, fixed amplitude and unlimited duration. Such a wave is called a continuous wave. In reality a wave can be considered continuous when its amplitude variation is lower than a given value (e.g. 5%) and its duration is very long with respect both to its period and to the response time of any interacting system.

Non-continuous waves may be amplitude modulated waves or pulsed waves. In the first case the amplitude varies periodically in time, whereas in the second it periodically goes to zero.

Pulsed waves are characterized by several parameters. The time duration of each pulse is known as the pulse length or pulse width. The pulse repetition period (or pulse period) is the time interval between two consecutive pulses, and the pulse repetition frequency (or pulse frequency) is the number of pulses propagated per second. In general, the pulse period is much longer than the wave period. Finally, the ratio of the pulse width to the pulse period, i.e. the fraction of pulse period where the amplitude differs from zero, is termed the duty cycle, or duty factor.

In order to obtain pulses of finite width, the source must be damped, so that the *oscillations disappear after the required number of waves has* been propagated. As shown in Fig.1, the heavier the damping, the further are the waves from the condition of a pure tone, and the larger is the number of components involved in the Fourier analysis. Therefore, pulsed waves are constituted by oscillations which do not take place at a single frequency, but at frequencies extending over a continuous range, known as the frequency bandwidth. Any increase of the damping results in an increase of the frequency bandwidth.

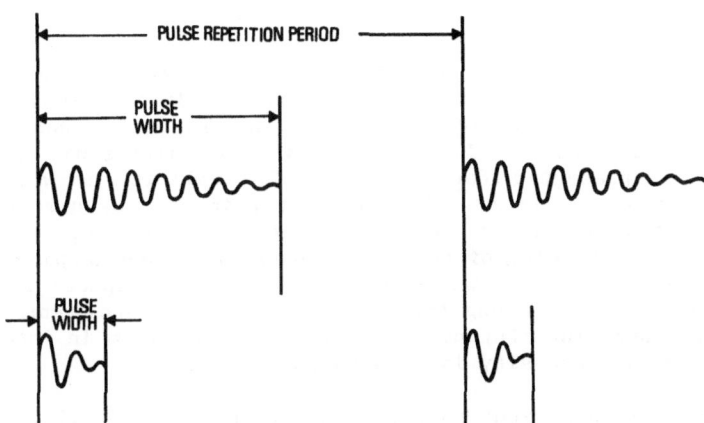

Fig.1 - Example of pulsed waves having the same pulse period, but different dampings.

SOUND PROPAGATION

Since both optics and acoustics deal with wave propagation, the corresponding physical laws are in many respects analogous. Some differences exist which are related to the different nature of physical systems and to the wavelength (for sound it is several orders of magnitude longer than for light). The latter is responsible for the fact that in acoustics the concept of "ray", and the "geometric" representation of sound propagation are seldom exploited. It is well known that such representation is satisfactory only when all physical systems interacting with the radiation (obstacles, limiting surfaces, slits) have linear dimensions much greater than the wavelength.

As shown in Table 2, human dimensions are much larger than optical wavelengths, but are comparable with acoustic wavelengths. For ultrasound, the case may occur where the ratio of the dimensions of objects of interest (in particular the human body or its parts) to the wavelength is such that geometric laws are satisfied to first approximation. In this case one can speak in terms of sound rays, or beams, propagating in straight lines and obeying laws similar to those governing geometric optics.

Table 2. Typical wavelengths of some acoustic and optical radiations propagating in air (meters)

Grave tone (audibility limit)	16
Shrill tone (audibility limit)	1.6×10^{-2}
Ultrasound in medicine	$2 \times 10^{-5} - 3 \times 10^{-4}$
Red light	8×10^{-7}
Violet light	3.5×10^{-7}

The propagation of a sound beam may be described rather simply at large distances from the source, but is complex in its proximity because of the finite dimensions of any transducer. To better understand this point, let us consider in some detail the ultrasonic field of a transducer, represented for the sake of simplicity as a cylindrical oscillating piston (Fig.2a). As already mentioned, the ultrasonic field may be described as the overlapping of elemental spherical waves emitted in phase from each point of the piston base. This overlapping gives rise to interference of sound waves in the surrounding space: moving along the piston axis, i.e. along the direction of the sound beam, points are encountered where interference gives rise to a maximum in intensity, and points where the intensity is reduced to zero.

The intensity distribution pattern is as shown in Fig.2b. The position of the last maximum depends on the piston diameter D and on the wavelength through the relation:

$$x = \frac{D^2 - \lambda^2}{4\lambda} \qquad (22)$$

and divides the space into two regions. The one nearer to the source, where interference effects occur, is called the near field, or Fresnel, region; the farther one is called the far field, or Fraunhofer, region.

In the far field region the sound intensity, measured along the propagation axis, attenuates (apart from possible absorption and obstacles) because of the diffraction. This effect causes the sound beam to spread

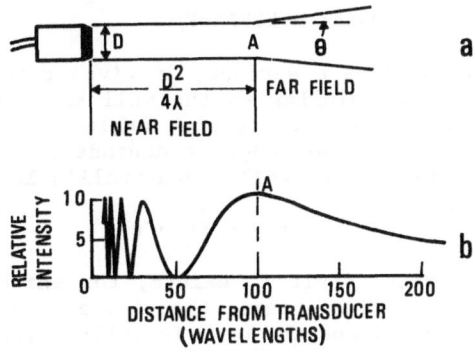

Fig.2 – The ultrasonic field produced by a cylindrical source (a) and its intensity vs.distance (b).

out or diverge; apart from a number of lobes of very much reduced intensity, the main part of the beam travels within a cone whose aperture is called the divergence of the beam. The divergence depends on the diameter of the transducer and on the wavelength through the relationship:

$$\sin \theta = 1.22 \ \lambda /D \qquad (23)$$

Thus if the diameter is small compared to λ , then the waves diverge at very short distance from the source, giving rise to spherical waves. On the other hand, when the diameter of the transducer is a large number of wavelengths, the beam is highly directional and keeps nearly parallel over long distances.

Since the cross-section of a cone is proportional to the square of its height, the beam intensity in the far field attenuates with distance according to the classical inverse-square dependence.

PEAK VALUES AND AVERAGE VALUES

It has been shown that sound intensity, as well as other acoustic quantities, depends on space and time variations, sometimes in a very complicated way. Thus one frequently resorts for practical measurements to space and/or time averaging. One can define and measure a spatial peak intensity I(SP) as the intensity measured along the beam axis or a spatial average intensity I(SA) as the ratio of the total beam power to its area of cross section. With regard to time, one distinguishes between a time peak intensity I(TP) and a time average intensity I(TA); the average is performed over a time interval much greater than the wave or pulse period. In the case of pulsed waves, time average may be referred to a single pulse and the sound intensity is therefore referred to as pulse average intensity I(PA).

In practice one specifies both characteristics for any intensity measurement, indicating for example I(SATA) an intensity averaged over both space and time, or I(SPTA) the time averaged axial peak intensity, etc. When this specification is missing, it is generally assumed a time- and space-averaged intensity, i.e. I(SATA).

REFLECTION AND TRANSMISSION AT A SURFACE

When a sound wave strikes a surface, it gives rise to reflection and refraction phenomena very similar to the well known effects of optical radiation; in particular, the reflection angle r equals the incidence angle i, whereas the refraction angle t depends on the values of sound speed in both media through the well known Snell's law:

$$c_1/\sin i = c_2/\sin t \qquad (24)$$

If $c_2 > c_1$, a critical angle i_c exists, for which t is equal to 90 degrees. For incidence angles greater than i_c, no refracted wave can pass through the second medium, and the beam is fully reflected. The critical angle is immediately deduced from eq.(24):

$$\sin i_c = c_1/c_2 \qquad (25)$$

Since c_1 and c_2 may be significantly different, as in the case of an air-solid interface, total reflection may occur even at small incidence angles.

The extent to which the sound intensity is reflected or transmitted depends on the characteristics of both media: the intensity ratios can be expressed in terms of a quantity characteristic of each medium, which is called acoustic impedance and is defined as:

$$Z = p/v = \rho c \qquad (26)$$

where v and c are the velocity of molecules and the sound propagation speed in the medium, respectively. The acoustic impedance is much greater in liquids than in gases, and even greater in solids, since both the density and the sound speed are progressively greater in the three cases. Some typical values, both of biological and inorganic materials, are listed in Table 3.

Table 3. Acoustic impedance of some materials (kg/ms)

Steel	4.7×10^7
Aluminium	1.7×10^7
Perspex	3.2×10^6
Bone	7.8×10^6
Muscle	1.7×10^6
Water	1.4×10^6
Air	430
Hydrogen	110

At normal incidence, the intensities I_i, I_r and I_t of incident, reflected and transmitted beams are related by the expressions:

$$\frac{I_r}{I_i} = \frac{\cdot(Z_2 - Z_1)^2}{(Z_2 + Z_1)^2} \qquad \frac{I_t}{I_i} = \frac{4\,Z_1 Z_2}{(Z_2 + Z_1)^2} \qquad (27)$$

The reflection is high if the impedances of the two media are very different, and is zero if they are equal. The opposite is true for the transmission. This is especially important in the case of airborne ultrasound beams, which are almost completely reflected by the surface of any solid or liquid. Only about 0.1% of the airborne ultrasound intensity is transmitted into the human body.

The practical importance of eqs.(27) is evident. Impedance matching is needed to transfer energy from a transducer into a medium, in particular into a biological tissue. In practice, good contact between the surfaces of the transducer and of the absorbing body is difficult to achieve, since a layer of air separates them. This results in very little sound energy being transmitted. To overcome this difficulty, a commonly used technique is to insert between the transducer and the body a thin layer of a material with suitable impedance (a gel, oil or water), in order to maximize the energy transfer.

The introduction of a third medium, however, presents some difficulties, and the resultant transmission coefficient may not necessarily be equal to the product of the coefficients for each boundary. Much depends on the thickness of the intervening layer and on the wavelength. If the thickness of the layer is equal to an integer number of half-wavelengths, then sound will be transmitted as though the intervening medium did not exist. This optimum condition is difficult to realize in ultrasound applications because the very short wavelengths require an extremely high degree of precision in determining the layer thickness. Moreover, the transmission does not take place at a single frequency, but over a band of frequencies, which extends to both sides of a centre frequency and may be very wide, especially for pulsed waves. Under these conditions, a perfect coupling is impossible, since a given thickness will be equal to an exact number of half-wavelengths for only one of the frequencies in the band. However, where the frequency band is quite narrow and the impedance of the intervening layer is close to the value of those of the outer media, a departure of not more than one or two decibels from the ideal case my be expected.

A very interesting phenomenon is observed when a beam of longitudinal waves strikes the interface between a fluid and a solid at an oblique angle i. In this case part of the beam is converted into transverse waves, which propagate in the solid. This effect is usually called mode conversion, and may give rise to a double refraction or a double reflection when the incident beam travels in the fluid and in the solid, respectively. In the first case, since in a solid the speed of transverse waves is always less than the speed of longitudinal waves, Snell's law leads to different refraction angles. Referring to Fig.3a, we have:

$$c_1/\sin i = c_2/\sin r = c'_2/\sin r' \qquad (28)$$

Here, the subscripts 1 and 2 refer to the solid and the fluid, respectively, and the prime indicates the transverse waves. Two distinct beams are therefore transmitted into the solid, the longitudinal waves being refracted away from the normal more than the transverse waves. The critical angle is obviously different for either beam. If the incidence angle is greater than the first critical angle i_{c_1}, only transverse waves can pass through the solid. Increasing the incidence angle still further, the second critical angle i_{c_2} is reached, for which the transverse waves are refracted at an angle of 90 degrees: in this case surface waves are

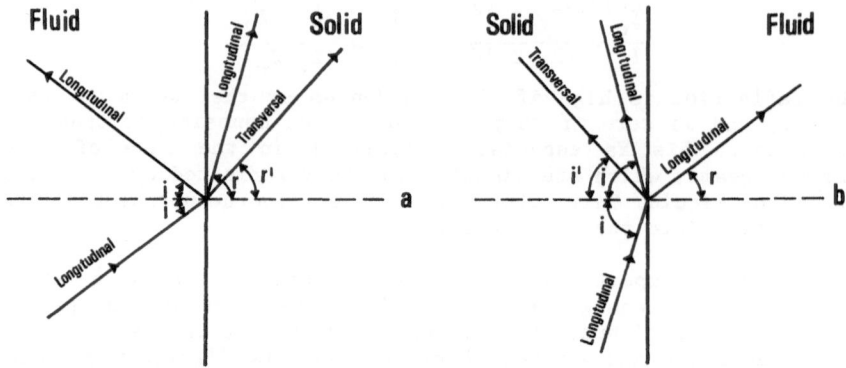

Fig.3 - Mode conversion at a fluid-solid interface. Longitudinal waves are partially converted into transverse waves giving rise to a double refraction (a) or to a double reflection (b).

propagated, whose properties differ from those of bulk waves. For incidence angles more than i_{c2}, no wave propagation in the solid occurs.

In the case of a longitudinal wave travelling in a solid and striking a boundary with a fluid at an incidence angle i, a beam of longitudinal waves passes into the fluid at some angle r to the normal, and two beams are reflected back into the solid (Fig.3b). The incidence, reflection and refraction angles are related in this case by the expressions:

$$c_1/\sin i = c'_1/\sin i' = c_2/\sin r \qquad (29)$$

Because of the different sound speeds, the beam of transverse waves is always closer to the normal than the incident beam.

The phenomena of reflection and refraction are exploited to create acoustic images of objects which are opaque to light by means of acoustic mirrors and lenses, i.e. selected materials shaped to reflect or refract sound waves in suitable directions.

STANDING WAVES

When a beam of sound waves strikes at normal incidence a boundary between two media, part of the waves are reflected backwards along the same axis of the incident beam. If the incident and reflected beams are continuous, they will interfere giving rise to standing waves (also called stationary waves). These waves correspond to a solution of the wave equation built up with two terms, describing waves travelling in the positive and negative direction, respectively.

In terms of displacement of the particles, we have:

$$u = u_1 \sin k(x-ct) + u_r \sin k(x+ct) \qquad (30)$$

In the special case of perfect (100 per cent) reflection, this corre-

24

sponds to $u_r = u_i$ and may be written as:

$$u = 2u_i \cos kx \sin kct = u(x) \sin kct \qquad (31)$$

This expression describes a situation where each particle of the medium oscillates sinusoidally with time, the amplitude of the oscillation being time-independent and sinusoidally distributed along the x-axis: waves do not propagate in either direction. The same is true also in the case of partial reflection ($u_r < u_i$), although the mathematical expression of the resulting wave is more complicated than eq.(31).

Standing waves are characterized by the appearance of fixed and equally spaced positions of minimum and maximum amplitude, called nodes and antinodes, respectively (Fig.4). The waveform varies with time, but always lies within the envelope shown in Figure 4. Perfect nodes of zero amplitude would appear only in the ideal case of 100 per cent reflection and no absorption; correspondingly, the amplitude at the antinodes would be twice the amplitude of the incident travelling wave. In practice, there will always be some finite value of amplitude at the nodes, and some reduction at the antinodes; the displacement from the ideal condition is expressed by the standing wave ratio (SWR), defined as the

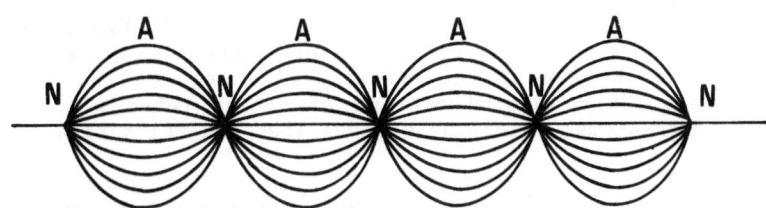

Fig.4 - Structure of standing waves in the case of perfect reflection (N:nodes, A:antinodes).

amplitude at an antinode relative to that at a node:

$$SWR = (u_i + u_r)/(u_i - u_r) \qquad (32)$$

It is seen that the standing wave ratio can never be less than unity. A value of 1 for the SWR would correspond to no reflection, a value of infinity to 100 per cent reflection.

For longitudinal waves, the SWR can also be expressed in terms of pressure:

$$SWR = (p_i + p_r)/(p_i - p_r) \qquad (33)$$

It is interesting in this case to note that nodal positions of pressure correspond to antinodes of displacement, and viceversa.

Standing waves are actually found in any medium of finite size. Due to reflections at the end boundaries, sound waves travel forward and back, while the intensity attenuates because of energy losses on reflection and absorption, unless sustained by an external device.

SCATTERING

An obstacle in the path of a sound beam causes reflection and refraction as described above, only if its dimensions are large relative to the wavelength. When, however, the obstacle dimensions are comparable with or less than one wavelength, scattering takes place, and secondary sound spreads out in all directions.

Scattering may be caused by particles diffused in a liquid or a gas: an important example is given by red cells in blood. Scattering is also responsible for the spreading of a sound beam which reflects from a rough surface. In particular, at high ultrasonic frequencies, scattering may take place in a solid having a polycrystalline structure, i.e. a solid consisting of a large number of tiny single crystals tightly packed together and oriented at random.

Scattering causes energy to be diverted from a sound beam, so that its intensity attenuates. In low-frequency scattering (or Rayleigh scattering), when the dimensions of the obstacle are much smaller than the wavelength, the amplitude of the scattered wave is proportional to the square of the frequency. The scattered intensity is therefore proportional to the fourth power of the frequency. Thus scattering increases significantly with increasing frequency.

ABSORPTION

In addition to the energy losses due to reflection, refraction, divergence, and scattering effects, the intensity of a sound beam attenuates because part of the vibrational energy of the particles is converted into heat. This absorption of energy takes place through a variety of mechanisms, mainly by viscous loss and relaxation processes.

The occurrence of absorption can be accounted for by introducing an absorption coefficient in the solution of the wave equation:

$$p(x,t) = p_0 \; e^{-\alpha x} \sin k(x-ct) \tag{34}$$

α is called the amplitudes absorption coefficient. The attenuation of intensity may also be expressed in terms of α; an intensity absorption coefficient is however frequently used, whose value is twice the value of α :

$$I = I_0 \; e^{-2\alpha x} = I_0 e^{-\mu x} \tag{35}$$

The absorption coefficients of a material increase with increasing frequency. If viscosity is the only mechanism responsible for absorption of a plane longitudinal wave, then α and μ are proportional to the square of the frequency. In the most general case, the absorption coefficients vary according to the general expressions:

$$\alpha = \alpha_0 \; (f/f_0)^n \qquad\qquad \mu = \mu_0 \; (f/f_0)^n \tag{36}$$

where f_0 is an arbitrary reference frequency, and n is a parameter which in turn depends on frequency. Within limited frequency ranges it may be assumed as a constant, ranging for most materials between 1 and 2.

The unit currently used for absorption coefficients is the decibel per centimetre (dB/cm).

THE DOPPLER EFFECT

The Doppler effect consists of a frequency (and consequently of a wavelength) shift of the waves emitted by a source moving relative to the receiver, with a non-zero component of velocity along the axis of the sound beam. The observed frequency increases when the source and the receiver approach each other, and decreases when they move away. The effect is easily explained if we consider that in the first case compression and rarefaction waves arrive at the receiver at a higher frequency, and in the second at a lower frequency, with respect to the condition where the source and the receiver are stationary. Motion of either causes a decreasing or increasing path that each wave must travel.

The phenomenon is clearly depicted in Fig.5 for a moving point source radiating spherical waves. The successively generated spheres are closer together ahead of the source, and farther apart behind it. Since the frequency is determined by the number of waves passing a stationary receiver per unit time, it is clear that the frequency is higher ahead of the source and lower behind it. By simple geometric considerations, it may be deduced that, if a source moves relative to a receiver with velocity V, the perceived frequency f is related to the emitted frequency f_0 by the relation:

$$f = \frac{f_0 c}{c - V \cos\theta} \qquad (37)$$

where θ is the angle between the direction of the velocity vector $\vec{V}$ and the vector joining the source and the receiver. The frequency shift therefore depends on the velocity component directed towards the receiver. The Doppler shift at a given time and position only depends on the source velocity and frequency at the instant of generation of the wave.

In clinical diagnostic applications the Doppler effect is used to determine the speed of a moving target, such as flowing blood.

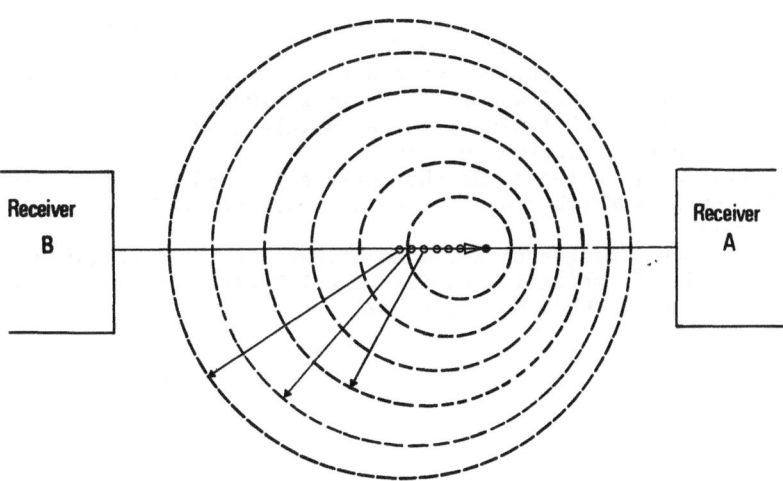

Fig.5 - The Doppler effect. Frequencies experienced at receivers A and B are respectively higher and lower than the frequency emitted by the source.

Sound waves received from a source are subsequently reflected back towards the receiver at rest relative to the source. Under these conditions, a double frequency shift occurs: the first during transmission, with the target acting as a receiver, and the second during reflection from the target, when it acts as a source.

CAVITATION

In fluid mechanics, the term cavitation indicates the formation of gas- or vapour-filled cavities in a liquid by mechanical forces. A typical example is observed in boiling water. Cavitation is in response to an alternating pressure field. From an acoustic field, it is called acoustic cavitation.

During the rarefaction phase of the acoustic cycle, the local pressure becomes lower than the ambient pressure, and any bubbles preexisting (called "nuclei") in the liquid may begin to grow; during the next half of the cycle the local pressure rises above the ambient pressure, and the bubbles growth reverses. The degree of growth, and the lifetime of bubbles depend on several factors: the acoustic pressure amplitude, the value of the ambient pressure, the frequency of the waves and the duty cycle (if pulsed), and obviously the characteristics of the liquid and the dissolved gases.

Where the acoustic pressure is sufficiently high, the bubbles will collapse suddenly on compression, and will release a large amount of energy almost istantaneously. The minimum acoustic intensity required for the onset of this collective phenomenon is called the cavitation threshold (or threshold intensity). The cavitation threshold increases with increasing frequency and ambient pressure. It also varies with temperature, because of the temperature dependence of the surface and of the saturation vapour pressure of the bubbles.

REFERENCES

1. B. Brown and D.Gordon (Eds.), "Ultrasonic Techniques in Biology and Medicine", London Iliffe Books, London (1979).
2. P.E.Edmonds (Ed.) "Ultrasonic". Methods of Experimental Physics, vol.19, Academic Press, New York (1981).
3. A.D.Pierce, "Acoustics. An Introduction to its Physical Principles and Applications", McGraw-Hill, New York (1981).
4. M.H.Repacholi and D.A.Benwell, "Essentials of Medical Ultrasonics", Humana Press, Clifton, NJ (1981).
5. M.H.Repacholi, "Ultrasound: characteristics and Biological Action", National Research Council Canada, Publication N°.NRCC 19244, Ottawa (1981).
6. J.P.Woodcock, "Ultrasonics", Adam Hilger Ltd, Bristol (1979).
7. World Health Organization Environmental Health Criteria Document 22, "Ultrasound", WHO, Geneva (1982).

SOURCES AND APPLICATIONS OF ULTRASOUND

Deirdre A. Benwell, and Stephen H.P. Bly

Radiation Protection Bureau, Health and Welfare Canada, Room 233, Environmental Health Centre, Tunney's Pasture Ottawa Ontario, K1A 0L2, Canada

INTRODUCTION

Ultrasound is a form of mechanical energy having frequencies above the human hearing range (20 kHz). Among the earliest known sources of ultrasound are those emanating from the animal kingdom. Dogs, birds, crickets, and bats are amongst those creatures whose communication signals extend beyond the range of human hearing. In addition bats use ultrasound as a guidance system between 50 and 100 kHz. This latter fact is reputed to have been first postulated by Spallanzani, an Italian Scientist, in 1794 (Health and Welfare 1980a).

Most modern applications of ultrasound utilize sources which are either piezoelectric or magnetostrictive. The discovery of the piezoelectric effect (mechanical stresses on specially cut quartz crystal produce surface charges), was first made by the Curie brothers in 1880 (Curie 1880). The discovery of the phenomenon of magnetostriction (that certain materials have the property that an application of a magnetic field causes a change in physical dimensions, and vice versa), was first reported by J.P. Joule in 1847 (Mason 1976). One of the early practical applications of ultrasound was a device constructed by Chilowsky and Langevin during and after World War I for the underwater detection of submarines (Mason 1976). Since then ultrasound has found increasingly wide-spread application, especially in the medical field.

This paper reviews the various types of ultrasound sources available today and describes briefly their principle of operation. Applications in medicine and industry are then described.

DESCRIPTION OF TYPES OF ULTRASOUND SOURCE

Aerodynamic Generators

The simplest and most efficient emitters designed for operation in a gas medium are aerodynamic systems of various types, in which the source of acoustic energy is a gas jet. Aerodynamic generators may be divided into two classes, differing according to the principle of sound generation: 1) aerodynamic sirens, based on the mechanical interruption of a gas flow by means of moving (usually rotating) surfaces, and 2) whistles of various kinds, which utilize certain types of jet instability. The former are however distinguished by one drawback: they include rotating parts, which means a certain complication of their manufacture and utilization. However, whistles are, as a rule, extremely simple in their construction: they do not require attention during their periods of operation and therefore have unquestionable advantages over sirens.

The Hartmann type acoustic gas jet generator. The Hartmann generator is small in size, simple in construction, and is capable of producing considerable output power (up to several hundred watts at frequencies up to about 40 kHz) (Rozenburg 1969). A diagram of the Hartmann generator is given in Figure 1. It consists of a nozzle with a connecting pipe for the injection of air, and a cylindrical cavity. A wire clamp insures coaxiality of the nozzle and cavity and permits their displacement relative to one another. The generation of sound in Hartmann generators is closely related to the effects that occur in supersonic jets.

Magnetostrictive Transducers

Magnetostrictive transducers are widely used in industrial applications of ultrasound. They have acquired a special reputation as radiators in equipment for the application of ultrasound in the frequency range from 15 to 60 kHz (Rosenburg 1969).

The materials used for these transducers are usually metals and alloys having magnetostrictive properties: iron-colbalt alloys, iron - nickel alloys, and iron - aluminum alloys. In addition ceramics with magnetostrictive properties, namely, special types of ferrites have been developed. These are efficient, inexpensive, relatively simple to use, and do not require hard-to-get raw materials. The relationship between the mechanical strain and the applied magnetic field strength and flux density is illustrated for three common magnetostrictive materials, in Figure 2 (Wells, 1977). Δ is the change in length per unit length, H is the magnetic field and B is the flux density. The graphs indicate a square-law relationship. A magnetostrictive material is composed of magnetic domains which are oriented at random in the absence of a magnetic field. Electron spins are more or less parallel within a domain, giving rise to its magnetism. The application of an external magnetic field tends to change the orientation of the spins by the rotation of the domains, and it is this rotation which causes the change which occurs in the dimensions of the material. The mechanical strain depends on the square of the magnetic field. The ability of a magnetostrictive transducer to convert electrical to mechanical energy, and vice versa, is measured by its magneto mechanical coupling efficiency (Wells, 1977) k_m. This is defined by $k_m^2 =$(stored mechanical energy)/(total stored energy).

In practice, an oscillating magnetic field is superimposed on a d.c. current (steady field) to obtain displacements proportional to the oscillating field. To get suitably large vibration amplitudes the transducer is always operated at resonance (continuous wave). The resonance frequency (f) is determined by

$$f = c/2l$$

where c is the speed of sound in the magnetostrictor and l is its length. Hence, from size restrictions, magnetostrictive transducers are limited to less than 60 kHz. They are therefore particularly useful for the production of intense cavitation required in ultrasonic cleaners (see Table 3 under Industrial and Consumer Ultrasound Applications section).

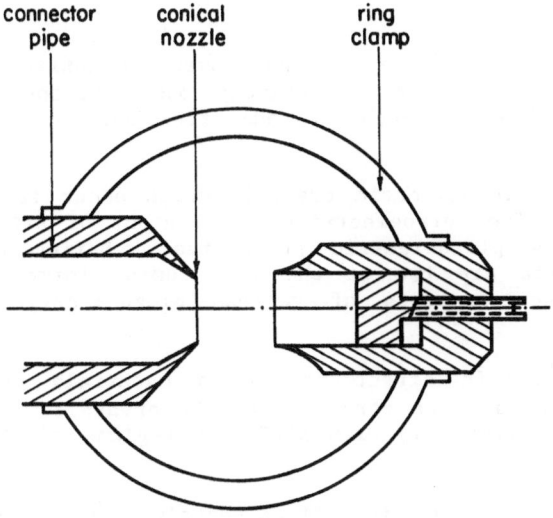

Figure 1.   Diagram of Hartmann Generator,
(From Rozenberg, 1969).

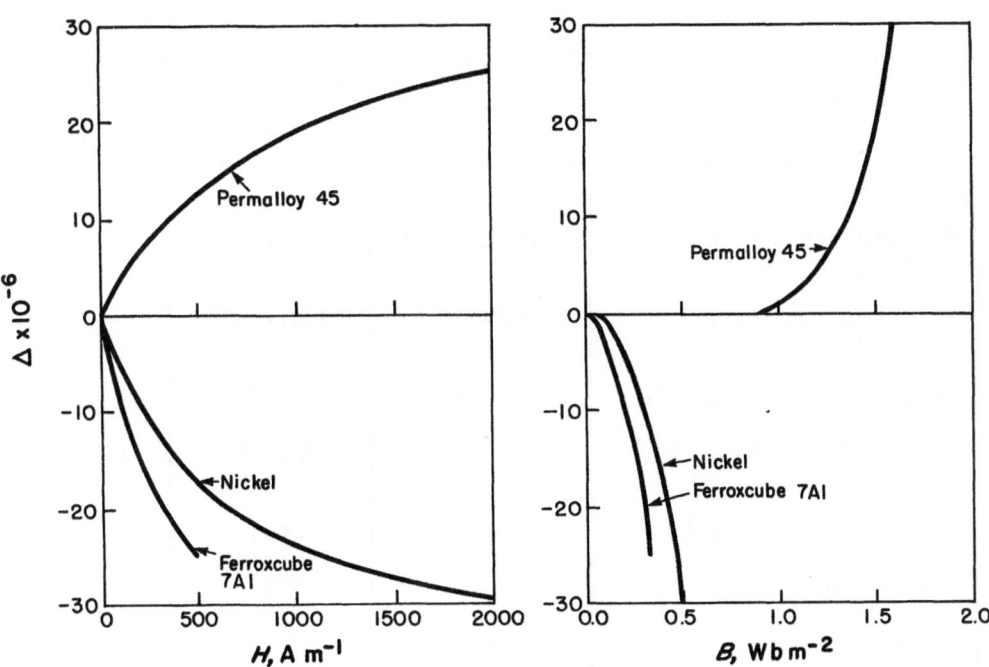

Figure 2.   Characteristics of some Typical Magnetostrictive
Materials, (Wells 1977).

Piezoelectric Transducers

Piezoelectric transducers are used over the entire span of ultrasonic frequencies and are used exclusively in ultrasonic diagnostic and physiotherapy devices at Megahertz (MHz) frequencies. An example is shown in Figure 3.

Examples of piezoelectric crystals which occur in nature are quartz and tourmaline. The ferroelectrics are a group of artificial materials, possessing strong piezoelectric properties. Barium titanate and lead zirconium titanate are two of the more common ferroelectric materials. Table 1 contains constants of various piezoelectric materials (Wells 1977).

The piezoelectric effect arises in materials essentially due to asymmetries in the lattice structure of the crystals. Hence, an electric field interacts differently with different regions of the crystal causing it to deform.

Transducer output functions often contain many frequencies. However a transducer is generally designed to oscillate around a principal or central frequency. The thickness of a transducer is thus designed to equal one-half a wavelength, causing a resonance situation to exist in the crystal element for sinusoidal vibration. At the resonance frequency, constructive interference occurs within the crystal element, producing a fairly strong output. However, unless the excitation is sinusoidal (also known as continuous wave or c.w), transducers do not generally vibrate precisely in a sinusoidal fashion at the fundamental frequency. For

TABLE 1   Properties of Some Typical Piezoelectric Materials
(from Wells 1977).

	Quartz, x-cut	PZT-4	PZT-5A
Tensor subscript	11	33	33
Transmitting constant, d $[mV^{-1}]$	2.31×10^{-12}	289×10^{-12}	374×10^{-12}
Receiving constant, g $[VmN^{-1}]$	5.78×10^{-2}	2.61×10^{-2}	2.48×10^{-2}
Coupling coefficient, ke	0.10	0.70	0.71
Dielectric constant, ε^T $[Fm^{-1}]$	4.00×10^{-11}	1150×10^{-11}	1500×10^{-11}
Wave velocity, $c[ms^{-1}]$	5740	4000	3780
Density, $p[kg\ m^{-3}]$	2650	7500	7750
Characteristic impedance $Z[kg\ m^{-2}s^{-1}]$	1.52×10^7	3.00×10^7	2.93×10^7
Mechanical Q	25000	500	75
Curie temperature $[°C]$	573	328	365

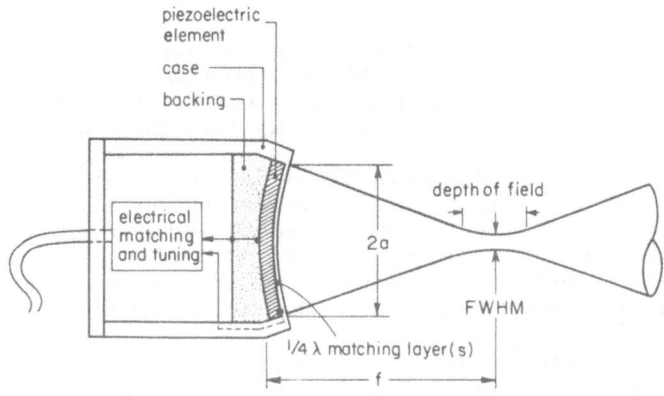

Figure 3. The General Components and Beam Properties of Focused
Piezoelectric Circular Transducers, (Hunt 1983).

example, if the voltage profile applied to the crystal is a sharp spike
then a broad band of frequencies is available. However, the frequency
response will depend on the way in the crystal's vibration is dampened.
The damping depends on the crystal, the load, the backing material, and
electrical tuning (see Figure 3). The quality factor (Q) of a transducer
system characterizes the frequency response of the the transducer; eg. a
transducer with a low Q is said to be a broad-banded transducer, compared
to a high Q transducer, whose output is narrow-banded and more critically
dependent upon frequency. With a spike excitation, the pulse from a
broad-banded transducer therefore contains many more frequencies and is a
sharper pulse than one from a narrow-banded tranducer.

A simple ultrasonic transducer is shown in Figure 4. It consists of a
piezoelectric crystal plus the holder in which the crystal is housed. The
piezoelectric crystal is housed in the forward portion of the case with a
backing material behind it and a face plate in front of it.

The purpose of the face plate shown in Figure 4(b) is to protect the
crystal. To be transparent to ultrasound, it must be an odd multiple of
one half of a wavelength. The remainder of the transducer housing is
dependent primarily on the application of the transducer. For instance, an
immersion-type transducer would require a waterproof case to protect the
internal components from moisture.

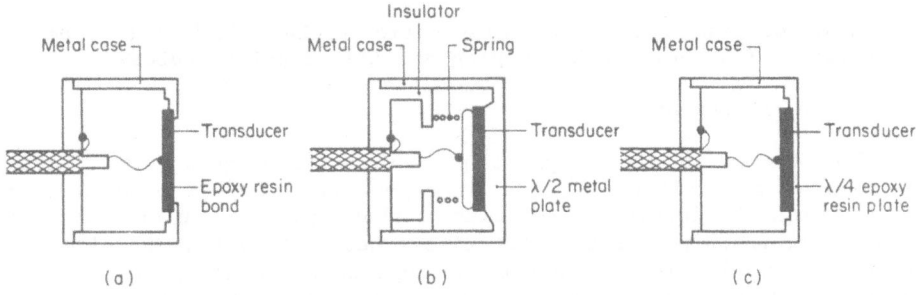

Figure 4. Typical Piezoelectric Transducer Construction, (Wells 1977).

For a cw excitation, air provides a low impedance backing, so that almost all of the energy is available for transmission into the load (see Figure 4(b)). A plate of quarter wave length thickness (Figure 4(c)) provides for maximum transmission efficiency into the load.

The development of transducers for medical diagnosis has given rise to a wide variety of transducers. An important subset of these rely on the generation and detection of short pulses which echo from reflecting or scattering structures of the body. The efficient generation of short pulses has been essential to the development of ultrasonography. It is not simple to generate a short pulse, even when the excitation is an impulse.

If a piezoelectric crystal element is sandwiched between two isotropic materials as shown in Figure 5 and a voltage spike is applied to the crystal, the crystal will oscillate or ring about it's undeformed position until all of the energy is dissipated. During this process, four waves will be generated, two at each of the crystal interfaces. One wave from each interface will propagate to the outside material, the other wave will propagate inward into the crystal. The inward wave will traverse the crystal and strike the opposite interface and several internal reflections may take place within the crystal until all the energy is dissipated. The output of the ultrasonic crystal in either of the two side materials due to the electrical spike is therefore not a single waveform but actually a series of waveforms.

To get a short pulse some of these extra signals must be eliminated. This is done with a matching but lossy backing. This gives the desired short (~1μS) pulse but means that most of the energy is lost to the backing. By using multiple ¼ (wavelength) layers of epoxy for impedance transforming, the transmission efficiency is increased.

ULTRASOUND GENERATORS DESIGNED FOR MEDICAL DIAGNOSTIC APPLICATIONS

In the last two decades, the advantages of techniques using ultrasound have become widely recognized in diagnostic medicine. In most diagnostic techniques the ultrasound beam is transmitted into the body of a patient and directed toward a region of interest. The portion of the reflected or scattered signal that returns to the transducer contains information on the structure of the tissue examined. Some typical ultrasonic transducers are shown in Figure 6 (Rose 1979). Diagnostic ultrasound has been adopted by the medical profession at a astonishing rate, its usage now being comparable to that of X-rays and nuclear medicine. Although the major reason for this exponential increase in use is because of the tremendous technological advance in electronic devices on the market it is also partly because of the desire of physicans to reduce dependence on X-rays where there is a question of safety.

Most medical ultrasonic diagnostic probes fall into one of two categories: (i) pulse-echo imaging and (ii) doppler probes.

Pulse-Echo Instruments

The A-scan is the simplest pulse-echo technique. It yields a one dimensional scan along the line of sight, or axis, of a transducer. An A-scan image is formed by emitting a short pulse of ultrasound from the transducer, which passes into the tissue being examined, and simultaneously starts the bright spot of an oscilloscope to sweep along the X-axis of the screen. During the sweep, acoustic echoes returning to the transducer (which acts both as transmitter and receiver) are applied to the oscilloscope to deflect the bright spot along the y-axis. These echoes

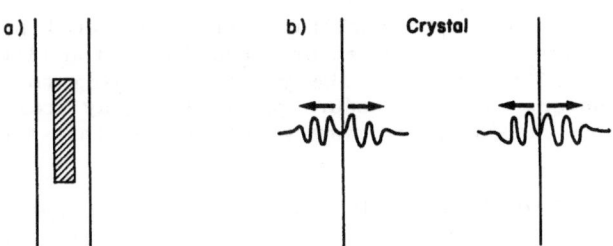

Figure 5. Piezoelectric Element Sandwich Effect,
(Rose 1979).

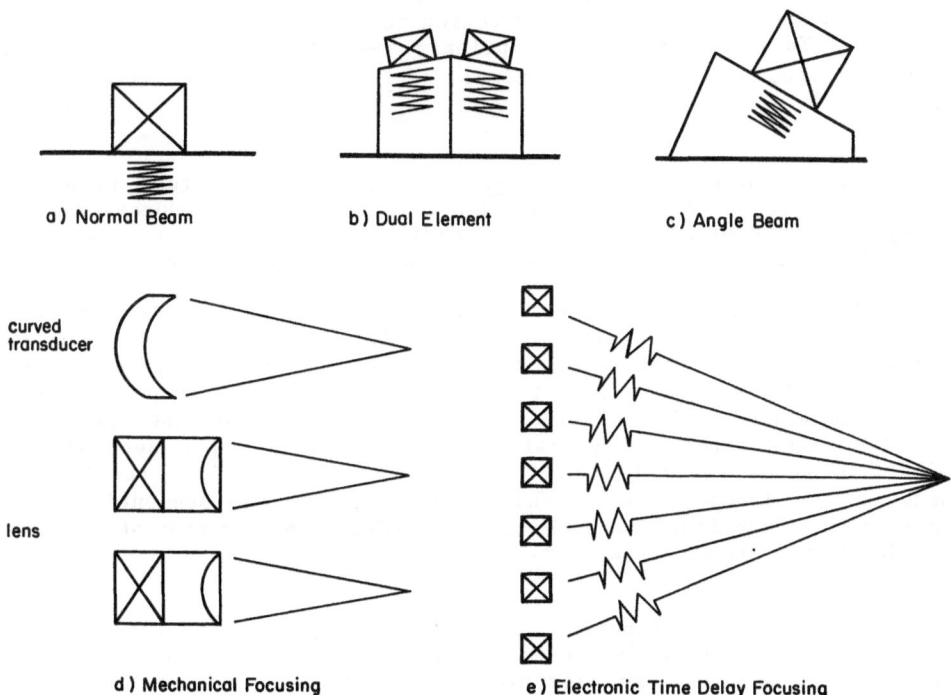

a) Normal Beam   b) Dual Element   c) Angle Beam

curved
transducer

lens

d) Mechanical Focusing   e) Electronic Time Delay Focusing

Figure 6. Typical Ultrasonic Transducers, (Rose 1979).

come from reflecting surfaces, such as tissue interfaces, in the patient's body. The distance of a deflection on the screen from a reference point is proportional to the time between the initiation of the pulse and the return of its echo to the transducer and therefore it is proportional to the distance of the echoing surface from the transducer.

An A-scan with an ultrasound beam which intercepts the moving object such as a beating heart, produces repetitive echoes from a surface whose representations on the screen constantly change position. The time-motion technique, or M-scan, provides a record of this motion with time. For an M - scan, returning echoes are caused to brightness-modulate the bright spot of of the oscilloscope trace (rather than to deflect it), which moves along the x-axis and the entire trace is moved at a constant speed along the y-axis. M-mode patterns can thus give information on heart-valve function.

In a B-scan, returning echo amplitudes are registered by brightness modulation, but the transducer is moved or scanned over the tissue, and the oscilloscope trace positioned along the y-axis according to the line of sight of the transducer. This procedure produces a gray scale image of a plain section through the body, and many variations of this technique have been developed.

Until the early 1970s, virtually all B-mode imaging systems required several seconds to produce an image. Consequently, these systems were limited to imaging static targets.

Now rapid 2-dimensional B-mode imaging known as "real-time scanning" enables visualization of moving targets within the body. In order to image the moving targets within the body, means have been developed to rapidly move the acoustic beam throughout a region necessary to image the organs of interest. To this end, three primary methods have been developed: sequential linear arrays, mechanical sector, and phase array sector scanners.

Sequential Linear Array Scanners. A linear array (see Figure 7), consists of a number of narrow individual rectangular transducers arranged side by side in a single assembly. Two-dimensional images are produced in a sequential linear array scanner by transmitting on a group of elements and receiving the echo information with the same group for each B-mode line on the final display. The first group (say elements 1-8) is pulsed and echoes from the insonification are received. At the completion of this transmit-receive operation, the next group (elements 2-9) is pulsed, and so on throughout the display. As a result of the electronic scanning in these systems, as well as the relatively low number of image lines per frame, very high frame rates are possible (eg. 160 frames per second) (Ramm 1983). In these systems, the field of view is identical to the total length of the linear array. This feature limits the sequential linear arrays in some applications such as echocardiography because of the small acoustic windows between the ribs.

Mechanical Sector Scanners. Mechanical sector scanners include one or more spherically focussed transducers which are rocked or rotated about a fixed axis by means of an electric motor. Usually the transducers are contained in a liquid-filled housing with an acoustic window, and the entire assembly is placed directly onto the skin surface to produce the resulting image in a circular sector format, as illustrated in Figure 7. Individual B-mode lines are scanned radially from a common point corresponding to the centre of rotation. Rocking sector scanners are reported capable of producing images at the rate of 30 per/sec with a maximum field of view advertised to be up to 90°. The larger fields of view can be obtained with rotating head transducer systems which have the additional advantages of minimal vibration, reduced patient discomfort, and a more uniform line density in the image.

Phased Array Sector Scanners. Phased array scanners are the most sophisticated real-time systems. These utilize a small array transducer which readily allows visualization of anatomic structures through restricted acoustic windows. Phased array systems produce images by rapidly steering the acoustic beam through the target organ by electronic rather than mechanical means. In contrast to the sequential linear arrays, all of the array elements in a linear phased array system are utilized in producing each individual B-mode line which comprise the final 2-dimensional image.

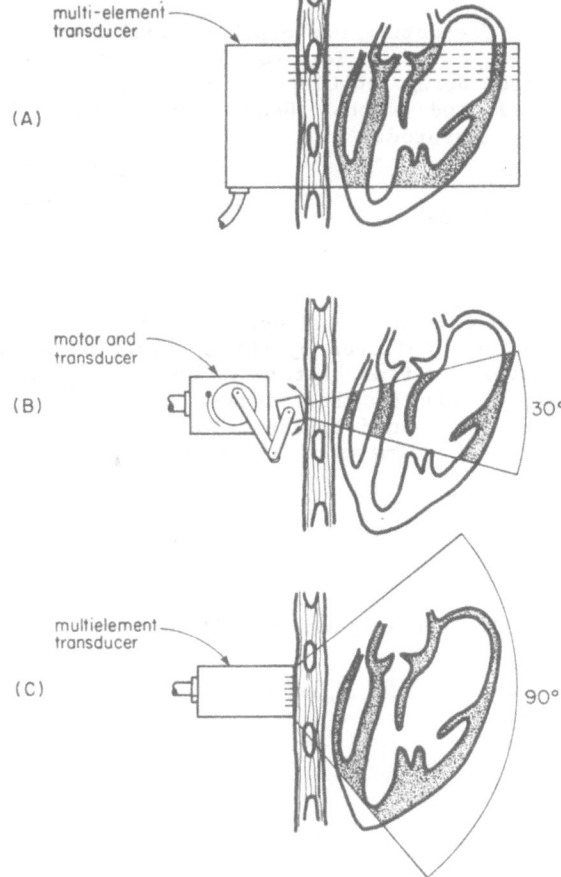

Figure 7. Diagrams Showing:
          A) Sequential Linear Array Scan,
          B) Mechanical Sector Scan,
          C) Phased Array Sector Scan Techniques.
          (Ramm 1983).

    Each of these last three real time techniques have proven to be
diagnostically useful and have enjoyed commercial success (Ramm 1983).
Although there are advantages and disadvantages for each, the phased array
approach offers intrinsic signal processing capabilities which cannot be
realized with the single transducer or a simple sequential array.

Doppler Instruments

    The doppler effect can be defined as a change in observed frequency of
a wave because of the motion of source or observer. Medical instruments
utilize this effect for the purpose of measuring blood flow or detection of
fetal heart beat. Instruments usually have two separate, though adjacent,
D-shaped transducers; a transmitter which sends a continuous beam into the
body, and a receiver which picks up scattered ultrasound returning from the
tissue or blood. The simplest doppler instruments for fetal heart
detection or monitoring (CW) employ continuous wave low power beams of
ultrasound with long dwell times often resulting during monitoring
procedures. Blood flow measuring devices require higher power to see the
weak signals from blood. One drawback with CW doppler analysis is that
many motions or flows could actually exist below a transducer, and there is

no way of selecting some pre-determined depth to analyze the motion or flow rate at that particular point. To over come this difficulty, pulsed doppler instruments are being developed that can accept only echoes produced at some pre-selected depth. Hence blood flow within a selected deep lying vessel can be measured.

MEDICAL ULTRASOUND APPLICATIONS

Introduction

The main application of ultrasound during World Wars' I and II was in the use of sonar. This was followed by the application of ultrasound for ultrasonic flaw detector systems later to become commonly known as non-destructive testing in its broadest sense. Since that time there has been a proliferation of ultrasound applications in industry, medicine and on the consumer market. A summary of these is given in Table 2. This

Table 2. Applications of Ultrasound.

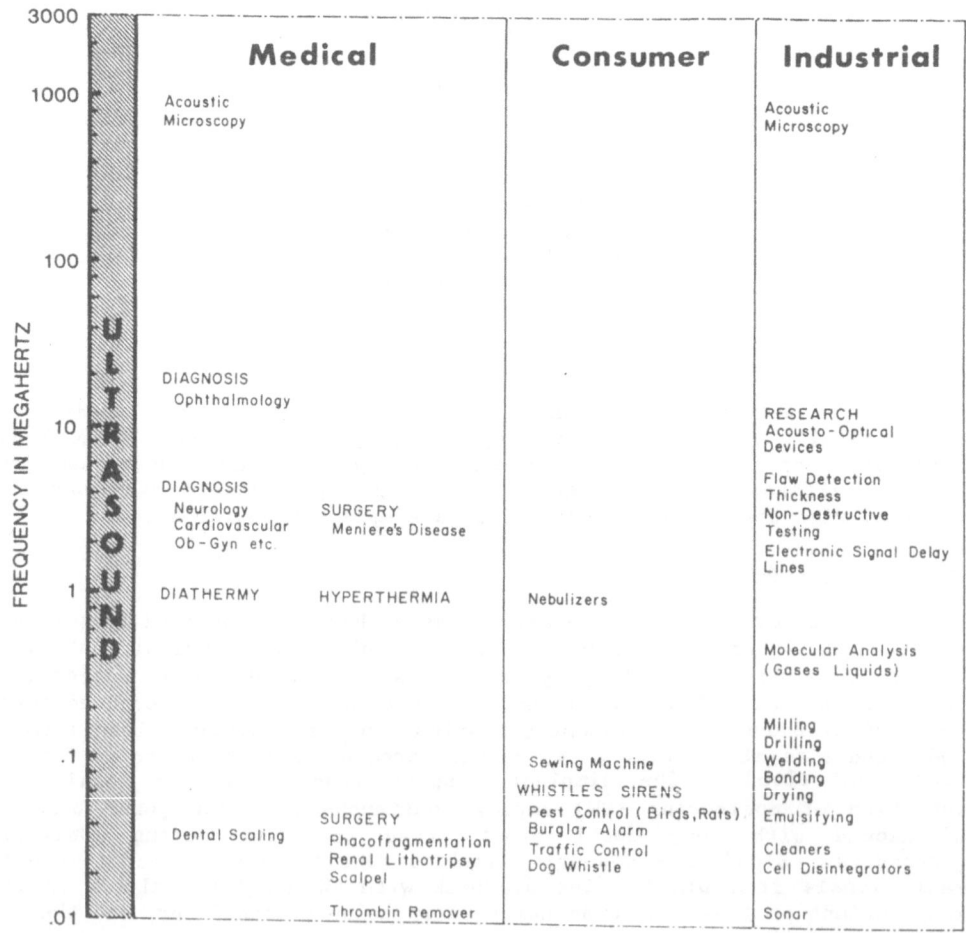

section deals with medical ultrasound applications and the following section deals with industrial and consumer applications. Each section briefly describes the various applications of ultrasound and relates them to the basic principles of the ultrasound sources involved.

Medical applications can be divided into six categories. Nearly all of the medical applications use sound within the frequency range of 0.5 to 15 MHz (NCRP 1983). The choice of frequency used in any specific application is based on considerations of sound absorption, adequate penetration and, in diagnostic applications, adequate resolution.

Diagnosis

Ultrasound has been commonly used in medical diagnosis for over 15 years (NCRP 1983). The first type of diagnostic ultrasound used in medicine was A-mode echo ranging techniques. Today ultra--sonography is used in every major medical centre and even in many private physicians offices. The types of diagnostic techniques have been described in Section 3. This section outlines specific clinical applications of these different diagnostic ultrasound source types.

Ultrasound has been used diagnostically for many regions of the body. In some cases ultrasound is the method of choice and in some cases it is the only technique available. A brief review of the various clinical applications taken from NCRP Report #74 (NCRP 1983), and an "Overview of Ultrasound" (Stewart and Stratmeyer 1982) is as follows.

Head. Brain scans are conducted of neonatal and infant brains where the fontanelles provide acoustic windows.

Eyes and Orbit. Ultrasound can be effectively employed to provide high-resolution B-mode imaging of the eye at about 10 MHz. Accurate measures of the thickness of the cornea and the lens and the axial length of the eye are readily performed with A-mode scans at 10-20 MHz. Foreign body localization, mass evaluation, and retinal detachment may also be detected.

Neck. Thyroid scanning may be accurately performed at frequencies above 5 MHz for the diagnosis of thyroid cysts. Cystic lesions are distinguishable from solid tumors. Cystic and solid tumors may also be identified in other parts of the neck.

Chest. A number of important ultrasound applications apply to cardiology and to the heart. M-mode echocardiography is the technique of choice for many applications including quantitative measurements of heart chamber size and wall thickness. Real time imaging can detect aneurysms, wall motion abnormalities and lesions.

Breast. Ultrasound is an excellent tool for visualizing the various soft tissues of the breast. It can differentiate simple cysts from solid masses, the latter requiring surgical biopsy. Ultrasound may be particularly valuable in the dense fibrous breast of younger women in which examination by X-ray mammography is poor.

Abdomen. There are a number of applications of ultrasound in the abdomen as it is an excellent non-invasive technique for the evaluation of soft tissue. In the liver, kidneys, pancreas, and spleen it is used to evaluate size, as well as to differentiate between cystic and solid lesions. Ultrasound is used in the gall bladder for stone detection, and to evaluate the size of biliary ducts. It is used to measure aneurysmal dilation of the aorta. Other applications include the diagnosis of ascites and abesses in the peritoneal space.

Pelvis. Ultrasound is widely used in the practice of obstetrics. A very large number of fetal abnormalities and diseases have been detected by the use of diagnostic ultrasound on the pregnant uterus. Some of the main applications include amniocentesis guidance, estimation of fetal age, diagnosis of multiple pregnancy, localization of placenta, fetal heart monitoring, fetal growth rate measurement, molar pregnancy diagnosis, ectopic pregnancy diagnosis, and detection of congenital abnormalities.

Ultrasound is also used in gynecology on the non-pregnant uterus for the evaluation of size of masses and in ovaries for ovulation timing. In addition diagnostic ultrasound is used in the pelvis and in the bladder for tumor assessment and in the prostate for tumor detection.

Extremities. Ultrasound is used for vascular studies and for peripheral vascular flow measurements in arteries and veins.

Ultrasonic Guidance Procedures. Diagnostic ultrasound is used as a guidance technique for amniocentesis, needle biopsy, cyst location, and placement of ionizing radiation therapy fields.

Physical Therapy

Diathermy or therapeutic ultrasound differs fundamentally from diagnostic ultrasound in that diathermy involves putting enough energy into the body to cause a healing biological effect whereas diagnostic applications are designed to obtain information without causing any biological effect.

Ultrasound therapy devices generally operate in the frequency range 0.5 to 3 MHz. The different frequencies are used as a means of achieving different penetration depths into the tissue. The hand-held transducers are usually 2-4 cm in diameter. Typical spatial-average temporal-average intensities used for treatment range from 0.1 to 3.0 W/cm^2 (Health and Welfare Canada 1980a, NCRP 1983). Treatment consists of moving the applicator over the area to be treated for between 5 and 15 minutes, a gel or oil being used between the applicator and the skin to provide good acoustic coupling. Pulse and CW modes may be used. The 'pulse' mode (typically with 2-3 ms on time and 10-20 ms off time) allows a higher intensity to be used during the pulse without increasing the temperature.

The aims of ultrasound therapy are to relieve pain, decrease soft tissue stiffness, and accelerate healing. (NCRP 1983, Stewart and Stratmeyer 1982, Dyson et al 1976).

Ultrasound is useful as a therapeutic agent because of its ability to heat tissues selectively and because it can cause cell-stimulating non thermal effects (Lehmann et al 1978, Lehmann 1982). In addition, ultrasonic heating of peripheral nerves and free nerve endings increases the pain threshold without interfering with other sensory or motor functions (Lehmann et al 1978; Lehmann 1982). Heating in combination with exercise also increases the extensibility of collagen tissues and thereby is useful in reducing joint stiffness and in treating soft tissue contractures. According to Lehmann and Guy (1972), the effective temperature range for physical therapy is 40-45 °C at the site of the

40

treatment. Cell stimulating non-thermal effects are believed to be of importance to the application of ultrasound to wound healing (Dyson 1982).

Surgery

Surgical applications use high intensity ultrasound to destroy tissue. The destruction alleviates the diseased state. Typically 10 W/cm^2 and greater intensities are used at the site of application. Amongst the advantages of ultrasonic surgery are: (i) the lesser risk to both patient and surgeon, (ii) the ability to reach parts of wounds otherwise only accessible with difficulty, and (iii) the localized heat effect at the active site leading to the formation of a very thin layer of necrotic tissue and within that layer the sealing of blood vessels and lymph vessels resulting in an operating area largely free of blood.

One of the earliest and best known surgical treatments is that used for Meniere's disease. This disease is a disorder of the vestibular organ in the ear, and causes severe vertigo. Conventional surgical treatment may result in deafness. Ultrasound irradiation of up to 25 W/cm^2 applied to the lateral- semi-circular canal has resulted in cessation of vertigo in 85% of patients and partial improvement in 10% (James 1963).

Ultrasound is also frequently used in the surgical treatment of cataracts. The ultrasound magnetostrictive device used has a vibrating needle oscillating at 20 to 40 kHz which is introduced into the eye and used to emulsify the diseased lens. The debris is removed by applying suction through a special chamber contained within the device. Phaco-emulsification and aspiration are the terms used for this process. They are described by Kelmann (Kelmann 1964). More recently the surgical aspirator technique has been used successfully in other applications such as in urologic surgery (Addonizio 1984), where the procedure has been used in the management of renal stones by ultrasonic shattering.

Surgical techniques for cutting and welding of tissue using low frequency ultrasonic probes have been used mainly in Eastern Europe (Wehner 1981). Compared to conventional oscillating saws, ultrasonic saws are generally inferior with respect to performance. However, it is reported by Wehner that the tendency for the patient to bleed is greatly reduced and that the ultrasonic scalpel provides a simple method for the removal of scar tissue from surrounding healthy tissues (Wehner 1981).

Dentistry

Ultrasound dental scalers were first developed in the United States in the mid to late 50's. They are used for removal of calculus from both root and crown surfaces of teeth and for other purposes, (Forrest 1967). The ultrasonic dental scaler acts through a small hard object attached to a magnetostrictive transducer that usually vibrates at frequencies in the 20 and 40 kHz range in a sliding fashion against dental tissue surfaces, at small excursions of 10-40 microns (Frost 1977). One of the features of an ultrasonic dental scaler is an adjustable water stream or mist to cool the tool tip at tissue surface. Cooling dissipates heat that has developed through energy lost within the transducer and through friction contact with the tooth at the tool tip (Stewart and Stratmeyer 1982).

Hyperthermia

One of the more recent applications of ultrasound in medicine is in the treatment of cancer by hyperthermia. This application is still in a research and development stage. Ultrasound as a technique for hyperthermia has the significant advantage over other modalities such as radiofrequency and microwave heating due to its ability to localize heat. Ultrasound may be used alone or in combination with either radiotherapy or chemotherapy. An excellent review of the subject is given by (Kremkau 1979). A number of the versatile ways in which ultrasound transducer technology can heat required volumes in soft tissue are described by ter Haar (1981). The main limitation with ultrasound heating lies in its inability to traverse bone or air. If large volumes of tissue are to be heated either mechanical or electronic beam steering is necessary.

Acoustic Microscopy

Acoustic microscopes have frequencies varying from 100 MHz to 3 GHz. They are used to analyze various materials including tissue samples. The main advantages of acoustic microscopy over conventional microscopy are the ability to visualize through optically opaque objects, to determine the mechanical properties of the object under study, and the lack of need to use contrast stains on optically transparent objects. A review of acoustic microscope techniques and applications is given by Kessler and Yuhas (1979).

INDUSTRIAL AND CONSUMER ULTRASOUND APPLICATIONS

Applications of ultrasound in industry have been divided into high and low power applications. In the former case ultrasound is applied at a high enough level that its appplication is the effect of ultrasound, on the medium involved. In the case of low power ultrasound on, the other hand, no temporary or permanent changes occur in the material on which the ultrasound acts. The main low power applications are non-destructive testing and signal processing.

High Power

The applications of high power ultrasound generally depend on complex vibration induced effects occurring in matter. These are:

1. cavitation and microstreaming in liquids,
2. surface instability occuring at liquid-liquid, liquid-gas interfaces,
3. heating and the induction of fatigue in solids, and
4. heating in liquid and liquid like media.

Table 3 lists a number of industrial applications of high power ultrasound. The data was taken from Shoh 1975 and Michael 1974.

Non-destructive Testing

Ultrasound is used in the non-destructive testing of jet liners, nuclear power plant components, automotive components, and many other devices, in order to find, locate, and define flaws in various materials.

Other applications of low power ultrasound obtaining information about systems are listed in Table 4. The data was adapted from Lynworth 1975.

Most equipment in use involves intrusive probes but there are also non-invasive externally mounted transducers. Both pulse and resonance techniques are widely used. A fuller account is given in Lynworth 1975.

42

Table 3. Industrial Applications of High-Power Ultrasound.
(WHO 1982)

Application	Description	Frequency (kHz)	Power or intensity range
cleaning and degreasing	cavitating cleaning solution scrubs parts immersed in solution	18 – 100	usually below 10 W/cm^2 but up to 100 W power
soldering and brazing	displacement of oxide film to accomplish bonding without flux	approx. 30	2 – 200 W/cm^2
plastic welding	welding soft and rigid plastic	20 – 60	usually 20 – 30 W/cm^2 but power below 10 000 W output
metal welding	welding similar and dissimilar metals	10 – 60	up to 10 000 W/cm^2
machining	rotary machining, impact grinding using abrasive slurry, vibration-assisted drilling	usually 20	
extraction	extracting perfume, juices, chemicals from flowers, fruits, plants	approx. 20	about 500 W/cm^2
atomization	fuel atomization to improve combustion efficiency and reduce pollution; also dispersion of molten metals	20 – 30 000	up to 800 W
emulsification, dispersion, and homogenization	mixing and homogenizing liquids, slurries, and creams	–	–
defoaming and degassing	separation of foam and gas from liquid, reducing gas and foam content	–	–
foaming of beverages	displacing air by foam in bottles or containers prior to capping	–	–
electro-plating	increases plating rates and produces denser, more uniform deposit	approx. 20	30 W

Table 4. Low-Power Applications of Ultrasound in Industry.
(WHO 1982)

Application	Principle	Frequency
Measurement of:		
flow	determining flow rates for gases, liquids, and solids – Doppler technique	1 – 10 MHz
elastic properties	relating speed of sound to resonance modes of polarization	25 kHz – 300 MHz
temperature	response to temperature dependence of sound, speed, or attenuation	up to 30 MHz
thickness	timing round trip interval of pulse	2 – 10 MHz
density, porosity	resonant and non-resonant probe transmission	up to 50 kHz
grain size of metals	ultrasound attenuation	few MHz
pressure	frequency of quartz crystal resonator changes with applied pressure	0.5 – 1 MHz
level	attenuation of ultrasound beam or measure sure travel time (pulse echo technique)	around 100 kHz
Counting	beam interruptions counted	40 kHz
Gas leaks	detection of ultrasonic "noise"	36 – 44 kHz
Flaw detection	observe discontinuities in reflected beam	25 kHz to 25 MHz (mW power)
Delay lines	transform electric signal into ultrasound and back again after ultrasound has travelled a well-defined path	few MHz
Burglar alarms	ultrasound beamed into room and a certain level of reflected beam is monitored; if this level changes (with intruder) alarm sounds.	18 – 50 kHz (mW powers)
Pest control	frequency and intensity of ultrasound bothersome to pests-inaudible to human	18 – 50 kHz (mW powers)
Sonar	Doppler method determines presence and velocity of object	5 – 50 kHz
Acoustic microscope	observe phase shift and attenuation of ultrasound beam by the specimen	100 – 3000 MHz

Electronic Signal Processing

Electronic signal processing refers to the processing of electrical signals by ultrasound. It therefore includes devices such as Surface Acoustic Wave (SAW) transducers which can be used to make amplifiers and filters, and delay lines for communications signal processing.

Consumer Applications

One of the more recent consumer applications is in the area of atomizers or ultrasonic nebulizers. Ultrasonic nebulizers work on the principal that when a beam of ultrasound of sufficient intensity is passed through a liquid and directed at an interface, "atomization" of the liquid may occur. Under suitable conditions, very fine dense fogs may be produced. Miller et al describes the maintenance of humidity using an ultrasonic nebulizer (Miller 1968).

Ultrasonic sewing machines are rarely met on the consumer market. They essentially use the welding techniques also used in industry. Commercial whistles or sirens use the acoustic gas jet generator. Most other consumer applications such as remote controlled ultrasound burglar alarms, use ultrasound that is propagated through air, generally between 20 and 40 kHz, the source being a piezoelectric transducer similar to that used to produce audible sound.

SUMMARY AND CONCLUSIONS

A number of sources and a variety of important applications of ultrasound exist today. However two of the most significant and widely used civilian applications at present seem to be medical diagnostic ultrasound and non-destructive testing, both of which are designed to image structures without causing effects from the ultrasound exposure itself. It is impressive to realize that these common place techniques are based on the piezoelectric effect, discovered only just over 100 years ago. Of the many other applications, medical therapeutic ultrasound and sonar are two other applications that hold an established and useful position in our society. If the technological revolution of the 1980's continues, it is difficult to imagine how the applications of ultrasound will evolve and progress over the next hundred years. It is clear, however, that ultrasound has a position of established usefulness today.

REFERENCES

Addonizio, J., Choudhury, M.D., Bayegh, N., and Chopp, R.T., 1984, Cavitron Ultrasonic Surgical Aspirators, Applications In Urologic Surgery, Urology, May XXIII 5:417-420.

Curie, J. and Curie, P., 1880, Sur l'electricté polaire dans les cristaux cristaux lémiedrès à faces inlinées, C.R. Acad. Sci., (Paris), 91:383.

Dyson, M., Franks, C., and Suckling, J., 1976, Stimulation of healing of varicose veins by ultrasound, Ultrasonics, 14:232-236.

Dyson, M., 1982, Non-thermal Cellular Effects of Ultrasound, Br. J. Cancer, 45 Suppl. V, pp. 165-171.

Forrest, J.O., 1967, Ultrasonic scaling: A 5 year assessment, Br. Dent. J., 122:9-14.

Frost, H.N., 1977, Heating under ultrasonic dental scaling conditions, In: "Symposium on biological effects and characterizations of ultrasound sources", HEW Publn. (FDA) 78-8048, pp. 64-76, Washington, U.S.A.

Health and Welfare Canada, 1980a, "Safety Code-23. Guidelines for the safe use of ultrasound. Part I: Medical and Paramedical applications", 80-EHD-59, Information Directorate, Health and Welfare Canada, Brooke Claxton Building, Ottawa, Ontario K1A OK9.

Health and Welfare Canada, 1980b, "Safety Code 24. Guidelines for the Safe Use of Ultrasound: Industrial and Commercial Applications", 80-EHD-60, Information Directorate, National Health and Welfare, Brooke Claxton Building, Ottawa, K1A OK9.

Hunt, J.W., Arditi, M., and Foster, F.S., 1983, Ultrasound transducers for pulse-echo medical imaging, IEEE Trans-Biomedical Engineering, Vol. BME-30, pp. 453-481.

James, J. A., 1963, New developments in the ultrasonic therapy of Menieres disease, Ann. R. Coll. Surg., 33:226.

Joule, J.P., 1847, On the effects of magnetism upon the dimensions of iron and steel bars, Phil Mag. Series, Vol. 3 (30), pp. 76-87.

Kelman, K.A., 1964, Phaco-emulsification and aspiration. Am. J. Ophthalmol., 67: 464-477.

Kessler, L.W. and Yuhas, D.E., 1979, Acoustic Microscopy, Proc. IEEE, 67: 526-536.

Kremkau, F.W., 1979, Cancer therapy with ultrasound: A historical review, J. Clin Ultrasound, August 7, pp. 287-300.

Lehmann, J.F., and Guy, A.W., 1972, Ultrasound therapy, in: "Proceedings of Ultrasound and Biological Tissues", HEW Publication (FDA) 73-8008, pp. 141-152, Washington, D.C., U.S.A.

Lehmann, J.F., Warren, C.G., and Guy, A.W., 1978, Therapy with continuous wave ultrasound, Chapter 10 in: "Ultrasound: Its Application in Medicine and Biology, Part II", Fry, F.J., Ed. (Elsevier Scientific Publishing Co., New York).

Lehmann, J.F., Ed., 1982, "Therapeutic Heat and Cold, 3rd Edition", (Williams & Wilkins, Baltimore).

Lynworth, L.C., 1975, Industrial applications of ultrasound - A Review. II. Measurements, Tests, and Process Control using Industrial Ultrasound, IEEE Transactions on Sonics and Ultrasonics", Vol. SU-22, No.2, March, pp. 71-101.

Mason, Warren P., 1976, Sonics and Ultrasonics: Early history and perspectives, in: " Proceedings of 1976 Ultrasonic Symposium sponsored by IEEE Group on Sonics and Ultrasonics", pp. 610-617.

Michael, P.L., Kerlin, R.L., Bienvenue, A.R., and Prout, J.H., 1974, An evaluation of industrial acoustic radiation above 10 KHz. Prepared for NIOSH under contract no. HSM. 99, 72-125 Feb., Physical Agents Branch, 1014 Broadway, Cincinatti, Ohio, 45202, USA.

Miller, W.F., Johnston, F.F., and Tarkoff, M.P., 1968, Use of ultrasonic aerosols with ventilating assister, J. Asthma Res., 5:335-354.

NCRP, 1983, "Biological effects of ultrasound: Mechanisms and clinical implications", NCRP Report No. 74., National Council on Radiation Protection and Measurements, NCRP Publications, 7910 Woodmount Ave, Suite 1016, Bethesda, Md. 20814, U.S.A.

Ramm, O.T. von, Smith, S.W., 1983, Beam steering with linear arrays, IEEE Transactions on Biomedical Engineers, Vol. BME-30, No. 8, pp. 438-452.

Rose, J.L., and Goldberg, B.B., 1979, "Basic Physics of Diagnostic Ultrasound", Wiley.

Rozenberg, L.D., (Ed.), 1969, Sources of high-intensity ultrasound, Volume 1, Plenum Press, New York.

Shoh, A., 1975, Industrial applications of ultrasound - a review. 1 High-Power Ultrasound, IEEE Transactions on Sonics and Ultrasonics, Vol. SU-22 (2), March, pp. 60-71.

Stewart, H.F., and Stratmeyer, M.E., (Eds.), 1982, "An overview of ultrasound: theory measurement, medical applications, and biological effects", HWS Publication FDA 82-8190, FDA, Rockville, Maryland 20857, USA.

ter Haar G., and Hand, J.W., 1981, Review article, Heating techniques in hyperthermia, III Ultrasound, 54 (642), pp. 459-642.

WHO, 1982, Environmental Health Criteria 22, Ultrasound, World Health Organization, Geneva Switzerland.

Wehner, W., Mueller, T., Mueller, W., Neuman, A., 1981, Grundlagenunter-suchungen zur Ultraschall chirugie. 1 Mitt. Prinzip, Stand und Perspektiven der Chirurgie mit Leitungschall, Z. Exper. Chirurg., 14 (6): 357-365.

Wells, P.N.T., 1977, "Biomedical Ultrasonics," Academic Press.

APPLICATIONS OF ULTRASOUND IN MEDICINE -

COMPARISON WITH OTHER MODALITIES

Marvin C. Ziskin
Professor of Radiology and Medical Physics
Temple University Medical School
3400 N. Broad St.
Philadelphia, PA 19140

There exist a large variety of important applications of ultrasound in medicine today. The applications can be divided into three major categories: surgical, therapeutic, and diagnostic. For these categories, an important distinguishing physical feature is the intensity level utilized. Nearly all these applications employ sound in the frequency range of 0.8 - 15 MHz. The choice of frequency used in any specific application is based on considerations of sound absorption, adequate penetration and, in diagnostic applications, adequate resolution.

Surgical Applications and Hyperthermia

Surgical applications employ high intensity ultrasound for the purposeful destruction of tissue. Typically 10 W/cm^2 (SATA) and greater intensities are required at the site of application. In order to avoid destroying intravening tissue, it is sometimes necessary to use a multiple transducer arrangement in which all the transducers are focused onto the same target.

A number of specific surgical applications have been found very useful. It has been especially successful in the treatment of Meniere's disease. This disease is a disorder of the vestibular organ in the inner ear and causes servere vertigo. Conventional surgical treatment may result in deafness. Ultrasound irradiation of up to 25 W/cm^2 has been applied to the lateral semi-circular canal and has resulted in cessation of vertigo, clinical improvement, and greatly reduced incidence of facial nerve paralysis.

Ultrasound has also been very helpful in the surgical treatment of cataracts. In this application, an ultrasound instrument (phacoemulsifier) employing a vibrating needle oscillating at 20-40 kHz is introduced into the eye and used to emulsify the diseased lens. The debris is removed by applying suction through a special chamber contained within the instrument. This technique provides a faster, less traumatic method than conventional surgery and results in a shorter convalescent period.

Other surgical applications of ultrasound have included hypophysectomy, ablation of the substantia nigra in the treatment of Parkinson's disease, removal of warts, and the treatment of laryngeal papillomatosis. However, these latter applications have either not been very successful or have not been as advantagious as conventional surgical techniques and have not received wide exceptance.

A new development which is showing much promise is the ultrasonic renal lithotriptor. This device is inserted into the renal pelvis, and when placed in contact with kidney stones and energized, is capable of breaking the stones into small pieces which can be suctioned out and removed. This procedure, when successful, eliminates the need of surgical operation for removal of kidney stones and is becoming popular. In one version of this approach, the patient is placed into a water bath and subjected to multiple sonic shock waves generated by external transducers focused onto a internal kidney stone. Although an elaborate and expensive procedure, this transcutaneous instrument is engendering a great deal of interest and appeal because its use obviates the need for any surgical procedure.

There has been a renewed interest in the use of ultrasonic hyperthermia in the treatment of cancer. A number of studies has revealed that when various types of rodent, rabbit, and human tumors are heated to 42 C° and above, there occurs a selected and irreversible inhibition of metabolism that correlates with a loss of biological malignancy, and ultimately tumor regression. These findings consititute the underlying basis for employing hyperthermia for the treatment of malignancy. A excellent review of this topic can be found in the chapter on hyperthermia in this volume written by Dr. P. P. Lele.

Applications in Physical Therapy

Ultrasound has been employed in physical therapy for over 40 years. It is used in the treatment of a number of joint and soft tissue ailments such as arthritis, bursitis, muscle spasms, traumatic soft tissue injuries, and certain collagen diseases. The aim of this technique is to relieve pain, decrease soft tissue stiffness and accelerate healing. Most of the benefits of ultrasound as a therapeutic agent reside in its ability to heat deep tissues selectively. Heating causes vaso-dilatation and subsequent increased blood profusion, thereby ensuring adequate delivery of metabolites needed in tissue repair and in adequate removal of waste products. Heating also increases the rate of many, if not most, biochemical reactions and accelerates the diffusion rate across biological membranes. In addition, ultrasonic heating of peripheral nerves and free nerve endings increases the pain threshold without interfering with other sensory or motor functions. Heating in combination with excercise also increases the extensibility of collagen tissues and therefore is used for reducing joint stiffness and in treating soft tissue contractures.

In contrast to other forms of heating, such as with microwaves or short-waves, ultrasound can selectively heat areas where pathological conditions which respond to heat therapy are frequently found. This selective heating is due to the differing acoustic absorption properties of tissue, which are related in large measure to the collagen (protein) content. Thus, greater heating occurs in tendons, periosteum, myofascial interfaces, joint capsules and scar tissues. Please refer to the chapter entitled " Recent Advances and Techniques in Therapeutic Ultrasound" by Dr. G. ter Haar appearing in this volume.

Applications in Dentistry

Ultrasound is widely used in removal of calculus and other deposits from teeth. The ultrasonic instruments used in dental scaling operate by moving a smaller scraper at oscillatory frequencies from 18-40 kHz with a vibration amplitude of a few micrometers. In usage, water is sprayed against the vibrating tip for cooling purposes, and cavitational effects on the water reinforce the mechanical effects of the vibrations in removing deposits. It is estimated that in the United States alone, there are approximately 100,000 ultrasonic units in use today in dental offices.

Diagnostic Applications

Ultrasound has been used in medical diagnosis for over 25 years. Ultrasonography started as a very specialized laboratory tool for measuring depths of internal surfaces by A-mode echo-ranging techniques. It has shown remarkable growth and progress, and today is employed in every major medical center and even in many private physicians' offices. Perhaps the most important reasons for the popularity of ultrasound, are its excellent capability for visualizing and differentiating soft tissue, its non-invasive nature (compared to surgical methods), and its apparent safety.

The following listing of applications, though impressive by any measure, is not intended to be complete, but rather to illustrate the range of successful usages.

Diagnostic Techniques

Diagnostic techniques can be grouped into three basic types: pulse-echo, Doppler, and through-transmission. The pulse-echo technique is by far the most commonly used.

In the A-mode (amplitude modulation), echoes are displayed as vertical deflection occurring at various positions along a horizontal oscilloscope baseline, with the height of the deflection being proportional to the amplitude of the detected echo. This display is used primarily for making internal distance measurements and is especially valuable in measuring the width of intraocular structures.

The M-mode (motion) display employs brightness modulation and is used in observing the movements of anatomic structures. This technique has been extremely valuable in studying dynamic changes in the heart. Much of this information, so easily obtained with ultrasound, is not possible to obtain with any other diagnostic technique. For example, the individual leaflets of cardiac valves are readily identified, and their excursions and velocities readily measured.

The B-scan provides a two-dimenisional cross-sectional visualization of anatomical structures. It is obtained by moving the transducer over the surface of the body and displaying the echoes in brightness modulation, with the location and direction of the baseline accurately following that of the transducer. Instruments providing 15 or more internal structures. B-scanning is widely employed in many medical applications. It is of special value in obstetrics where its use helps to keep x-ray examinations to a minimum, and where the B-scan provides more information than radiographs of the abdomen or fluoroscopy.

Doppler instruments detect frequency changes in returning echoes and provide the clinician with information on the motion of internal structures. The most important application of the Doppler technique is the detection and semi-quantification of blood flow. It is also used to monitor fetal heart rate during labor where the motion of the fetal heart wall is responsible for the Doppler signal.

Through-transmission techniques measure sound which has completely transversed the body or object under investigation. New developments in two-dimensional through-transmission imaging techniques are just beginning to be evaluated in clinical settings. Laboratory studies have produced dynamic images on submerged objects such as embryos, fish, and human extremities. There is also active interest in ultrasonic computerized tomography, particularly for breast imaging. However, there are no commercially available through-transmission instruments and clinical usefulness of the techniques remains to be proven.

Specific Clinical Applications

Ultrasound has been employed diagnostically for virtually every region of the body, and with few exceptions has met with great success. Perusal of any one of a number of textbooks on diagnostic ultrasound reveals the extent and usefulness of this technique. For diagnosing some diseases, ultrasound is the method of choice and in some diseases it is the only technique available. What follows is a very brief review of the various clinical applications.

Brain

A-mode echoencephalography provides a convenient technique for detecting a shift of midline intracerebral structures and thereby diagnosing a space-occupying lesion. Two-dimensional ultrasonic examination of the brain is currently limited primarily to the newborn in which excellent anatomical visualization through the fontanelles is not blocked by thick skull bone as in the adult. Hydrocephalus, intracranial hemorrhages, aneurysms, and other malformations are readily identified. Intra-operative ultrasound examination of the adult skull has been helpful in the placement of intracerebral shunts and in localizing brain tumors.

Eye

The eye lends itself admirably to ultrasonic examination. Because of its superficial location and low attenuation, high frequency (10-12

MHz) ultrasound can be effectively employed to provide high-resolution imaging. Accurate measurements of the thicknesses of the cornea and lens and the axial length of the eye are readily performed. Foreign body localization is valuable, particularly for nonradiopaque objects such as wood or glass.

The ultrasonic examination of intraocular pathology is of special value in cases of opaque corneas or mature lenses where funduscopic examination is impossible. With ultrasound, it is possible to detect detached retinas and retinal tumors. Retrobulbar tumors can also be detected with ultrasound.

Neck

Thyroid scanning is performed at frequencies above 5 MHz with great clinical accuracy for the diagnosis of thyroid cysts. Cystic lesions are distinguishable from solid tumors. The relationship of the carotid artery and jugular vein to a thyroid mass can be determined before a surgical procedure or an aspiration is attempted.

Salivary glands may be investigated for cystic and solid tumors. Calculi of sufficient size will cast an acoustic shadow. Lymphadenopathy may be located and studied for suppuratin in inflammatory conditions.

Heart

The practice of cardiology has been profoundly affected by ultrasound. M-mode echocardiography is the technique of choice in obtaining quantitative measurements of heart chamber size and wall thickness. It can measure accurately the range and velocity of valvular motion. Mitral stenosis is readily diagnosed by the reduced velocity of the valve leaflets during opening and closure.

Two-dimensional echocardiography can detect wall motion abnormalities and aneurysms. It is also useful in evaluating complicated congenital heart lesions such as tetralogy of Fallot, pulmonary atresia, or persistent truncus arteriosus. With the injection of an ultrasonic contrast agent, it is possible to diagnose left-to-right and right-to-left shunts at the arterial level.

Breast

Ultrasound is an excellent tool for visualizing the various soft tissues of the breast. It is of great value in differentiating simple cysts from solid masses which require surgical biopsy. It is particulary valuable in the dense fibrous breast of younger women in which examination by x-ray mammography is poor.

Abdomen

Ultrasound provides a simple method of confirming the presence of ascites. Palpable abdominal masses can be evaluated for size, compositon, and organ of origin. Benign and malignant solid tumors, cysts, abscesses, and hematomas can be diagnosed.

The size and contour of the liver can be evaluated as well as tissue texture. The portal venous system and hepatic veins are well demonstrated. The intrahepatic bile ducts can be seen when dilated. Some hepatic masses that can be found with ultrasound include simple hepatic cyst, hydatid cyst, abscess, metastases, hepatoma, hemangioma, or lymphoma. Ultrasonically guided biopsy of an abnormal liver mass can be easily performed for definitive diagnosis when indicated.

The size, shape, and internal consistency of the spleen can be determined by ultrasound. Solid or cystic intrasplenic masses as well as surrounding hematoma can be detected.

Ultrasound is an excellent, noninvasive technique for evaluation of the normal an abnormal pancreas. The size, shape, texture of the gland, and the status of the pancreatic duct can be evaluated. Acute or chronic pancreatitis can be detected as well as the size and location of pseudocysts. Malignant tumors of the pancreas can be diagnosed.

Ultrasonically guided biopsy of pancreatic tumors may preclude the need for diagnostic surgery. Ultrasound is also an excellent method for evaluating the bile-filled gallbladder since there is no contrast agent necessary, as there would be for x-rays, and, therefore, no delay in performing the study. Recent advances in real-time instrumentation allow the option of replacing oral cholecystography by high-resolution, real-time instrumentation allow the option of replacing oral cholecystography by high-resolution, real-time sonography as the primary screening method for gallstones. The entire biliary tree can be evaluated for evidence of dilation. In many cases, particularly with real-time equipment, the exact level and nature of an obstructing lesion can be found. The diagnosis of gallstones and the differentiation of obstructive versus nonobstructive jaundice can be made with a high degree of accuracy and with few technical failures, using real-time equipment.

Renal size, shape, position, and tissue texture can be evaluated by ultrasound without regard to renal function. Ultrasound is used when there is nonvisualization on intravenous pyelography, when there is a mass present on a pyelogram, in patients who are allergic to radiological contrast agents, or in cases of anuria. Renal cysts can be easily detected by ultrasound, thereby eliminating the need for angiography or other invasive procedures. Ultrasound can confirm polycystic kidney disease, solid tumor masses, and perinephric fluid collections. It is used to distinguish between obstructive uropathy and renal parenchymal disease in patients with anuria. Ultrasonically guided antegrade pyelography or percutaneous nephrostomy can be performed on obstructed patients for diagnostic and therapeutic purposes.

Ultrasound is the procedure of choice to detect and measure an aortic aneurysm. Thrombosis within the aneurysm can also be identified. Adenopathy due to lymphoma or metastatic disease can be diagnosed.

Obstetrics

Ultrasound is widely used in the practice of obstetrics. Its popularity arises because it yields excellent anatomic visualization, and because physicians have observed no harmful effects from its use. Real-time B-scanners with frame rates greater than 15 per second are most desirable for evaluation of the fetus. Obstetrical uses of ultrasound are numerous. Sonography can be used to confirm an intra-uterine pregnancy, determine fetal viability, assess fetal anatomy, and evaluate for congenital anomalies. The growth and development of the fetus can be monitored by ultrasound, and gestational age can be assessed. Fetal position and multiple gestation can be easily determined. Hydramnios and oligohydramnios can be diagnosed.

The site of placental implantation can be identified, placenta previa can usually be diagnosed, and abruptio placenta can sometimes be detected. Molar pregnancies can always be recognized as being abnormal, but can occasionally be mistaken for missed abortion. Ultrasound has also been used for guidance in the performance of amniocentesis. Also, ultrasound is used very frequently to monitor fetal heart rate during labor.

Gynecology

The pelvic organs can be demonstrated by using a full urinary bladder as an acoustic window. When there is a pelvic mass present, ultrasound can be used to determine whether the mass is solid or cystic in nature, and whether it originates from the uterus or ovaries. Common pelvic masses that may be demonstrated by ultrasound include fibroid, ovarian cyst, dermoid cyst, hemorrhagic cyst, tubo-ovarian abscess, hydrosalpinx, ectopic pregnancy, endometrioma, cystadenoma, and cystoadenocarcinoma. Non-gynecological masses can also be seen in the pelvis such as appendiceal or diverticular abscess, colonic carcinoma, neurogenic tumors, and lymphadenopathy. Ovarian follicular development can be followed with serial ultrasound examinations, and this facilitates the administration of medical therapy to infertility patients.

Peripheral Vascular System

Doppler ultrasound is useful in evaluating the presence of deep venous thrombosis, one of the major causes of hospital death in the United States. Doppler ultrasound is also important in detecting reduced or altered blood flow, and when coupled with B-scanning, becomes an invaluable technique for diagnosing arterial occlusive disease. B-scan imaging is frequently utilized to find smaller, potentially ulcerated plaques.

Superficial Structures

Size, location, and possible abscess formation of non-radiopaque foreign bodies, such as wood or plastic, may be exmained. Tears of major tendons can be quickly diagnosed. Tendon cystic lesions, neuromas, and popliteal masses have characteristic ultrasound appearances.

The testes can be examined ultrasonically. It is possible to

diagnose testicular cysts and solid tumors, and peritesticular
conditions such as hydrocoeles, varicocele, and spermatic cysts.

OTHER IMAGING MODALITIES

Imaging of the body has become a indispensible aid for medical
diagnosis. In the past several years there has been a dramatic
increase in the technology and number of imaging modalities available
to the practicing physician. In addition to the various ultrasound
technologies, a physician may chose to use radiography, fluoroscopy,
x-ray computed tomography (CT scans), radioisotope scans, positron
emission scan (PET scans), and magnetic resonance imaging. Each of
these techniques have important and considerable benefits and tend to
complement diagnostic information obtainable from each other. The
choice of which technology or technologies employed for any given
patient depends on the pathology that is expected to be present. A
secondary, but important consideration is also the cost and
availability of each technology. The salient points of each of the
imaging modalities will now be discussed.

Radiography

Radiography has been the standard imaging modality in medicine
ever since its discovery in 1895 by Wilhelm Roentgen. This remains
today as the most commonly performed imaging procedure in medicine. In
radiography a broad beam of x-rays is sent through the body. The
transmitted photons expose a photographic film. The image on the
radiograph is then a distribution of the x-ray attenuation through the
body. The energy of the x-ray photons utilized varies from 10-120 kilo
electron volts. At these energies the primary mechanism of
interaction is the Compton effect. The incidence of Compton reactions
depends most directly on the electron density which in turn depends
upon the density of materials. Thus, the most pertinent tissue
property relative to x-ray imaging is tissue density. In contrast, for
ultrasound the pertinent tissue property is acoustic impedance, or the
product of density and acoustic velocity. There is approximately a 4%
variation of densities amongst soft body tissues and approximately 8%
variation of acoustic impendances amongst the tissues. Thus,
ultrasound is intrinsically twice as sensitive in distinguishing one
soft tissue from another.

The theoretical limit for resolving capability of a diagnostic
modality is of the order of magnitude of the wavelength. Whereas the
wavelengths utilized in ultrasound vary from 0.1-1.0 mm, those of
x-rays vary from 0.1-1.0 Angstrom units or 10 million times smaller.
As a consequence ultrasonic techniques are limited in resolution by
wavelengths of ultrasound but there is no practical limit on x-ray
resolution because of wavelength. Limitation on x-ray imaging
resolution stems from factors such as focal spot size of the x-ray tube
and, grain size of the photographic emulsion. Therefore, radiography
is by far the preferred imaging modality whenever there is sufficient
tissue contrast and when ionizing radiation hazards are not of major
concern.

Fluoroscopy is the technique for real-time imaging of the x-ray
image. Instead of capturing x-ray photons on a photographic film, the

x-ray photons are made to enter an image-intensifying tube in which a series of transformations from light photons produces an image on a phosphorous screen which is either viewed directly or viewed via television. This permits the viewing moving structures as they move. It's primarily used today in the study of the digestive tract. Swallowing difficulties are readily observed by means of barium swallow studies. Intestinal spasmodic regions are readily detectable, again with the swallow of barium. These gastrointestinal pathologies have not been amenable to ultrasound techniques.

Computerized Tomography (CT)

X-ray computerized tomograms (CT scans) have been available for the past 10 years. They have made a major impact in that they have added to x-ray imaging the ability to see tomographic slices (cross sectional images at right angles to the long axis of the body) with excellent spatial and contrast resolution. As with standard radiography, the pertinent tissue property is density, but whereas standard radiography can only distinguish five different radiographic densities (air, fat, water and soft tissue, bone, and metal), CT scans can distinguish differences in x-ray attenuation as small as 0.5%. A spatial resolution is limited primarily by the pixel size on the reconstructed image. This is of the order of 1mm and is approximately at the same spatial resolution as ultrasound. CT scanning has been particularly valuable in viewing regions containing bone such as the skull and the spine. It is also excellent in the pelvis. The former is important because ultrasound has not been very good in visualizing bone. In fact, because of the high acoustic impendance of bone relative to surrounding soft tissue, very little sound gets transmitted into bone; and that which is transmitted into bone is very heavily attenuated by absorption. Also, ultrasound has not been very successful in imaging within the skull because of the heavy skull bone and its refractive and absorbing affect on the ultrasound beam. CT scanning and ultrasound scanning are somewhat competitive in the abdomen. Even within the same organ, different pathologies may appear better on the CT scan or on the ultrasound scan. A frequent distinguishing guideline for which modality to use is the obesity of the patient. Ultrasound is prefered for thin patients with small amounts of intestinal gas and CT scanning is preferred for obese patients and those who have considerable intestinal gas present.

Radioisotope Scanning

Radioisotope scanning consist of injecting relatively short lived radioisotopes into a patient and imaging the resulting distribution of radioactivity within regions of the body. The radioactive isotopes are chemically attached to molecules which have a prediction for localizing in various organs of the body.

This permits the imaging of specific functioning tissue within the body. In general the spatial resolution of this technique is considerably inferior to the other modalities previously mentioned. However, this modality provides significant physiological information in addition to anatomic distribution. For example, two thyroid nodules can have essentially identical morphologic appearance, but one may be metabolically very active and produce a hot spot on the nuclear scan whereas, the other would nonfunction and appear cold. The clinical significance of being able to distinguish these two nodules is of utmost importance. A particularly valuable use of nuclear scanning is in the survey of cancer metastasis and its spread to bone. Another is the identification of the sites of intestinal bleeding. Both of these are impossible to image by any other modality.

Magnetic Resonance Imaging

Magnetic resonance imaging (MRI), previously called nuclear magnetic resonance imaging, is the latest newcomer to this array of imaging modalities. It is the most costly and probability the most complex, but does offer a great deal.

Hydrogen nuclei posses a magnetic moment and when placed in a magnetic field move from their otherwise randomly oriented positions to attempt to align themselves with the direction of the applied field. The nuclei begin to precess and the angular frequency of the precession of the magnetic moment is the product of the magnetic field applied and the magnetogyric ratio a fundamental physical constant for each nuclear species. When a superimposed electromagnetic field is applied at right angles and at the proper frequency, nuclei will flip from the low energy parallel orientation to the higher energy antiparallel position. The change in energy between these orientations is related to the resident frequency. When the superimposed radiofrequency energy pulse is removed, the protons tend to realign themselves with the magnetic field. This requires a finite period of time and is referred to as a relaxation time or more specifically the spin−lattice relaxation time (T_1). In pure water, the proton spinlattice relaxation time at room temperature is approximately 3 seconds. In biological tissue it varies between a few hundred milliseconds and about 2 seconds. The variation amongst soft tissues is quite large. In general, the greater the water content of the tissue the longer the T_1 time. The spin−spin relaxation time, also called T_2, is a measure of how rapidly a transverse component of magnetization returns to its rest state. The T_2 time results from interaction with nuclei themselves and is tissue specific with an even greater variability than T_1 amongst soft tissues.

Both T_1 and T_2 times can be utilized as the bases for imaging tissue properties. Images can be reconstructed by computer in a manner almost identical to that of CT scans. Spatial localization within the body is provided by applying a magnetization gradient superimposed upon the applied field. This gradient causes any point along the gradient to have a different magnetic strength and consequently a different resonance frequency from its neighboring locations. By carefully tuning the receiving antenna, it is possible to select the position for sampling of the NMR signal. This is all performed under computer control and the reconstructed images are very impressive.

MRI has been particularly valuable in imaging the brain and spinal cord. Here grey and white matter are readily differentiated better than with any other modality. The images appear on a par with actual cadaver specimens. MRI has not proven to be as valuable in the abdomen, and certainly will not replace CT scanning or ultrasound. Additionally, MRI has the ability to image blood vessels by virtue of the absence of a signal coming from the region of the blood. The reason for this is that the protons that are irradiated within any sample of blood are transported out of the field prior to the completion of the imaging process.

Additional Comments on the Comparison of Modalities

An important concern of which modality should be utilized is that of cost. Of the techniques mentioned, ultrasound is usually the cheapest, the most transportable, and when everything else is equal should be the modality of choice. On the other hand magnetic resonance imaging is by far the most expensive and the least available. However, with time these units should become more available and should become competitive with CT scanners.

The dependence of image quality on the operator obtaining the images, varies with the different techniques. That of ultrasound probably requires the greatest skill. Most of the x-ray techniques are more a matter of correct positioning and selection of the appropriate exposure factors and then effectively pushing a button. Ultrasound, on the other hand, has to be applied manually with a transducer and the body is then searched until all the pertinent pathology is revealed and displayed in the most effective manner. In any event, the interpretation of any of the images requires a high degree of medical knowledge and should be performed by individuals who have the appropriate training and expertise.

Safety concerns do have a role in the choice of imaging modalities. In general x-rays, because of their ionizing capability and potential for carcinogenesis, are considered to be more dangerous than ultrasound. When everthing else is equal, the one producing the least hazard would certainly be the one chosen. To date no known hazard has ever resulted from diagnostic ultrasound nor from magnetic resonance imaging. Nevertheless, we must remain vigilant for any possible adverse affect no matter how subtle or how delayed.

Summary

Today, more than ever, the physician is presented with tremendously powerful imaging modalities. These have become, and will continue to be, vital in the medical care of patients.

ASPECTS OF NONLINEAR ACOUSTICS

WHICH ARE IMPORTANT IN BIOMEDICAL ULTRASOUND

Edwin L. Carstensen

Department of Electrical Engineering
University of Rochester
Rochester, New York 14627

.   In most applications of ultrasound in medicine, it is satisfactory to assume that tissue behaves as a linear medium. It has become apparent within the last few years, however, that there are enough exceptions to this position that it is desirable for research scientists and development engineers to be aware of the basic concepts and implications of finite amplitude acoustics.

This overview presents the concepts of shock generation, with harmonic production and saturation, and considers the effects which this has on the absorption of ultrasound and ways in which nonlinearities are involved in the study of biological effects of ultrasound.

NONLINEARITIES OF BIOLOGICAL MEDIA

To derive an equation which will adequately describe the propagation of an acoustic wave we must have an equation of state which characterizes the relationship between stress and strain or pressure and density for the medium through which the wave passses. For linear acoustics, this equation can be a simple linear relationship - Hooke's Law. Most of the interesting nonlinear aspects of sound propagation can be treated by expressing the equation of state as a power series and using only the first (linear) and second order terms in this equation. The degree of nonlinearity of a medium is commonly expressed in terms of a quantity B/A which is related to the ratio of the second and first order terms in this expansion. For water at $3^{O}C$, B/A is 5.2. For tissues with high water content such as liver, brain and muscle, B/A ~ 6.5 - 7.5. Fat has a value of B/A of approximately 11. The nonlinearity parameter appears to increase in proportion to the solute concentration in biologically interesting materials. There is little to suggest that it depends strongly on the nature of the molecular constituents or the structure of soft tissues (Law *et al.*, 1985; Cobb, 1982; Sehgal *et al.*, 1985). At the present time, there are no precise methods for measurement of the nonlinearity parameters B/A *in vivo*. However, the insensitivity of B/A to small differences in tissue constituents provides little motivation for the development of imaging techniques based on this property of tissues.

SHOCK FORMATION

In any real medium, the instantaneous velocity of propagation of an acoustic disturbance is a function of the local pressure. Thus, the wave becomes "supersonic" during the compressional phase of the wave, and "subsonic" during the rarefaction phase, i.e. the "crest" advances more rapidly than the "trough" of the wave and, in the extreme case, this produces a pressure discontinuity or a "hard" shock. After propagating through the medium at high intensity the signal contains a rich spectrum of harmonics instead of a pure sine wave that was generated by the piezoelectric source. When the shock wave is fully formed, the amplitude of the harmonic components of the wave are inversely proportional to the harmonic number i.e. the amplitude of the second harmonic will equal half of the fundamental.

The degree of waveform distortion depends upon the source intensity, the distance which the wave has propagated and the frequency as well as on the nonlinear properties of the medium. It is possible to characterize the degree of shock development in terms of a single *shock parameter* σ which combines the influence of all of these interacting parameters. For spherically converging waves,

$$\sigma = \beta \epsilon k r \ln(r_0/r) \tag{1}$$

where r_0 is the focal distance and r is the distance from the center of curvature to the field point. Here, $\beta = 1 + B/2A$, $k = 2\pi/\lambda$ is the acoustic wave number and $\epsilon = u_0 c_0$ is the acoustic Mach number, where u_0 is the particle velocity amplitude at the source. It can be shown (Muir and Carstensen, 1980) that

$$\epsilon = (2I_0 \cdot 10^7 / r_0 c_0^3)^{1/2}, \tag{2}$$

where I_0 is the r.m.s. source intensity measured in units of W/cm^2 and r_0 and c_0 are in cgs units. In the plane wave limit (i.e. $r_0 \rightarrow \infty$), Equation (1) approaches

$$\sigma = \beta \epsilon k x, \tag{3}$$

where x is the distance from the source. The theory upon which these relationships rests assumes a wave of uniform presure across a phase front and neglects diffraction anomalies which are associated with finite size sources and which will dominate the behavior of a converging wave near the focal region (Blackstock, 1966).

Two stages of shock formation can be defined which provide useful information about the degree of harmonic distortion (Muir and Carstensen, 1980). The shock parameter conveniently characterizes these key stages. The value $\sigma = 1$ characterizes the beginning of shock formation. At this value, the fundamental has lost 1 dB to harmonic generation. Although this is a fairly weak shock, the 2nd, 3rd and 4th harmonics have amplitudes which are 8, 12 and 15 dB below the fundamental, respectively. At $\sigma = 3$, a mature shock with a sawtooth waveform has formed. This wave can distort no further because nature does not permit multivalued waveforms. The tendency for further distortion is then balanced by dissipation at the shock fronts, greatly accelerating the normal rate of conversion of acoustic energy into heat. At $\sigma = 3$, the fundamental has lost 6 dB and the harmonic amplitudes are inversely proportional to the harmonic number, i.e. the 2nd, 3rd and 4th harmonic amplitudes are 6, 10 and 12 dB below the fudamental, respectively.

Above about $\sigma = 3$, increases in source intensity are compensated by losses in the medium and the field intensity approaches a limit. This is the phenomenon of acoustic saturation. It becomes evident first in the fundamental but eventually applies to the total intensity of the propagating shock wave.

OBSERVATIONS OF FINITE AMPLITUDE FIELDS

Recent developments in polyvinyl difluoride (PVDF) film hydrophones have made it possible to record the temporal aspects of finite amplitude propagation in the the medically interesting frequency range (Bacon, 1982, 1984). These devices have uniform response characteristics over a very wide frequency range and appear to be linear up to the maximum pressure levels for which tests have been performed. Even though the piezoelectric elements in these hydrophones are able to transduce the pressure response without distortion, care must be taken to avoid phase shifts in the cables which are used to couple the element to an oscilloscope. However, when this is done it is possible to obtain excellent pictures of waves even in hard shock. If one wishes to study the fundamental component of the wave almost any hydrophone can be used. One simply uses a low pass filter in the output to eliminate contamination of the signal by harmonics. Observations of the fundamental component alone can provide significant information on the behavior of the wave under nonlinear conditions. For $\sigma > 3$, the finite amplitude absorption of the fundamental component is the same as that for each of the harmonic components.

A small spherical radiometer is very useful for direct measurements of the total intensity in a finite amplitude wave (Carstensen et al., 1980). The force on a steel sphere is essentially independent of frequency for values of ka > 1 (Dunn et al., 1977), where a is the radius of the sphere. The "sensitivity" of the radiometer can be adjusted by pulsing the source, using an appropriate duty cycle and making certain that the transient response of the source is a negligible contribution to the total energy in each pulse. Streaming artifacts must be avoided in any use of a radiometer for intensity measurements. However, they become particularly troublesome with finite amplitude waves. Streaming is directly related to the absorption of acoustic energy from the wave (Nyborg, 1965). If a radiometer is used in a poorly absorbing medium such as water, streaming is usually so small that it can be ignored. At finite amplitudes, however, even water becomes absorbing as discussed below. We found that it was necessary to place a film window both in front and behind the steel sphere to break the streaming-induced flow.

ABSORPTION

In the common linear treatment of sound propagation, the absorption can be described as an exponential reduction of signal amplitude with distance as the wave progresses through the medium. The rate of decay of the signal depends upon the small amplitude absorption coefficient which is a property of the medium. In most tissues, this absorption coefficient is roughly proportional to the frequency, but at a given frequency it is a simple constant.

With finite amplitude waves, the rate of conversion of acoustic energy to heat depends upon the intensity, the distance traveled and the nonlinear properties of the medium as well as its small signal absorption coefficient. Thus, rather than the usual absorption coefficient, we must accept a more general definition of an *absorption parameter*

$$\alpha = -\nabla \cdot \mathbf{I}/2I, \tag{4}$$

where $\mathbf{I}$ is the local intensity.

Harmonic Absorption. There are two conceptually different, nonlinear aspects to the absorption of ultrasound. For illustration, we consider here the case of an ultrasonic wave propagating through the water where it undergoes nonlinear distortion, becomes rich in harmonics, and, upon penetration of the tissue sample, is absorbed. The physical processes are particularly clear in the context of this example but these two fundamental processes are involved in all cases of finite amplitude sound propagation even though the effects may be more subtly interrelated. Because the inherent frequency dependence of the absorption of the tissue

64

sample, the presence of harmonic components in the wave leads to a greater rate of heat deposition than for an equal intensity at the fundamental frequency. This is simply the classical absorption of nonlinearly generated harmonic frequencies. This nonlinear aspect of the absorption of ultrasound will be called *harmonic absorption*. For a medium which has a small amplitude absorption coefficient α_0 which is directly proportional to the frequency, harmonic absorption leads to an increase in the harmonic absorption parameter α_{har} as defined in Equation (3) by a factor of two. The transition takes place between weak and hard shock (i.e. for values of the shock parameter $1 < \sigma < 3$) (Carstensen *et al.*, 1982).

Finite Amplitude Absorption. The theory which has been most useful in the treatment of the nonlinear aspects of sound propagation begins with the assumption that the small amplitude absorption coefficient of the medium is negligible (Blackstock, 1966). In spite of that fact, it predicts attenuation of the wave and eventually saturation. This *finite amplitude absorption* α_{fin} is completely foreign to the concepts of linear acoustics and therefore is perhaps the most interesting aspect of nonlinear sound absorption. The shock forming process, which occurs in the weakly absorbing water path between source and sample (and which resulted in attenuation in that medium in spite of its very small absorption coefficient), will continue within the tissue for a short distance, leading to finite amplitude absorption in that medium as well.

Finite amplitude absorption is negligible at intensities below weak shock; it rises very rapidly above $\sigma = 1$; it becomes a constant for values above $\sigma = 3$. This upper limit to the finite amplitude absorption is greater in focused than in plane fields - the shorter the focal length of the source the greater the maximum value of α_{fin}. In focused fields, the finite amplitude absorption increases as the point of observation approaches the focus. With focused fields, much greater local intensities (but smaller source intensities) are required to produce a given magnitude of finite amplitude absorption than in a plane wave field. Under realistically attainable conditions, the finite amplitude absorption can approach values of the order of 1 neper/cm, a value somewhat greater than the small signal absorption coefficient of most soft tissues. Note that the finite amplitude absorption occurs in water and other similarly loss free materials as well as in tissues. Hence, finite amplitude absorption can be the dominant factor in the nonlinear absorption processes of such materials (Dalecki *et al.*, 1986).

The effects of focusing on absorption, which were mentioned above, can be generalized to the broad subject of finite amplitude effects. In focused fields, a given shock parameter requires a larger local intensity (albeit a smaller source intensity) than for plane wave fields. In focused fields, the wave travels over much of its path at relatively low intensity and hence requires a large amplitude to acquire the distortion which produces shock in a relatively short path length. When plane waves travel through highly absorbing materials such as tissue rather than water, the harmonic components of the wave may be absorbed almost as rapidly as they are generated and interesting examples of finite amplitude effects are unlikely to occur in those medical applications where an unfocused source is placed in direct contact with the skin of a patient. In an absorbing medium, finite amplitude effects may be more easily achieved using converging fields than with plane waves.

BEAM PATTERNS

There are two qualitatively different finite amplitude effects on the beam patterns of sound sources. First, under certain conditions, the distribution of the intensity of the sound itself is changed because of relatively greater attenuation (saturation) of the axial portion of the beam. This tends to broaden beam pattern when the axial portion of the beam approaches hard shock (Muir and Carstensen, 1980; Carstensen et al., 1980). Second, and perhaps more interesting, the "heating pattern" of the sound field is sharpened when the shock parameter for the axial portion of the beam is between weak and hard shock ($1 < \sigma_{axial} < 3$). This arises because the heating rate is a very strong function of intensity once shock formation begins. Thus, the large axial intensities lead to disproportionately greater heating rates than the lower, off-axis portions of the beam. When the axial intensities reach hard shock, the axial heating rates saturate and the "heating pattern" eventually becomes broader than the linear or low intensity beam pattern of the source.

BIOLOGICAL EFFECTS OF FINITE AMPLITUDE ULTRASOUND

Biological Effects Experiments. There are several ways in which nonlinear processes enter into biological effects experiments – frequently in subtle ways that may not be immediately obvious unless the investigator is alert to the possibility.

It is common to calibrate a sound field at low intensity and assume that the fields can be linearly extrapolated from those values when source power is increased. In view of the discussions above, it is apparent that this could lead to serious errors. Not only will the total intensity potentially be in error but also the subject may be exposed to a broad spectrum of frequencies rather than the single frequency in the source signal. If heat production is the mechanism of action of the ultrasound, this could enhance the effect. If cavitation is involved, the shift in pressure to higher frequencies could reduce the magnitude of the effect.

In a study of the effects of pulsed ultrasound on plant roots about ten years ago (Child et al., 1975), we wanted to have a comparatively uniform sound field over the root tip. With this in mind, we exposed the roots in the farfield (13 cm) of a 2 MHz source. The local intensity was 10 W/cm^2 In measuring the beam pattern of the transducer, we observed a distorted wave form in the output of a ceramic probe hydrophone. We simply blamed the receiving system for the "poor" wave form, but the probe was trying to tell us, within its limited ability, that we were exposing the roots not simply to 2 MHz sound waves but also to a significant level of nonlinearly generated harmonic frequencies. As the scientific community directs more of its attention to the possible biological effects of the high intensity, short-pulse- length exposures which are used in diagnostic ultrasound, errors of this kind are likely to increase. In order to avoid contamination of the acoustic field with higher harmonics it may be necessary in some experiments to expose the subjects in the near field or perhaps in a focused sound field.

As discussed above, nonlinear phenomena can make materials, such as water or aqueous gels, which are normally considered to be lossless, into relatively good absorbers. For this reason, unanticipated heating may become important in certain experiments. As mentioned above, streaming in fluids depends upon the momentum transferred to the medium by absorption. In calibration of sound fields by radiometry, it may be possible to ignore the effects of streaming at low c.w. intensities but not at the same temporal average intensity with pulsed fields in which the temporal peak intensities are in shock. These concepts may be important in the physical processes which lead to biological effects as well as in calibration of the sound fields for the experiments.

Ultrasonic Imaging. In pulse echo diagnostic ultrasound, there appears to be a trend toward the use of ever greater temporal peak intensities. This may improve signal-to-noise ratios in certain applications. There is no clear indication that these levels are associated with adverse biological effects in human subjects. However, it is important that the designers are aware of the nonlinear phenomena which may be taking place under these conditions. Nonlinearly generated harmonics have been demonstrated in the fields of some commercial devices (Parker, 1985; Duck and Starritt, 1984). In techniques which deliberately use harmonic signals (e.g. for the detection of bubbles) finite amplitude harmonics could introduce significant errors. However, in many applications, harmonic generation may be no more important than the associated loss of energy. Eventually, acoustic saturation sets an upper limit to the amount of acoustic power which can be used effectively in ultrasonic imaging.

Ultrasonic Diathermy. After nearly one half century of use, ultrasound is still medicine's most effective method of producing heat deep within the tissues of the body. Because of the modest intensities and relatively short path lengths normally used in ultrasonic diathermy it is unlikely that nonlinear effects need be considered in this application of ultrasound in medicine.

Ultrasonic Surgery. In ultrasonic surgery, however, it is probable that, either inadvertantly or by design, finite amplitude phenomena may be involved. Nonlinear processes may evidence themselves in rather different ways. Because of saturation, it may be impossible to produce tissue damage under certain conditions. On the other hand, enhanced absorption under shock conditions may lower the thresholds at which lesions are produced in tissues.

Our experience during ultrasonic surgery of an autotransplanted kidney illustrates the former. In this procedure, the organ is removed surgically from the animal for treatment and then replaced. We found that an unfocused 5 MHz source could produce a lesion in the kidney with an intensity of 1-2 W/cm^2 when it was nearly in contact with the organ but that with a 10 cm water path between the source and the tissue, no amount of input to the transducer could effect a lesion. Although it was not immediately apparent to us at the time, we had encountered the phenomenon of acoustic saturation.

The observed threshold for lesion production in cat brain and in other mammalian tissues by focused ultrasound can be represented empirically over a wide range of source intensities I_0 and times t by $I_0 t^{-1/2} =$ constant (Fry et al., 1970). It now appears that this simple relationship hides a fairly complex combination of non-thermal and thermal biophysical mechanisms involving nonlinear aspects of sound propagation and arising in part from an artifact which results from failure to recognize the effects of finite amplitude phenomena on the local intensity in the propagating medium. That non-thermal mechanisms are involved comes from the observation by Fry and colleagues (1970) that at the highest intensities used in their study, the lesions were diffuse, suggesting to them that cavitation was a probable mechanism for the action of ultrasound under those conditions. There is little doubt that heating is also important. At the low intensity extreme of the exposures, lesion formation can be explained by a linear heating process. In fact, for relatively low intensities and long exposure times, thermal diffusion from the narrow focused sound beam makes the thresholds nearly independent of exposure time (i.e. for long exposure times, threshold intensities have less than a $t^{-1/2}$ slope) (Lerner et al.,. 1973). For intermediate local intensities (of the order of 500-1000 W/cm^2), it has been clear for some time that a simple linear heating model was not a satisfactory explanation of the observed lesion thresholds (Carstensen et al., 1974).

The importance of nonlinear phenomena in the formation of lesions in tissue has been demonstrated recently (Carstensen et al., 1981). That study used unfocused sound fields. The nonlinear absorption parameters which were used in those lesion threshold predictions were shown to arise from a combination of "harmonic" absorption and "finite amplitude" absorption processes. In focused sound fields, however, the nonlinear contributions to heating can be more pronounced than with plane waves (Dalecki et al., 1987). For this to occur, much larger local intensities (but smaller source intensities) are required for focused than for plane waves.

Early studies of focal ultrasonic lesion production in in tissues have assumed a linear relationship between source and focal intensities. Of course, at finite amplitudes, this is not true. Thus, generalizations such as the $It^{-1/2}$ = constant relationship mentioned above and the frequency "independence" of thresholds which has been observed are really statements about source intensity and not, in general, the intensity of the ultrasound at the site of the lesion. Another important phenomenon from the standpoint of focal lesion production is the influence which finite amplitudes have on the effective heating patterns of the focused sound field. Although axial heating is accentuated under some conditions, it is counterbalanced partially by increased heat diffusion from the relatively narrower heating pattern.

In summary, nonlinear effects appear to explain in part the magnitudes of thresholds which have been observed for production of ultrasonic lesions in tissues. However, in arriving at an understanding of the physical processes involved, it has become apparent that the qualitative nature of the threshold curves depends upon whether the sound fields are specified in terms of source intensities or the intensities at the focus in the tissue.

PROBLEM AREAS

Blackstock's (1966) theory has made a major contribution to the understanding of fundamental nonlinear processes in sound propagation. It has been particularly useful in introducing finite amplitude acoustics to biomedical ultrasound. It deals with both plane and spherical waves. With any real source, the converging (or diverging) aspects of the sound field must be considered to obtain quantitative predictions of finite amplitude effects. This is true even for plane piston radiators (Carstensen et al., 1980). However many of the sources which are used in diagnostic and surgical applications of ultrasound are deliberately focused. Present theory tells us that, under appropriate conditions, the most dramatic effects of finite amplitude sound propagation may be experienced in the focal region. Yet, it is in the focal region that the quantitative usefulness of present theory becomes limited. Thus, from the standpoint of biomedical ultrasound, it will be particularly important to include the effects of diffraction. A start in this direction has recently been made (Lucas and Muir, 1983; Saito and Muir, 1984; Swindell, 1985).

Finite amplitude effects are profoundly modified by propagation in media with small signal absorption coefficients which are comparable in magnitude to those of typical body tissues (Haran and Cook, 1983). For general applications of finite amplitude ultasound in medicine, it will be important to include relaxation absorption processes in the characteristics of the media. Some theoretical work has been published on nonlinear propagation in relaxing media (Poltakova *et al.*, 1962; Swindell, 1985). It will be essential that future theory be able to deal with converging waves and include the effects of diffraction as well as relaxational absorption.

ACKNOWLEDGMENTS

This work has been supported in part by Public Health Service Grant No. 39241.

The basic phenomena summarized here are abstracted in part from a paper by Carstensen and Muir (1986).

REFERENCES

Bacon, D. R., 1982, Characteristics of a PVDF membrane hydrophone for use in the range 1-100 MHz, *IEEE Trans. Son. Ultrasonics* SU-29:18-25.
Bacon, D. R., 1984, Finite Amplitude distortion of the pulsed fields used in diagnostic ultrasound, *Ultrasound Med. Biol.* 10:189-198.
Blackstock, D. T., 1966, Connection between the Fay and Fubini solutions for plane sound waves of finite amplitude, *J. Acoust. Soc. Am.* 39:1019-1026.
Carstensen, E. L., Miller, M. W. and Linke, C. A., 1974, Biological effects of ultrasound, *J. Biol. Phys.* 2:173-192
Carstensen, E. L., Law, W. D., McKay, N. D. and Muir, T. G., 1980, Demonstration of nonlinear acoustic effects at biomedical frequencies and intensities, *Ultrasound Med. Biol.* 6:359-368.
Carstensen, E. L., Becroft, S. A., Law, W. K. and Barbee, D. B., 1981, Finite amplitude effects on the thresholds for lesion production in tissues by unfocused ultrasound, *J. Acoust. Soc. Am.* 70:302-309.
Carstensen, E. L., McKay, N. D., Dalecki, D. and Muir, T. G., 1982, Absorption of finite amplitude ultrasound in tissues, *Acustica* 51:116-123.
Carstensen, E. L. and Muir, T. G., 1986, The role of nonlinear acoustics in biomedical ultrasound, *in* "Tissue Characterization with Ultrasound," J. G. Greenleaf, ed., CRC Press, Boca Raton, Fla., pp. 57-79.
Child, S. Z., Carstensen, E. L. and Miller, M. W., 1975, Growth of pea roots exposed to pulsed ultrasound, *J. Acoust. Soc. Am.* 58:1109-1110.
Cobb, W., 1982, Measurement of the acoustic nonlinearity parameter for biological media, Ph.D Dissertation, Yale University, New Haven, CT.

Dalecki, D., Carstensen, E. L., Parker, K. J. and Muir, T. G., 1987, Absorption of Focused, Finite Amplitude Ultrasound, in preparation.

Duck, F. A., and Starritt, H. C., 1984, Acoustic Shock Generation by Imaging Equipment, *Br. J. Radiol.* 57:231-240.

Dunn, F., Averbuch, A. J. and O'Brien, W. D., 1977, A primary method for the determination of ultrasonic intensity with the elastic sphere radiometer, *Acustica* 38:58-61.

Fry, F., Kossoff, G., Eggleton, R. C. and Dunn, F., 1970, Threshold ultrasonic dosages for structural changes in the mammalian brain, *J. Acoust. Soc. Am.*, 48:1413-1417.

Haran, M. E. and Cook, B. D., 1983, Distortion of finite amplitude ultrasound in lossy media, *J. Acoust. Soc. Am.* 73:774-779.

Law, W. K., Frizzell, L. A. and Dunn, F., 1985, Determination of the nonlinearity parameter B/A of biological media, *Ultrasound Med. Biol.* 11:307-318

Lerner, R. M., Carstensen, E. L. and Dunn, F., 1973, Frequency dependence of thresholds for ultrasonic production of thermal lesions in tissue, *J. Acoust. Soc. Am.* 54:504-506.

Lucas, B. G. and Muir, T. G., 1983, Field of a finite-amplitude focusing source, *J. Acoust. Soc. Am.*, 74, 1522-1528.

Muir, T. G. and Carstensen, E. L., 1980, Prediction of nonlinear acoustic effects at biomedical frequencies and intensities, *Ultrasound Med. Biol.* 6:345-357.

Nyborg, W. L., 1965, Acoustic streaming, *Ch. 11 in* "Physical Acoustics" Vol. II, Part B, W. P. Mason, ed., Academic Press, 1965.

Parker, K. J., 1985, Observation of nonlinear acoustic effects in a B-scan imaging instrument, *IEEE Trans. Sonics and Ultrasonics* SU-32:4-8.

Poltakova, A. L., Soluyan, S. I., and Khokhlov, R. V., 1962, Propágation of finite disturbances in a relaxing medium, *Sov. Phys. Acoust.* 8:78-82.

Saito, S. and Muir, T. G., 1984, Second harmonic component in a finite-amplitude sound focusing system, *Proc. Acoust. Soc. Japan*, Spring Meeting, (In Japanese).

Sehgal, C. M., Bahn, R. C. and Greenleaf, J. F., 1984, Measurement of acoustic nonlinearity parameter B/A of human tissues by the thermodynamic method, *J. Acoust. Soc. Am.* 76:1023-1029.

Swindell, W., 1985, A theoretical study of nonlinear effects with focused ultrasound in tissues: An 'Acoustic Bragg Peak', *Ultrasound Med. Biol.* 11:121-130.

INTERACTION MECHANISMS: HEATING

Wesley L. Nyborg

Physics Department
University of Vermont
Burlington, Vermont 05405 USA

INTRODUCTION

When ultrasound of a given frequency is transmitted into a medium (e.g., a liquid, a solid, or biological tissue) a fraction of the acoustic power is converted into heat. If effects of shear viscosity are not important the time-averaged rate Q at which heat is produced per unit volume is given by the following expression (Nyborg, 1981; Cavicchi and O'Brien, Jr., 1984):

$$Q = (2\alpha/\rho c) \ \langle p^2 \rangle \ , \tag{1}$$

where α is the absorption coefficient at the specified frequency; ρ and c are the density and velocity of sound, respectively, for the medium; p is the acoustic pressure (total instantaneous pressure less the mean value) and $\langle p^2 \rangle$ denotes the time average of p^2. If the ultrasound source is driven at frequency f, and if the approximations of linear acoustics hold, the pressure at any point will be given by

$$p = p_0 \cos(\omega t + \beta), \quad \omega = 2\pi f \ . \tag{2}$$

Here the pressure amplitude p_0 and the phase β are each independent of time but (in general) vary in space. When Eq. 2 holds one obtains from Eq. 1 that

$$Q = \alpha p_0^2 / \rho c \ . \tag{3}$$

In a plane traveling wave the expression $p_0^2/\rho c$ is just twice the intensity I and Q is equal to $2\alpha I$; however, this simple relationship between Q and the intensity does not hold generally. The units of α in Eq. 1 or 3 are nepers (Np) per unit length, the neper being 8.7 decibels (dB). Values of α have been measured in mammalian tissues over a range of the frequency f. The most extensive and reliable data are for "soft" tissues, including liver, brain and kidney. Recent results (Parker, 1983) show that the simple formula

$$\alpha = 5.0 \ f \tag{4}$$

gives values which are roughly typical for liver tissues; here α is in Np/m when f is in MHz. For example, at a frequency of 3 MHz one obtains $\alpha = 15$ Np/m from Eq. 4. Other tissues have widely differing absorbing properties. (NCRP, 1983). For testis the coefficient α is less than half as large as would be obtained from Eq. 4, while for bone α exceeds values from Eq. 4 by a large factor, betweem 10 and 60. In body fluids the absorption coefficient is relatively small: for blood α is less than obtained from Eq. 4 by a factor of about three, while for amniotic fluid α is about one-tenth as large as for blood.

In applications of ultrasound to physical therapy heat is produced for beneficial purposes. The field is typically unfocused and is applied continuously or in a series of repeated pulses. In a pulsed regime the peak duration may, for example, be 1 ms and the interval between pulses 4 ms. Fig. 1 shows the field for a specific situation. Here the source transducer is a circular disc with diameter 1.2 cm and vibrates uniformly (like a piston) at a frequency of 3 MHz; there is no focusing. The medium is assumed to have acoustical characteristics similar to those of soft tissue, the absorption coefficient α being 0.15 Np/cm (1.3 dB/cm). The velocity of sound is approximated as 1500 m/s and the density as 1 gm/cm^3. In preparing Fig. 1 approximate equations were used, as discussed by Nyborg and Steele (1985).

The field quantity plotted in Fig. 1 is proportional to $p_o{}^2$ (the square of the pressure amplitude) and hence, when Eq. 3

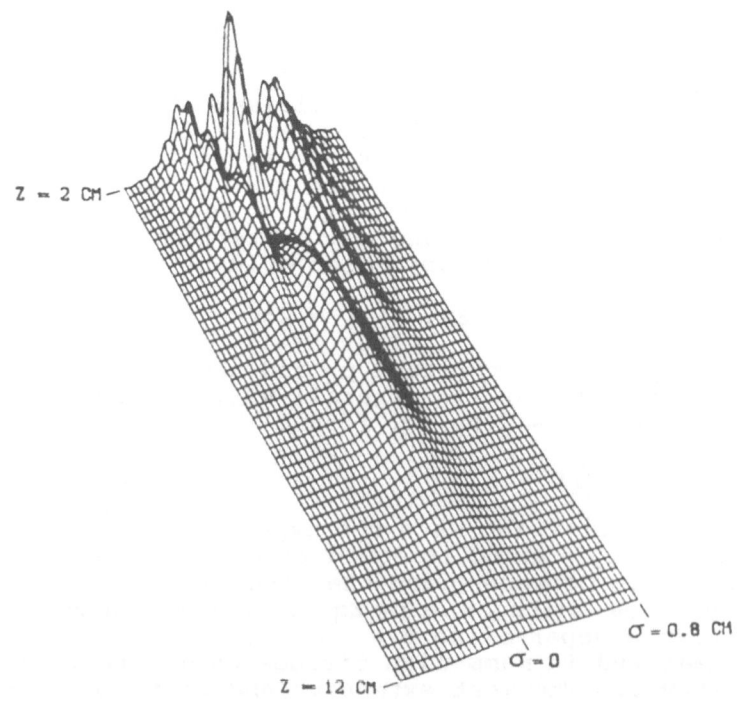

Fig. 1. Distribution of $p_o{}^2$ in the field of the piston source discussed in the text. From Nyborg and Steele (1985)

applies, is proportional to Q, the rate of heat production per unit volume. The region selected for display lies between planes at 2 cm and z = 12 cm, where z is distance from the source, and extends outward from the axis a distance of 0.8 cm. It should be realized that the field is symmetrical about the axis; Fig. 1 applies to any plane passing through the axis.

It is obvious in Fig. 1 that the spatial distribution of $p_0{}^2$ is highly nonuniform, especially at small values of z. Peaks and valleys are closely spaced near the source but are more widely spaced at larger distances. The peaks tend to decrease in height as z increases, because of absorption.

Just after the sound field is turned on the temperature at any point begins to rise linearly with time, the temperature T after a small time t being given by

$$T = T_0 + Qt/c_v \quad , \tag{5}$$

where T_0 is the temperature at t = 0, Q applies locally at the point in question and c_v is the heat capacity of the medium per unit volume. However, because of heat conduction, Eq. 5 is valid for only a very short time in a sound field like that shown in Fig. 1, especially near the transducer where the p_0 distribution is highly nonuniform.

In discussing the temperature-time dependence further, we consider a particular point in the field, namely the point at the highest peak in Fig. 1. This point is on the axis at a distance z = 2.35 cm from the transducer; we shall refer to the point as $P_{2.35}$. Some detailed information on the maximal region (symmetrical about the axis) whose peak is at $P_{2.35}$, is contained in the plots of Figs. 2 and 3; these are along perpendicular lines passing through $P_{2.35}$.

Figure 2 contains an axial plot; here the quantity Q (in normalizing units) is plotted along the axis, versus distance

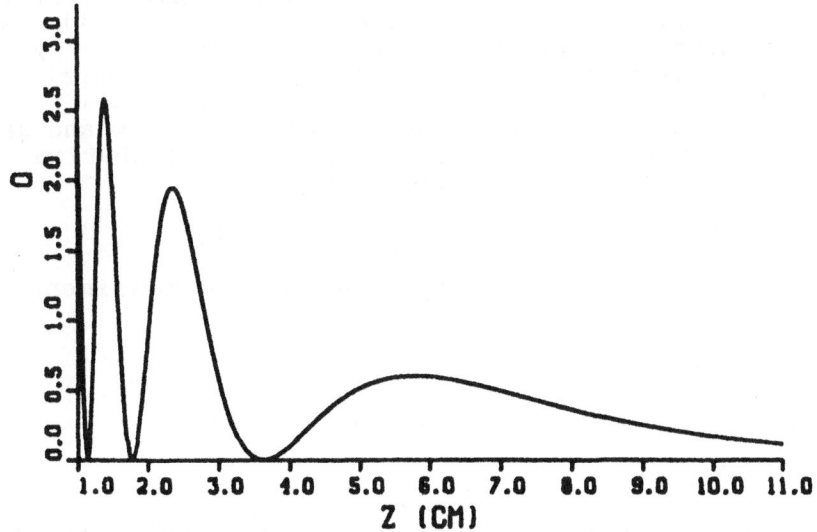

Fig. 2.   Plot along the axis of the piston source, showing Q versus distance z from the transducer. From Nyborg and Steele (1985).

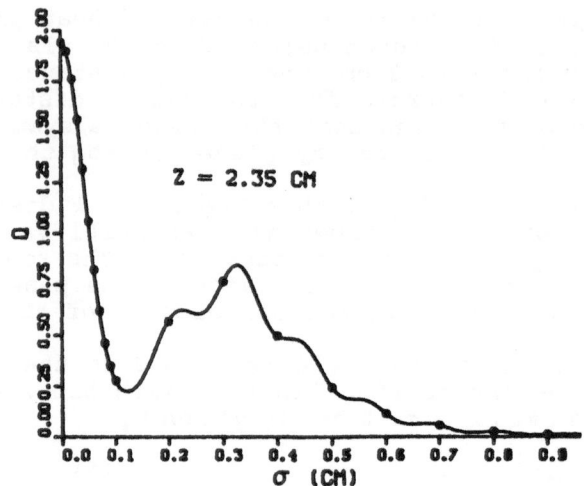

Fig. 3. Plot transverse to the axis of the piston source, showing Q versus distance from the axis in the plane z = 2.35 cm. From Nyborg and Steele (1985).

z from the transducer. Figure 3 is a transverse plot, showing Q versus distance from the axis along any direction in the plane at z = 2.35 cm. It is seen from Figs. 1-3 that the maximal region at $P_{2.35}$ extends about 18 mm axially between minima at z = 1.8 cm and z = 3.6 cm) and only about 2.2 mm transversely in the plane z = 2.35 mm (the minimum in Fig. 3 being at 1.1 mm from the axis).

TEMPERATURE FIELD OF A SMALL SOURCE

One can regard the temperature history at $P_{2.35}$ as being determined by the heat flowing to that point from all parts of the field. Consider a volume element dv, i.e., a small part of the medium of volume dv, located at P*, which is at a distance r from $P_{2.35}$. See Fig. 4. At time t = 0 the sound field is turned on and heat generation commences everywhere in the sound field at a rate Q per unit volume. The spatial distribution of Q is as shown in Fig. 1. From theory for heat conduction in a medium of conductivity K (Carslaw and Jaeger, 1959) the temperature at $P_{2.35}$ receives a contribution dT from the small heat source at P* equal to

$$dT = (Q \ dv/4\pi Kr) \ erfc \ (R) , \qquad (6)$$

where Q is the local value at P* and R is the nondimensional quantity

$$R = r/2(\kappa t)^{\frac{1}{2}} \qquad (7)$$

and κ is the thermal diffusivity defined by

$$\kappa = K/c_V , \qquad (8)$$

with c_V the heat capacity per unit volume. For media with thermal properties similar to water we take

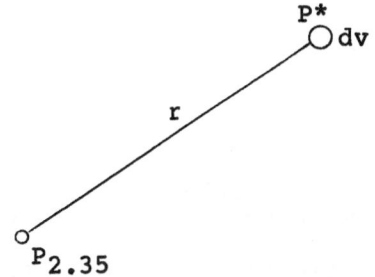

Fig. 4. A volume element dv, located at p*, is at a distance
         r from the point $P_{2.35}$.

$c_v = 4.2$ J/cm^3 ^{o}C

$K = 0.0060$ W/cm ^{o}C   (9)

$\kappa = 0.00144$ cm^2/s

The complementary error function erfc (R) is defined by

$$\text{erfc (R)} = (2/\sqrt{\pi}) \int_R^\infty e^{-u^2} \, du. \qquad (10)$$

A short list of values for erfc (R) versus R appears in Table 1.
In this table it is seen that erfc (R), a decreasing
function of R, is equal to unity when R = 0 and falls to zero
when R becomes large. Noting in Eq. 7 that R varies inversely
with the time t, we realize that for very small t the temperature at $P_{2.35}$ is little affected by heat generated in the
volume element dv at a distant point P*. However, as t increases, so does the temperature increment dT contributed by
the small heat source at P*; when t becomes very large the
contribution dT approaches but never exceeds a limiting (i.e.,
steady state) value

$(dT)_{lim} = Q$ dv/4πKr.   (11)

These trends are seen, together with more quantitative information, in Fig. 5. Here are plots of temperature rise versus
t, based on Eqs. 6-10 for three values of r, all for the same
value of Q dv. (The quantity Q dv is the thermal power, i.e.,
thermal energy per unit time, generated by the volume element
at P*).

     Examining the curves in Fig. 5 we see that these shift
downward with increasing r. This is expected from Eq. 11;
specifically, this equation states that the steady state temperature $(dT)_{lim}$, reached at large values of the time, varies
inversely with r.

     Also the curves in Fig. 5 shift to the right with in-
creasing r. This can be explained in terms of the theory as
follows. From Eqs. 6 and 11, the ratio of dT to $(dT)_{lim}$ is a
function of R alone and is, in fact, equal to erfc (R). From
Eq. 7 the time t corresponding to a given value of R is
proportional to r^2. Hence the time required for dT to reach a
given fraction of $(dT)_{lim}$ is proportional to r^2.

Table 1
The complementary error function

R	erfc(R)	R	erfc(R)
0.0	1.000	1.1	0.120
0.1	0.888	1.2	0.090
0.2	0.777	1.3	0.066
0.3	0.672	1.4	0.048
0.4	0.572	1.5	0.034
0.5	0.480	1.6	0.024
0.6	0.396	1.7	0.016
0.7	0.322	1.8	0.011
0.8	0.258	1.9	0.007
0.9	0.203	2.0	0.005
1.0	0.157		

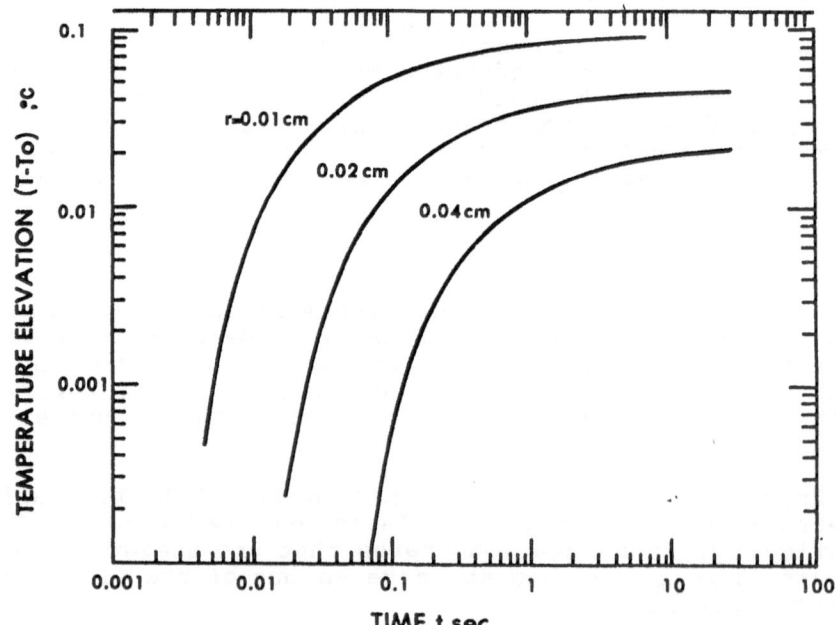

Fig. 5. Temperature elevation versus time at a several distances r from a point source of heat. From Nyborg (1977).

CALCULATION OF TEMPERATURE IN AN ULTRASOUND FIELD

We can now apply Eqs. 6-11 to calculation of the temperature T at $P_{2.35}$, relative to the original temperature T_0. If we consider the entire region of interest to be divided into small volume elements, the temperature rise $(T - T_0)$ is just the sum of contributions dT from all these elements, as given in Eq. 6. However, in view of the way these elementary contributions vary with time, an approximation can be made. In this approximation one ignores contributions from elements whose distance from $P_{2.35}$ is greater than r^*, a characteristic distance which varies with the time t. A specific expression for r^* is reached by noticing in Table 1 that erfc (R) is equal to 0.005 when R = 2. Thus contributions dT for which R is greater than 2 are less than 0.5% of the limiting value $(dT)_{lim}$. Assuming such contributions are negligible compared to contributions at smaller values of R, the characteristic value r^* is chosen so that R is equal to 2.0. From Eqs. 7 and 9 we are then led to

$$r^* = 0.15 \sqrt{t} \quad . \quad (r^* \text{ in cm}). \qquad (12)$$

A test calculation was carried out for a simplified situation in which Q was assumed constant throughout space. The above approximation, in which contributions for R > 2 were neglected, was found to give about 1 % error. The length r^* given by Eq. 12 can be regarded as the radius of a "sphere of influence", containing those volume elements which contribute significantly to the temperature rise at $P_{2.35}$.

Figures 6 and 7 show plots of the temperature rise $(T - T_0)$ at $P_{2.35}$ as a function of time t. These were generated by computing, at each value of t, the sum of contributions dT (given by Eq. 6) from heat sources throughout the sound field

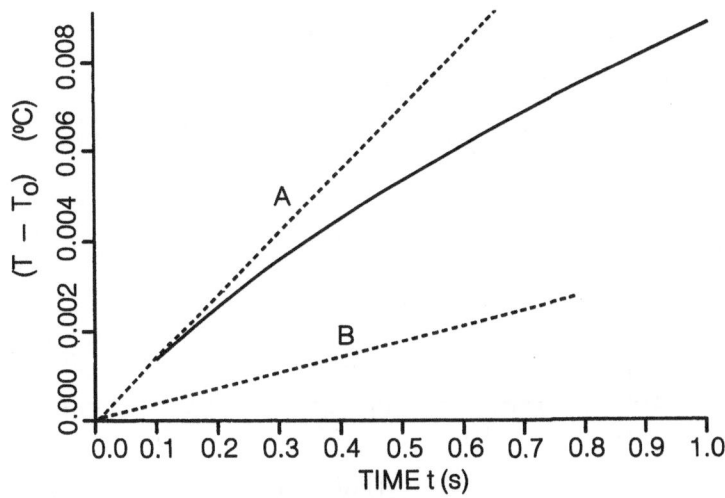

Fig. 6.   Solid curve gives computed temperatures elevation versus time at the point $P_{2.35}$ in the ultrasound field discussed in the text; during the first second. Dashed curves A and B are based on Eqs. 13 and 15, respectively.

under consideration. The frequency, radius and other parameters are as for Figs. 1-3. To determine the absolute values of Q the normalized values, such as those plotted in Figs. 2 and 3, are multiplied by 2 I_o; here I_o is equal to $cU_o^2/2$, where U_o is the velocity amplitude of the source. (Thus I_o is the intensity in a plane traveling wave with velocity amplitude U_o). For Figs. 6 and 7 the intensity I_o is 0.1 W/cm². To facilitate the computation, advantage was taken of axial symmetry; the elementary contributions dT were taken to be from rings with axes coinciding with that of the sound field. Figure 6 shows $T - T_o$ versus t for time t in the range 0 - 1 s. In the range 0.1 - 1 s the required numerical integration was carried out by summing contributions as described above, with Eq. 6 as the basis. For the range 0 to 0.1 s this method would have required choosing the volume elements to be very small; initially, only the elements very near the point $P_{2.35}$ contribute significantly to the temperature rise. Instead of doing this, integration was avoided entirely in this range, and use was made of the simple expression (Cf. Eq. 5)

$$T - T_o = Q_{2.35}\, t/c_v, \qquad (13)$$

where $Q_{2.35}$ is the value of Q at the point $P_{2.35}$. Equation (13) is just the expression which applies when the following condition holds: the time is so short that essentially no heat has been conducted away from the vicinity of $P_{2.35}$.

Another way of stating the condition for validity of Eq. 13 is to suppose that the integration method had been used, and refer to a characteristic of the Q distribution near $P_{2.35}$. We define a length $r_{2.35}$ as the radius of the largest

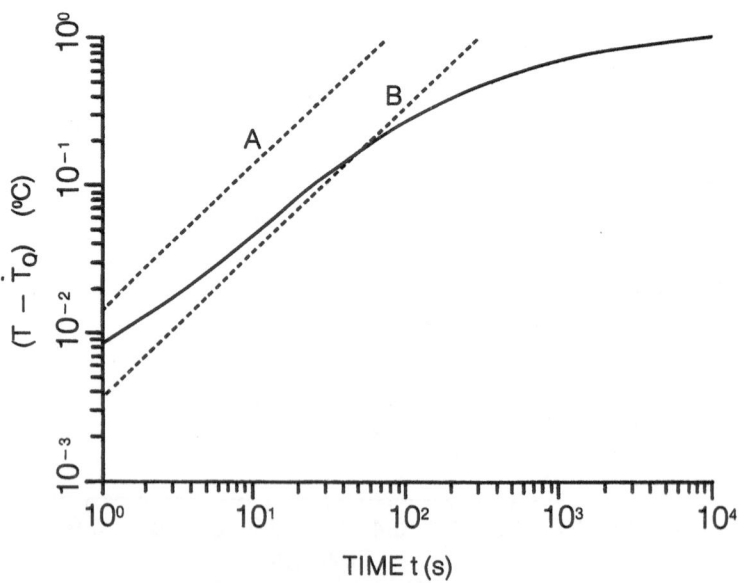

Fig. 7. Solid curve gives computed temperature elevation versus time at the point $P_{2.35}$ in the ultrasound field discussed in the text, during the interval 1. – 10⁴ s. Dashed curves A and B are based on Eqs. 13 and 15, respectively.

sphere centered at $P_{2.35}$ in which Q is essentially uniform, according to a suitable criterion. We expect Eq. 13 to apply when t is so small that most contributions to $T - T_O$ from surrounding volume elements come from elements within the distance $r_{2.35}$. Considering t to be related to $r_{2.35}$ according to Eq. 7, and regarding a contribution as negligible if $R > 1$ (a less stringent condition than was applied in obtaining Eq. 12), one obtains

$$t = 175 \ (r_{2.35})^2 . \quad (r_{2.35} \text{ in cm}). \quad (14)$$

This equation leads to the anticipated alternative statement of the condition for validity of Eq. 13: the latter equation applies if t is less than the value given in Eq. 14.

One obtains 0.1 s for t if $r_{2.35}$ is chosen as 0.25 mm. It appears consistent with the plot in Fig. 3 to consider Q as reasonably uniform out to 0.25 mm from the axis. Along the axis it is clear from Fig. 2 that Q is nearly constant over a range of 0.25 mm extending in either direction from the peak at $z = 2.35$ cm. Hence it is not unreasonable that 0.25 mm serves roughly as radius of a "sphere of uniformity" centered at $P_{2.35}$.

At times t greater than 0.1 s, the slope of the temperature-versus-time curve (Fig. 6) decreases with time. This can be explained by referring to the fact that heat flows away from the temperature peak, which is initially at $P_{2.35}$, and that the effect of this becomes more evident as time goes on.

An alternative explanation of the decreasing slope can be given by considering the contributions to the temperature $T - T_O$ from the surrounding volume elements, as given by Eq. 6. As time goes on, the temperature rise depends more and more on contributions from elements at distances greater than r^*. At these more distant elements the Q value is, on the average, less than in the near-vicinity of $P_{2.35}$, and the resulting rate of increase of temperature is correspondingly less.

As time t, and thus also the radius r^*, increases a point may be reached at which the average value of Q within the sphere of influence (the sphere of radius r^* centered at $P_{2.35}$) is equal to the average value of Q over the plane at $z = 2.35$ cm. Also, when this condition is reached it may be true that the average value of Q within the sphere of influence does not change rapidly with increasing time. If so, it would be expected that under these conditions the temperature rise would be given approximately by

$$T - T_O = \overline{Q}t/c_v, \quad (15)$$

where $\overline{Q}$ is the average of Q over the plane at $\underline{z} = 2.35$ cm. Equation 15 is the same as Eq. 13, except that $\overline{Q}$ replaces $Q_{2.35}$. In Fig. 6 the linear dashed curves A and B are based on Eqs. 13 and 15, respectively. It was pointed out earlier that curve A, which is based on the local value of Q at $P_{2.35}$, gives the temperature rise in agreement with the computed solid curve at values of the time in the range 0 - 0.1 s. At later times curve A gives values that are too high (relative to the computed solid curve), by an amount that increases with time. On the other hand, curve B, based on an average value of Q in the plane z = 2.35 cm, gives values of (T - T$_o$) that are too low in the range of Fig. 6.

In Fig. 7 the temperature rise (T - T$_o$) is plotted versus time t for the same conditions as in Fig. 6 except that the range of t is 1 - 10,000 s. To accommodate the large ranges of the variables, logarithmic scales are used. Thus log (T - T$_o$) is plotted versus log t. For comparison, two linear dashed curves (A) and (B) are shown in Fig. 7, each with 1:1 slope on the log-log scales used; as in Fig. 6, curve A is based on Eq. 13 and curve B on Eq. 15. We see that a trend noted in Fig. 6 is followed, in that the temperature rise given by the dashed curve A exceeds the computed value (solid curve) by an amount that increases with time. On the other hand, the dashed curve B lies below the solid curve at the lower values of time but crosses it at about 70 s, and lies above the solid curve thereafter. In the range 10 - 100 s, curve B, based on Eq. 15, gives values of the temperature rise which agree with computed values (solid curve) to within about 20%.

Other features can be noted for the computed solid curve in Fig. 7. The slope (dT/dt) increases with time until about t = 10 s, then is nearly constant until about t = 70 s. At this time the slope clearly begins to decrease, and becomes smaller as time goes on. A possible explanation of these features is as follows. The interval from 10 to 70 s is apparently one where the average value of Q in the "sphere of influence" (as defined earlier) is about equal to $\overline{Q}$, the average over the plane at z = 2.35 cm. One would expect the average to decrease when the radius of the sphere of influence exceeds the effective radius r_b of the beam, for then this sphere includes points outside the beam, where Q is relatively small. A criterion based on this idea (analogous to Eq. 14, choosing R = 1) gives

$$t = 175 \ r_b{}^2 \tag{16}$$

as the time at which the sphere of influence expands beyond the effective beam size. Taking r_b to be the transducer radius, 0.6 cm, one obtains 65 s for t from Eq. 16. This calculated time is consistent with the observation made earlier that the slope of the computed temperature versus time curve in Fig. 7 begins to decrease at about t = 70 s.

Figure 8 shows how the temperature rise varies with time to 10^5 s, and shows this for two positions on the axis. The upper curve applies at $P_{2.35}$, a position of maximum Q, and is an extension of the solid curve in Fig. 7. As time proceeds the rate of temperature rise approaches zero and the temperature approaches a limiting value. (This limiting value is not shown, but can be computed by letting erfc (R) equal unity in Eq. 6).

The lower curve in Fig. 8 applies at z = 3.62 cm; this is the position of minimum Q, as can be seen from Fig. 2. As expected, the two curves show that the temperature rise at the minimum is much less than that at the maximum at small values of time. It may be more surprising that the temperature at the minimum rapidly catches up, so that for time t greater than 100 s the temperature at z = 2.35 cm is greater than that

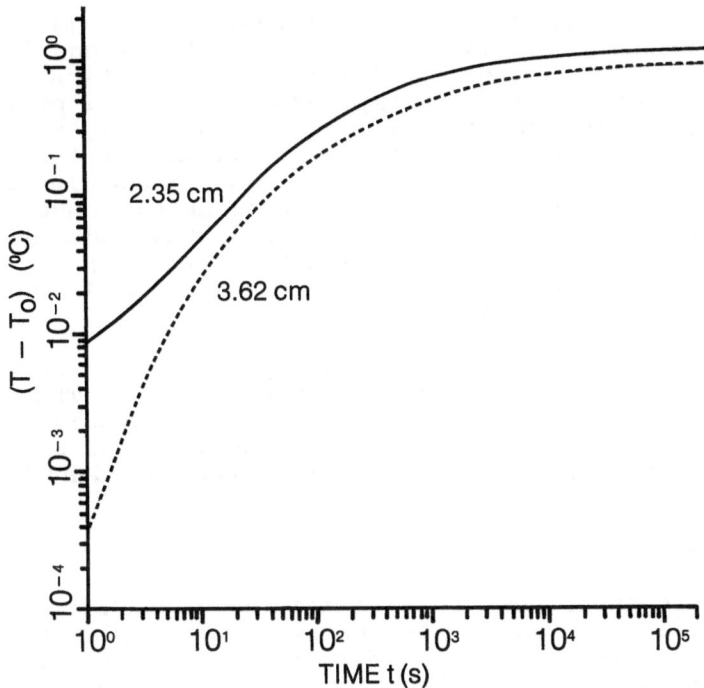

Fig. 8. Temperature rise versus time at two positions on the axis of the ultrasound field under discussion. The upper curve, for z = 2.35 cm, applies at a maximum of Q and the lower, for z = 3.62 cm, at a minimum. See Fig. 2.

at z = 3.62 cm by no more than 50%. The rather small difference that persists at large values of the time is less than would be accounted for from the attenuation caused by absorption along the path from 2.35 cm to 3.62 cm.

The near-convergence of the two curves in Fig. 8 at large values of t is consistent with the idea, discussed above, that the temperature at any point P is dependent on the average value of Q within the sphere of influence for that point. When the sphere has grown large enough to include a number of maxima and minima of Q, the average is not strongly affected by the value of Q at the point P itself.

In the integration procedure used in obtaining results such as those shown in Fig. 6-8, the basic volume element is a ring of radius a and volume 2πa da dz which generates heat at the rate 2πaQ da dz. Here Q is the value which applies at the location of the ring. Equation 6 gives the contribution of a ring to the temperature rise at an axial point (P) whose distance to any point on the ring is r. For rings lying in a plane at distance z from the transducer, summation with respect to a gives the total temperature rise at P produced by a sheet of thickness dz located at z. Preliminary findings suggest that the contribution of a sheet to the temperature rise at P can be found in a simpler way. According to these the contribution of the sheet is approximately equal to that which would come from a disc of thickness dz and radius equal to the transducer radius, in which Q is uniform; the value of Q is that which would apply at the distance z if a uniform plane wave propagated from the transducer.

If further work supports this approximation it will be possible to simplify temperature calculations. This simplification has already been used (in advance of detailed justification) to compute temperature distributions for a range of parameters; typical results have been published by the NCRP (1983).

DISCUSSION

In this paper some results have been described of temperature calculations in the near field of a piston-like ultrasound source and in a medium with acoustic properties resembling tissue. The situation is complicated by the non-uniformity of the near field but the task can be reduced somewhat by using simplifying approximations.

The analysis presented here serves to illustrate means by which temperatures can be predicted in some clinical situations,. It is only a beginning to a general procedure, however. In a more complete analysis, effects of perfusion must be considered. Also, for applications to diagnostic ultrasound, the theory must be extended to fields which are pulsed, focused and scanned.

A review of biological effects associated with temperature elevation is not attempted here. Other papers in this course will deal with this topic.

REFERENCES

Carslaw, H. S. and Jaeger, J. C., 1959, "Conduction of Heat in Solids", Clarendon Press, Oxford.
Cavicchi, T. J. and O'Brien, W. D., Jr., 1984, Heat generated by ultrasound in an absorbing medium, J. Acoust. Soc. Am., 76:1244.
NCRP, 1983, "Biological Effects of Ultrasound: Mechanisms and Clinical Implications," National Council of Radiation Protection and Measurements Report No. 74, NCRP Publications, 7910 Woodmont Ave., Suite 1016, Bethesda, MD 20814.
Nyborg, W. L., 1981, Heat generation by ultrasound in a relaxing medium, J. Acoust. Soc. Am., 70:310.
Nyborg, W. L. and Steele, R. B., 1985, Near field of a piston source of ultrasound in an absorbing medium, J. Acoust. Soc. Am., 78:1882.
Parker, K. J., 1983, Ultrasonic attenuation and absorption in liver tissue, Ultrasound in Med. & Biol., 9:363.

BIOLOGICAL EFFECTS OF ACOUSTIC CAVITATION

Edwin L. Carstensen

Department of Electrical Engineering
University of Rochester
Rochester, New York 14627
U. S. A.

Although there is no basis in present knowledge to indicate that human subjects have been harmed in diagnostic applications of ultrasound, there is clear evidence of damage to lower organisms with temporal maximum intensities somewhat less than those available from certain diagnostic devices. Where exposures of this kind have caused clear effects, the mechanism of action appears to be related to the phenomenon of cavitation. It now remains to determine whether these observations have relevance for medical practice.

Linear and second order analyses of the motion of spherical gaseous cavities in acoustic fields show that interaction of the elasticity of the gas within the cavity and the mass of the surrounding fluid give rise to resonance oscillation of bubbles which are much smaller than the wavelength of the sound; that damping from radiation, viscosity and heat conduction give the bubbles absorption-scattering cross-sections which can be many times greater than their geometrical cross-sections; that bubbles are subject to radiation forces which depend upon bubble size and position in standing wave fields; that there are forces on cells near oscillating bubbles which can be many times the force of gravity; and that oscillation of bubbles produce strong highly localized shear forces in the fluid near bubbles and localized fluid motion called microstreaming.

A requirement for cavitation to occur is the pre-existence of small stabilized gaseous nuclei. Once exposed to an acoustic field, these nuclei can grow and, in times of a millisecond or more, pass through resonance size. When acoustic pressures are of the order of one atmosphere or more, bubble oscillations become highly nonlinear. For appropriate combinations of acoustic pressure amplitude, frequency and size, bubbles may expand and collapse violently. The highly nonlinear transition from relatively stable oscillations where bubble radii change by less than a factor of two to the condition of violent collapse may occur with a relatively small change in acoustic pressure (e.g. as little as 10 per cent). Thus, it is useful to use the concept of a threshold for transient cavitation. Mechanical and chemical processes which take place above this threshold are quantitatively and qualitatively different than for stable, small oscillations of bubbles. During transient collapse, pressures in the gaseous cavities can be many thousands of atmospheres, leading to localized shockwaves and mechanical stress. During collapse, temperatures of many thousands of degrees Centigrade in the gas produce a wide range of chemical products some of which are potentially toxic. These violent processes can take place during the microsecond length pulses which are used in medical diagnosis but the requirements on the magnitudes of the temporal maximum intensities and the pre-existence of appropriate nuclei are more severe than with continuous exposures. Although transient cavitation can, in principle, occur with microsecond length pulses of ultrasound (Flynn, 1982), whether the appropriate conditions exist for this to take place in biological media is perhaps the most important aspect of the problem of the assessment of the safety of the use of ultrasound in medical diagnosis (Carstensen and Flynn, 1982).

With a few esoteric exceptions, known biological effects of ultrasound are caused either by heating or by cavitation or cavitation-related processes. When biological effects are reported for dilute suspensions of cells in saline solutions, it is reasonably safe to assume that cavitation is responsible since heating of this medium is very probably negligible. At the other extreme, for effects which have been observed in the tissues of mammals, there are very few cases in which heating can be ruled out as either the primary or a contributing factor. Some place between these two extremes, we have a number of particularly interesting and revealing studies of the effects of ultrasound on plant and animal materials which contain or are in contact with stabilized populations of small bubbles.

From our current knowledge of cavitation phenomena, it appears quite possible that effects from exposure to the microsecond length pulses used in diagnostic ultrasound are quantitatively and even qualitatively different than the effects of exposure to c.w. or long pulses. Out of the decades of investigation, only two or three studies have shown clear effects under conditions which are directly comparable to those used in diagnostic ultrasound. For this reason, most of the reports which are reviewed here have limited direct applicability to the question of clinical safety. Our overall objective is to learn as much as possible from the existing literature about the general phenomenon of cavitation but special attention is given to pulsed ultrasound at the end of this review.

CHEMICAL REACTIONS

Because of the very high temperatures in the gas during transient collapse, it has been inferred that free radicals would form. These products are so highly reactive that it is unlikely that they would exist for times or distances greater than that required for encounter with more than few molecules of the aqueous medium. Therefore, direct detection of the free radicals is difficult. However, several investigative groups recently have employed an intermediate molecule which traps the radicals long enough that they can be studied quantitatively by electron spin resonance techniques (Edmonds and Sancier, 1983). Evidence even has been obtained for free radical production by pulses as short as 6 µs in aqueous solutions (Riesz et al., 1985).

Even though free radicals may be created during transient cavitation, it does not follow that they interact directly with biological cells. In particular, it is unlikely that free radicals created during collapse of a cavity near a cell would last long enough to interact with the genetic material of the cell. However, the products which form through reaction with free radicals in the gas or at the liquid-gas interface may have a much longer lifetime. Henglein (1985) has recently demonstrated a wide range of such products in chemically defined media. As an example, when the fluid is saturated with carbon dioxide, one of the cavitation products is carbon monoxide (Henglein, 1985). No serious attempt has been made to study the chemistry of transient cavitation in media which may be said to be representative of biological materials. However, it is clear that a very wide spectrum of endproducts, in principle, could be produced in addition to free radicals themselves.

MACROMOLECULAR SOLUTIONS

A number of independent studies lend support to the concept that ultrasound - very probably through the mechanism of cavitation - can cause fragmentation and denaturation of DNA in solution. There is some disagreement among investigators on the levels required to produce these effects. Coakley and Dunn (1971) found no effects until reaching an intensity of 300 W/cm^2 whereas several studies report effects at levels at or below 1 W/cm^2 (e.g. Galperin-Lemaitre et al., 1975; McKee et al., 1977; Gupta and Wang, 1976).

Because these large molecules are found to be broken, it is tempting to ascribe the action of cavitation to mechanical shearing either from local microstreaming near stably oscillating bubbles or from the mechanical shock associated with the collapse of transient cavities. Although the dominant action probably is mechanical, Braginskaya et al. (1981) found evidence of the involvement of free radicals in the denaturation of DNA.

Although ultrasound can damage DNA in solution, there is little evidence to support the conclusion that this process occurs inside intact cells.

CELL SUSPENSIONS

Study of the effects of ultrasound on cell suspensions has been a popular pursuit. Reliable evidence for cell lysis, reduced cell survival and plating efficiency has been reported by many investigators. Since the effective cavitation sites are probably in the suspending fluid near the cells, it is not surprising that the surfaces and outer membranes of the cells are affected. This has been demonstrated as a change in surface charge as evidenced through studies of the electrophoretic mobility of cells after irradiation by ultrasound. Changes in the outer surface of cells are suggested in a qualitatively different way by the observations that exposure to ultrasound affects the way cells adhere to each other and to surfaces of the containers in which they are cultured. Other investigators have found evidence of potassium leakage from cells under conditions which have produced negligible lysis of cells, i.e. sublytic permeability changes in the membranes. There are rather convincing data showing changes in morphology of cells and spheroids which have been exposed to ultrasound under conditions where cavitation could have been active (Williams et al,, 1976; Sacks et al., 1981; Holmer et al., 1975).

It is less clear that cells which have survived ultrasonic radiation are affected in their internal structure or in their function. Almost all studies - with cell suspensions or with higher organisms - which have tested for genetic effects of ultrasound have had negative results. There have been many negative studies of the chromosomes of cells which have been irradiated with ultrasound. In principle, free radicals from acoustic cavitation could be mutagenic but experimental evidence to support this mechanism is very weak. At the present time, the weight of evidence is against the liklihood that the nuclei of cultured cells are altered by exposure to ultrasound (Thacker, 1973). On the other hand, as will be discussed later, there is a reasonable concensus that the nuclei of plant cells can be grossly changed after treatment with ultrasound. The physical and biological conditions are different in these two cases but, in view of the collective evidence, it would be wise to keep an open mind on the possible effects of ultrasound on nuclear material and cell function.

There is obviously much more to be learned from studies of cell suspensions but the available literature already has provided us with a rich collection of the effects of ultrasonic radiation at the cellular level. In general, cavitation provides us with an attractive physical mechanism to explain these biological effects. The intensities required to produce the effects are appropriate. Effects are frequently seen where standing waves help to stabilize bubbles in the sound field. In addition, enhancement of effects by rotation of the tubes which contain the cell suspensions is consistent with the cavitation postulate. In general, the application of an excess hydrostatic pressure of two or three atmospheres is enough to eliminate the effects. Low frequencies are, in general, more effective than high frequencies in producing biological effects. All of these qualitative characteristics are consistent with the cavitation postulate. Whether effects occur and what the magnitude of those effects are when they do occur depend upon both the magnitude of the sound field (intensity or pressure amplitude) and the time of exposure. At the present time, it is not possible to combine these two factors together in a universal ultrasonic "dose". In fact, it is clear from the nature of the exposure systems used in the study of cell suspensions that we would be able to make only the crudest estimates of either of these parameters for the studies which have been reported to date. The axial maximum intensities may be specified with some accuracy but there is no satisfactory way to describe the intensity-time combinations for all of the cells which are placed in an exposure chamber. At best, the data on exposures of cell suspensions and solutions of molecules suggest what could happen at intensities as great as the axial intensities used by each of the investigators. Furthermore, whether effects occur in laboratory exposures of cell suspensions depends in many cases critically upon the standing wave conditions in the exposure vessels. Standing waves are probably rare in medical uses of ultrasound.

Keeping these reservations in mind, we find that there is an interesting clustering of studies carried out under free field conditions which report effects in the range of intensities from 0.5 to 2 W/cm^2. This is probably the best order of magnitude estimate which we could make if we were forced to extrapolate from the available *in vitro* studies of cell suspensions in human subjects. Williams (1983) and his colleagues have made several different attempts to detect the effects of ultrasonic cavitation in the blood of human subjects and laboratory animals. Overall his results to date appear to be negative even though some of his studies employed intensities well above 2 W/cm^2.

STABILIZED BUBBLES

Perhaps the greatest mysteries and frustrations of cavitation research are the small gaseous bodies which serve as nuclei for cavitation events. Where they are stabilized before exposure to ultrasound, how they grow and generate new nuclei after exposure and what their lifetimes are after cavitation occurs, are difficult questions for the simplest media, but for the chemically and structurally complex material which makes up living tissues, the detailed answers may not become available to us even after many more years of study.

One exposure system deserves special treatment because of the simplification and control which it provides for cavitation nuclei. Nyborg, Miller and colleagues (e.g. Miller *et al.*, 1979) showed that it is possible to stabilize gas bodies small enough to be resonant in the biomedically interesting frequency range by using special membrane filters (Nucleopore, General Electric Company). The membrane material itself is thin and nearly transparent to ultrasound. The pore diameter for these filters is controlled by the manufacturing process and is highly uniform. If the membrane material is hydrophobic, the gas trapped in the pores is retained even when the membranes are immersed in water. When cell suspensions are exposed to ultrasound in the presence of these Nucleopore filters, the physical properties and location of the cavitation sites are known and, within limits, can be selected by the investigator as a part of the experimental design. At large acoustic pressures, there is a tendency for the bubbles to be dislodged and lost. Hence, the Nucleopore exposure system serves primarily as a model for stable, as opposed to transient, cavitation. However, since the bubbles are fixed in location, it is relatively easy to observe them microscopically and to watch the interaction of the biological cells as they approach and interact with the oscillating bubbles. Williams and Miller (1980) combined an unusually sensitive system for detection of ATP with the Nucleopore exposure system in a study of the effects of ultrasonic gas body activation on platelets and erythrocytes. The detection system literally counts individual ATP molecules. They report detecting ATP release from platelets at intensities as low as 4 mW/cm^2 (Williams, 1983). This appears to be the lowest intensity for which biological effects of c.w. ultrasound have been observed with reasonable certainty. The oscillating bubbles probably cause a shear stress on the red cell which in turn alters the permeability of the cell membrane to ATP. It is reasonable to infer from the ATP studies that other small molecules leak from the treated cells.

These studies have provided qualitatively and quantitatively new information about the biological effects of acoustic cavitation. Not only have new effects been revealed but details of the mechanisms of action of the bubbles on cells in suspension now are known. Furthermore, it is now clear that certain biological effects of ultrasound occur at extremely low intensities. It is reasonable to believe that these same effects could occur *in vivo* if somehow stable bubbles of appropriate size were present. This, of course, is the big question. Perhaps, the only way we will know whether nuclei are present will be through detection of the biological effects which result from their action. Knowing the biological endpoints to study and the required ultrasonic parameters to use should provide guidance in searches for effects *in vivo*. Also, these studies could be used in a "worst case" analysis of the effects of stable cavitation in mammals. Such an analysis would conclude that clumping of platelets and leakage from cells in the blood might occur at exposure levels of the order of

10 mW/cm². However, the frequency of these events or the magnitude of the effects very likely would be well below the natural occurrance of these processes and would be accomodated by the body's homeostatic repair processes.

PLANT TISSUES

Two rather different plant systems have been particularly useful in studies of the biological effects of acoustic cavitation: (1) the leaves of aquatic plants, notably *Elodea* and (2) root tips. In both, the sites of action of ultrasound almost certainly include the channels of gas which are stabilized in the spaces between the cells of the tissues. This assures us that air bodies are present and that the spatial relationship between the bubbles and the cells is stable. Furthermore, in contrast with cell suspensions, the spatial relationship between the sound beam and the tissue can be fixed so that it is possible to define the exposure of the cells both in intensity and time.

In contrast with the bubbles in the Nucleopore filters, plant root gas bodies are confined in three dimensions. This could make them relatively stable, but it is also probable that the maximum expansion of the bubble is limited by the confining tissue structure. Certainly, these nuclei are not physically equivalent to spherical bubbles in water. Miller (1979a) has modeled the of gas channels in plant leaves for small (stable) oscillations. However, the theoretical guidance which we have for the behavior of these bubbles at high intensities is limited.

The leaves of the aquatic plant, *Elodea*, have been used in studies of the effects of ultrasound by several investigators including the pioneers of bioultrasound, Harvey and Loomis (1928). Miller (1977, 1979a, 1979b, 1985) has used this tissue for a serious biophysical study of important aspects of acoustic cavitation. He considered the specific case of cylindrical gas bodies of the kind which are stabilized in the intercellular spaces of the leaves of *Elodea*. This model predicts oscillation of the cavity walls with resonant behavior at frequencies which depend upon the diameter of the air channels (Miller, 1979a). It is reasonable to infer from this that there must be corresponding frequency dependent biological effects from ultrasonic activation of these gas bodies. Miller reported thresholds for cell lysis with minima which correspond well with his theoretical predictions for the populations of bubble sizes found in his leaves (Miller, 1979b).

Root tips are rapidly dividing and differentiating tissues and provide a system for the study of the effects of ultrasonically induced cavitation on the growth and development of organized tissues. Near the tip of the root is a small, approximately spherical group of cells called the meristem which is responsible for generation of new cells. Each of these cells divides at a rate of roughly once per day. One of the daughter cells remains in the meristem and the other begins to elongate and differentiate. This process is responsible for growth of the root. In the garden pea (*Pisum sativum*), the meristem occupies the first millimeter of the plant root. The next 3 to 4 mm section contains elongating cells. There is relatively little growth or change in the rest of the root. Approximately 3 to 4 per cent of the space in the elongation region is gas (Carstensen *et al.*, 1981). The gas content of the meristem is less than 1%. From microscopic examination, it appears that most of this gas is divided among the spaces between the cells (Gershoy *et al.*, 1976). From histology, we can estimate that these channels are of the order of a few micrometers in diameter. Thus, it is reasonable to believe that these gas bodies could serve as nuclei for cavitation.

Exposures of the root tips of peas (*Pisum sativum*) for periods of one minute result in what appears to be an immediate reduction in growth rate followed by a gradual recovery over a period of several days. Roots of beans (*Vicia faba*) and corn (*Zea mays*) respond similarly. The threshold intensity for an effect on growth appears to be of the order of 1 W/cm^2. There are monotonic increases in the effects as intensity is increased. Exposure time also accentuates growth reduction. No simple dose-response relationship is apparent which could be used to summarize empirically all of the intensity-time observations nor have we a theoretical understanding of the processes involved which would provide the basis for such a parameter.

The rate of division of the cells in the meristem as measured by the mitotic index (the fraction of cells in mitosis) is reduced by exposure to ultrasound. However, this is not entirely a direct result of exposure of the meristematic cells. Using focused ultrasound, it was shown that irradiating at a point 4 mm up the root from the meristem was almost as effective as direct exposure of the observed meristematic cells (Law *et al.*, 1978). This demonstrates that the mitotic index can be affected indirectly either because of interference with the supply of nutrients to the meristem or by generation and transport to the meristem of toxic products from damaged cells.

In fact, all of these observations are consistent with a cavitation mechanism. Although the absorption coefficients of plant roots are very high, the diameters of the roots are small and heat exchange with surrounding water in the exposure system is excellent. Direct measurement of temperatures in exposed roots indicates that the primary mechanism of action of ultrasound is nonthermal (Eames *et al.*, 1975). The most sensitive sites of action are those which are known to contain a rich supply of gas bodies in the intercellular spaces of the root tissue. The intensities required to produce the effects are reasonable for a cavitation process. In addition, roots are more sensitive to frequencies below 2 MHz than above (Carstensen *et al.*, 1979). Excess hydrostatic pressure causes a marked reduction in the effectiveness of ultrasonic irradiation on root growth (Carstensen *et al.*, 1979). However, there is an interesting quantitative difference in the pressures required to suppress cavitation effects with cell suspensions and with roots. With cell suspensions, several investigators have shown that 2 to 3 atmospheres of excess pressure is sufficient to eliminate completely the action of ultrasound (Clarke and Hill, 1970; Ciaravino *et al.*, 1981). With roots, even at 30 atmospheres of excess hydrostatic pressure, some reduction in root growth was observed ($I = 4$ W/cm^2, $t = 1$ min, $f = 1$ MHz). The difference probably is a reflection of the nature of the interaction of the gas bodies with their respective stabilizing structures rather than a demonstration of a qualitatively new mechanism for the action of ultrasound. However, no direct tests of these postulates have been made.

What are the implications for mammalian tissues of the results of studies with plant tissues? Plant tissues have yielded a more detailed understanding of the mechanisms by which ultrasonic cavitation produces biological effects as well as better information on the nature of possible bioeffects and the physical conditions required to produce those effects. But, we know very little about the distribution of gas in mammalian tissues. In contrast with plants, mammalian cellular respiration ordinarily involves dissolved gases. We can be reasonably certain that the rich collection of small intercellular gas bodies found in parts of plant roots and *Elodea* leaves is not found in mammals. Therefore, direct extrapolation from plants to mammals is impossible. As with cell suspensions, we can use the data here for a worst case analysis. The available data show that effects may occur at intensities as low as 0.2 W/cm^2 at biomedically interesting frequencies if appropriate sizes of bubbles are present. The effects include lysis and sublytic perturbations of intracellular structures.

INSECTS

Insects are among the most rapidly developing of higher organisms. In a period of about 7 days, fruit flies (*Drosophila*) go from eggs to larvae, to pupae and, finally, to adult flies (imagos). During the pupa stage, a dramatic metamorphosis occurs in which nearly all of the tissues of the larva are transformed into completely new organs. The attractiveness of insects for studies of the biological effects of ultrasound has been recognized by a number of investigators. In the course of their studies, insects have been exposed to ultrasound at all four stages of development.

Fortuitously, in insect larvae, nature has provided us with a nearly ideal subject for studies of the effects of acoustic cavitation. Respiration, rather than involving the circulatory system as in higher animals, is accomplished in insects by bringing air directly to all of the tissues of the body. This is accomplished through tubes (trachae) which in larvae extend the length of the organism. In fruit flies (*Drosophila*), the diameter of these tubes is ranges from 10 to 50 micrometers depending upon age. Branching from the trachae are progressively smaller tubules which carry gases directly to the tissues. Thus, the organism contains a rich distribution of gas bodies which should serve as the nuclei required for transient cavitation.

Studies of *Drosophila* exposed in the larval stage have provided us with the most dramatic evidence available thus far that the exposures used in pulse-echo diagnostic ultrasound can cause adverse biological effects (Child et al., 1981). These studies show that there is a rather sharp threshold for killing between maximum intensities of 10 and 20 W/cm^2. For a significant fraction of exposed larvae, death is delayed until they have entered the pupa stage of development. That temporal peak rather than temporal average intensity is the relevant physical predictor for this biological effect was shown by an experiment in which the spatial average, temporal maximum intensity was 50 W/cm^2 throughout and the temporal average intensity was changed through the pulse repetition rate. Very significant killing occurred at average inensities as low as 3 mW/cm^2 and was only a litle greater at 100 times that average intensity. That there is a threshold for killing and that it depends upon temporal peak as opposed to temporal average intensity is strengthened by the experiments which showed that with a temporal maximum intensity of 4 W/cm^2 and pulse repetition rates great enough bring the temporal average intensities up to 80 mW/cm^2, there was no evidence of an effect even with exposures as long as 20 minutes.

In most of the experiments with *Drosophila*, even those involving relatively large c.w. exposures, it appears reasonably safe to exclude heating as the dominant factor (see Carstensen and Child, 1980). Hence, by default, cavitation is the probable mechanism of action. Transient cavitation can be expected even from very short pulses of ultrasound if the temporal peak intensities are above thresholds of the order of 10 W/cm^2 (Flynn, 1982). In fact, most observations are consistent with the predictions of this theory (Carstensen and Flynn, 1982). Profound effects on development have been observed at average intensities (<10 mW/cm^2) which are far too small to produce heating (Child et al., 1981). The frequency dependence of the effects is consistent with the cavitation mechanism (Berg et al., 1983). In a study of the effects of low average intensity pulsed ultrasound on eggs, it was found that the sensitivity of the organism increased dramatically at the stage of development when the respiratory apparatus of the fully developed larva within the egg shell fills with air (Child and Carstensen, 1982).

Because of physical and biological differences, it is not possible to extrapolate from insects to mammals particularly without a great deal more information about the mechanisms - biological and physical - which are involved. The most important result to come from studies with insects has been the unequivocal demonstration that, given the proper conditions, diagnostically relevant exposures can produce harmful effects. If similar effects occur in human beings, it could be a very serious concern. There appears to be little doubt that a cavitation related phenomenon is the primary mechanism of the action of ultrasound in most of the insect experiments. That information alone provides us with a significant advantage in the design of experiments which may someday give us answers to the nature of possible effects in mammals and estimates of the probabilities of their occurrence.

AMPHIBIAN EMBRYOS

As noted in the discussion of insects above, developing organisms are attractive subjects for biological effects studies. Development in itself is a prime public health concern. But, because developing tissue may magnify effects, it is potentially a very sensitive detector of damage. In particular, amphibian embryos exposed in an aqueous medium have excellent heat exchange. Thus, for reasonable exposures, we can assume that any observed effects may be attributed to cavitation.

Both microscopic and gross morphological changes have been reported as the result of exposure of developing amphibian eggs to ultrasound. There have been no serious attempts to independently confirm these studies. The recent paper by Sarvazyan and colleagues (1982) deserves special attention. In this study, frog embryos (*Rana temporaria, Ranan esculenta and Xenopus laevis*) and ectomesodermal explants from these embryos were exposed to 0.9 MHz continuous wave and pulsed (0.5 duty cycle) ultrasound with spatial average intensities less than 1 W/cm^2. Attempts were made to achieve free field conditions. Continuous wave exposures caused damage at intensities between 0.1 W/cm^2 to 1 W/cm^2 depending upon the stage of development. Pulsed exposures of explants at spatial, temporal average intensities of 0.025 W/cm^2 (i.e: approximately 0.1 W/cm^2 spatial, temporal peak intensity) produced damage over limited ranges of pulse repetition frequencies. Few of the data have been treated statistically. Although the scoring for damage is necessarily a qualitative judgment, the effects which are observed go monotonically with intensity from 0 to 100 %. These do not appear to be marginal or subtle effects. The authors present these results as examples of "non-cavitational and non- thermal" effects of ultrasound. Because of the small size of the subjects and the low average intensities used, it is very unlikely that heating is an important factor. Cavitation cannot be dismissed as easily. From studies with cell suspensions, we see that the thresholds for damage to frog embryos are comparable to our best estimates of the thresholds for cavitation under free field, continuous wave exposure.

AVIAN EMBRYOS

Several investigators have exposed avian embryos to ultrasound. Exposure conditions range from attempts to expose the organism through an intact shell (in spite of the fact that less than 1 % of the ultrasonic energy penetrates the shell) to exposures of isolated embryos in Petri dishes (where standing waves are very likely present). Perhaps the best compromise has been to remove a portion of the shell and outer membrane from the egg and expose the embryo via liquid coupling through the inner membrane. The embryo suffers little trauma from this preparation procedure. Reasonably good dosimetry is possible under these conditions. The highly absorbing material in the egg minimizes standing waves.

Gross malformations of the embryos have been reported by several investigators. For various reasons the only positive study which can be considered very seriously is that of Taylor and Dyson (1973) who reported that exposure of isolated chick embryos to pulsed ultrasound (20 µs on and 180 µs off, 25 W/cm² temporal maximum intensity) caused an increase in the rate of malformations. There were no observed effects with temporal peak intensities of 10 W/cm² Their threshold is interestingly close to that for effects of pulsed ultrasound on *Drosophila* larvae. Unfortunately the temporal average intensity used with the embryo study was high enough to produce heating. Thus, we cannot eliminate heating as at least a contributing mechanism. Furthermore, Barnett (1983), using 1 µs pulses and even higher temporal average intensities (4.5 W/cm², was unable to find any effects of ultrasound on development of chick embryos.

As with amphibian embryos, the available data are not strong enough to warrant attempts to extrapolate to human exposures. There is just enough information available to encourage us to explore further. Perhaps the most important lesson to be learned from the avian studies is that future experiments should be designed so that it is possible to differentiate clearly between thermal and cavitational mechanisms.

THE MAMMALIAN FETUS/EMBRYO

For obvious reasons, the mammalian fetus has been a favorite subject for bioeffects investigators. The comments about studies of avian embryos in the preceding section apply here as well. In spite of the fact that there are now more than 70 papers on this subject, there is no clear evidence in any investigation that effects will occur under conditions which are used in pulse-echo diagnosis. Exposures have employed intensities from a few milliwatts per square centimeter to temporal peak intensities greater than 1000 W/cm². About one half of the studies which have been reported have been negative, i.e. the investigators found no statistically significant effects. Curiously, these negative reports include high intensity exposures. There probably are some real effects but they appear to be small in magnitude. The most serious problem in interpreting this literature is that no clear effect has been reported where heating can be eliminated as at least a contributing mechanism.

EVIDENCE FOR CAVITATION IN MAMALLIAN TISSUES

Whether any of this discussion has anything to do with human subjects boils down to the fundamental question of whether appropriate nuclei exist in their tissues. We know that the fluids of the body are nearly saturated with dissolved gases, but firm evidence of the presence of gaseous nuclei are very difficult to obtain.

Instead of searching for nuclei, it may be more efficient to look for evidence of cavitation itself. There are a few studies which give us reason to believe that cavitation can occur in mammalian tissues. In the classic studies of thresholds for lesion production in the cat brain with focused ultrasound, Fry and colleagues (1970) observed that with intensities greater than 10,000 W/cm^2, the appearance of the lesion was qualitatively different than at lower intensities. Instead of a well defined thermal lesion, the damage appeared to involve massive mechanical disruption of the tissues at the microscopic level. Lehmann and Herrick (1953) reported highly localized lesions in tissues treated with intensities comparable to those used in therapy. Although the intensities in the Fry and the Lehmann studies differ by orders of magnitude, it is reasonable to infer that cavitation was responsible for each effect.

By using diagnostic ultrasound, ter Haar and colleagues (1981, 1982) were able to detect bubbles generated in hamster tissues which were irradiated at therapeutic levels of 0.8 MHz, c.w. ultrasound. They estimate that their detection equipment (an 8 MHz pulse-echo diagnostic ultrasound unit) was capable of resolving bubbles as small as 10-20 micrometers. These bubbles are probably too large to be very effective cavitation nuclei at the frequencies which they employed. However, Crum and Hansen (1982) note that it is very probable that under the conditions of the ter Haar experiments bubbles would grow by rectified diffusion to sizes great enough to be observed. They conclude that the observations with hamsters constitute indirect evidence that effective cavitation nuclei, although too small to be detected directly by this method, do exist in the tissues of these animals.

At the present time evidence for cavitation in mammalian tissues is very limited. As with studies of biological effects on other vertebrates, there is just enough information to be tantalizing but not enough to draw any firm conclusions.

PULSE-ECHO DIAGNOSTIC ULTRASOUND

Pulse-echo ultrasound has come to occupy a very important place in diagnostic medicine. Almost every part of the body is accessible to its probing beam. Only lung and bone are opaque to to the radiation. Some useful information can be obtained even in the brain. Modern obstetrical practice relies very heavily on the use of ultrasound in prenatal care and in delivery. A large fraction of the babies born today have been exposed to pulse echo ultrasound *in utero*. The use of pulse-echo ultrasound has grown rapidly in part because of its efficacy but also in large part because it is generally assumed to be safe and without biological effect. The rationale for this assumption has been based on (1) the fact that the intensities which are used normally are too small to produce significant increases in temperature in the exposed tissues, and (2) the tacit assumption that the pulses employed are too short to produce cavitation.

Several lines of investigation over the past five years have provided us with ample evidence that the second assumption is false under some conditions which are clinically relevant. First, a careful analysis of the theory of cavitation shows that cavitation should be expected to occur even with microsecond- length pulses if appropriate nuclei are excited by superthreshold levels of ultrasound. Second, Fawlkes and Crum (1985) have observed sonoluminescence from bubbles in water driven by microsecond length pulses of megahertz ultrasound. Evidence of free radical formation has been obtained with pulses as short as 6 μsec. Finally, short pulses of ultrasound at very low temporal average intensities have been found to kill the larvae of *Drosophila* and damage cells in the leaves of *Elodea*.

We are in the remarkable position at the moment where we know that pulsed ultrasound as used on occasion in clinical medicine can produce serious adverse effects in lower organisms. Yet, there is no solid evidence that the phenomenon occurs at all in mammals. But, there is nothing in our knowledge of the mechanism of the action of this radiation to suggest that it would not occur in the tissues of mammals if the appropriate conditions exist - most important, if appropriate nuclei exist within those tissues. Thus, the safety question is somewhat more clearly defined than it has been in the past. The research which extrapolates from the relatively known world of insects and plants to the unknown world of mammalian tissues will be challenging but at least it should be possible to avoid some of the unproductive approaches which have been used in earlier work.

The limited information available at the present time suggests that if cavitation occurs in mammals it is a rare event. In the end, we will want to know the probability of the occurance of cavitation injuries as well as the qualitative nature of those effects. This eventually should make it possible to balance risk and benefit quantitatively. Those probabilities are apt to be very small. Sensitive, perhaps qualitatively new methods of detection will be required. Careful control of conditions and thorough statistical analysis of the results will be necessary. Large sample sizes probably will be required to obtain significant results even with the best experimental designs. There is little hope that epidemiology can ever offer anything positive to this subject. Instead, any further knowledge will require the best combination of theoretical and experimental techniques and in the end it will be necessary to extrapolate from that knowledge to the human case.

IMPLICATIONS OF PRESENT KNOWLEDGE FOR SAFETY IN CLINICAL MEDICINE

In spite of several decades of research, there is no direct evidence that ultrasound as it is commonly used in diagnostic medicine causes any adverse effects in human subjects. This fact is remarkable when viewed in the light of the medical world where almost every benefit has some known associated risk. As long as diagnostic procedures do not produce significant heating, there is no firm basis in present knowledge to impose any limitation on the levels of ultrasound which are used.

As reassuring as this sounds, it must be recognized that the same exposure conditions which are used in medicine can produce deleterious effects in lower organisms through acoustic cavitation. In the light of the cavitation mechanism, these organisms admittedly are qualitatively and quantitatively different than human beings. The most important difference has to do with the distribution of cavitation nuclei. Whereas plants and insects have clearly defined, stabilized populations of small bubbles, almost nothing is known about the existence and nature of small gas bodies in the tissues of mammals. All we can do at present is to speculate on what might happen if bubbles of optimum size to exist.

Temporal maximum intensities in certain ultrasonic imaging devices exceed 1000 W/cm^2. This is well in excess of levels which are capable of producing transient cavitation in organisms where appropriate nuclei are present. However, if transient cavitation takes place, effects very probably would be highly localized, damaging only a few cells near the site of the collapsing cavity. From our best estimates of the numbers of small bubbles available as cavitation nuclei, the probability of such an occurrance in mammalian tissues is extremely small. Let us consider the risk benefit question under the assumption that a few cells would be damaged during the course of an ultrasound examination. If there was good reason to believe that the use of 1000 W/cm^2 as opposed to 1 W/cm^2 for the temporal maximum intensity would give a higher quality of diagnostic information, it would seem reasonable to use the higher level in almost any part of the body. It is difficult to see how the loss of a few cells in most organs or in the body fluids would have a significant effect on the health of the

patient.   Far   more   invasive and traumatic diagnostic
procedures are used in medicine   routinely.   The one possible
exception to this rationale concerns   the human generative
cells,   or the embryo or fetus at   sensitive   stages of
growth.   Damage to even a few cells,   if it were known   to
occur,   might not be acceptable.   The odds of such an   event
occurring,   of   course,   are   very   small.   Again,   if
the   diagnostician were   convinced that   1000   W/cm^2 would
provide   significantly   better   information than 1 W/cm^2,
s/he   might   be   willing   to play these very favorable odds.
Knowledge   of cavitation phenomena and the devices which are
used   in   biomedical ultrasound add an interesting twist   to
the   safety   question.   We can be sure that transient
cavitation will   not   occur   regardless of the presence of
nuclei if   the   maximum   intensities   remain   below
threshold   values   which for short   (microsecond length),
isolated pulses are of the order of 1 to 10   W/cm^2 depending
upon frequency.   Only a very small   fraction   of   the
diagnostic units   used in obstetrical practice   today   have
outputs   large enough that the fetus can be exposed to levels
of ultrasound which exceed the threshold for transient
cavitation.   For   routine   obstetrical   examinations,   a
very   conservative   approach   might be to hold exposures to
the fetus below threshold   levels.   This   would be true if
the maximum intensities for   the   devices as   calibrated in a
water bath were of the order   of   10   W/cm^2 or less.   It
must be emphasized that there   is   no   positive   basis in
studies with mammals for   such a limitation.   It is based
entirely   on   worst   case   extrapolations   from
theoretical   considerations and laboratory studies with lower
organisms.

THE PROBLEM

     Any future research which is motivated by concern for
safety   in   the   use of diagnostic ultrasound must focus
clearly   on   the   mechanism of acoustic cavitation.   Of the
two principle physical   processes   (heat and cavitation)
through which ultrasound   causes   biological effects,   only
cavitation   need be   considered in   normal   diagnostic
procedures.   We have evidence that adverse effects can   be
produced in lower organisms at acoustic levels comparable   to
those   used   by certain diagnostic   devices.   From   our
present   perspective,   the   outstanding problem is to bridge
the gap   from   this information to mammals and eventually to
human subjects.   A   summary   of   relevant literature shows
that there have been   some   tantalizing observations but
there are so many conflicting claims that   it   is   difficult
to be certain   which   of   several   subtle   effects   are real.
Unfortunately,   almost every study which has   reported
effects in higher organisms is tainted with the possible
contribution   of ultrasonic heating.   This confusion must
be   avoided in future research.   Physical models have been
developed   far   enough to guide biological investigations.
But since   the   rate of   occurrance of cavitation events in
mammals is   probably   very   small,   design   of   the
appropriate   experiments   for   the   qualitative and
quantitative assessment of risks under   realistic   conditions
is a worthy challenge to the basic scientists in   the
ultrasound community.

ACKNOWLEDGMENTS

This work has been supported in part by U. S. Public Health Service Grant No. 39241.

REFERENCES

Barnett, S. B., 1983, The Influence of Ultrasound on Embryonic Development, *Ultrasound Med. Biol.* 9:19-24.

Berg, R. B., Child, S. Z. and Carstensen, E. L., 1983, The Influence of Carrier Frequency on the Killing of *Drosophila* Larvae by Microsecond Pulses of Ultrasound, *Ultrasound Med. Biol.* 9:L448-L451.

Braginskaya, F. I. and Dunn, F., 1981, Some Aspects of the Effect of Ultrasound on Biological Structures, *Biophysics* 26:550.

Carstensen, E. L., Child, S. Z., Law, W. K., Horowitz, D. R. and Miller, M. W., 1979, Cavitation as a Mechanism for the Biological Effects of Ultrasound on Plant roots, *J. Acoust. Soc. Am.* 66:1285-1291.

Carstensen, E. L. and Child, S. Z., 1980, Effects of Ultrasound on *Drosophila*: II. The Heating Mechanism, *Ultrasound Med. Biol.* 6:257-261.

Carstensen, E. L.,Donaldson, T. L., Miller, M. W., Law, W. K. and Vives, B., 1981, Distribution of Gas in the Roots of *Pisum sativum*, *Env. Exp. Bot.* 21:1-4.

Carstensen, E. L. and Flynn, H. G., 1982, The Potential for Transient Cavitation with Microsecond Pulses of Ultrasound, *Ultrasound Med. Biol.* 8:L720-L724.

Child, S. Z., Carstensen, E. L. and Smachlo, K., 1981, Effects of Ultrasound on *Drosophila*: III. Exposure of Larvae to Low-Temporal-Average-Intensiy, Pulsed Irradiation, *Ultrasound Med. Biol.* 7:167-173.

Child, S. Z. and Carstensen, E. L., 1982, Effects of Ultrasound on *Drosophila:* IV. Pulsed Exposures of Eggs, *Ultrasound Med. Biol.* 8:311-312.

Child, S. Z., Davis, H. and Carstensen, E. L., 1984, A Test for the Effects of Low-Temporal-Average-Intensity, Pulsed Ulrasound on the Rat Fetus, *Expl. Cell Biol.* 52:207-210.

Ciaravino, V., Miller, M. W. and Kaufman, G. E., 1981, The Effect of 1 MHz Ultrasound on the Proliferation of Synchronized Chinese Hamster V-79 Cells, *Ultrasound Med. Biol.* 7:175-184.

Clarke, P. R. and Hill, C. R., 1970, Physical and Chemical Aspects of Ultrasonic Disruption of Cells, *J. Acoust. Soc. Am.* 47:649-653.

Coakley, W. T. and Dunn, F., 1971, Degradation of DNA in High- Intensity Focused Ultrasonic fields at 1 MHz, *J. Acoust. Soc. Am.* 50:1539-1545.

Crum, L. A. and Hansen, G. M., 1982, Growth of Air Bubbles in Tissue by Rectified Diffusion, *Phys. Med. Biol.* 27:413-417.

Crum, L. A. and Fowlkes, J. B., 1985, Cavitation Produced by Short Acoustic Pulses, *Ultrasonics International,* London, UK, July 2-5, 1985.

Eames, F. A., Carstensen, E. L., Miller, M. W. and Li, M., 1975 Ultrasonic Heating of *Vicia faba* Roots, *J. Acoust. Soc. Am.* 57:1192-1194.

Edmonds, P. D. and Sancier, K. M., 1983, Evidence for Free Radical Production by Ultrasonic Cavitation in Biological Media," *Ultrasound Med. Biol.* 9:635-639.

Flynn, H. G., 1982, Generation of Transient Cavities in Liquids by Microsecond Pulses of Ultrasound, *J. Acoust. Soc. Am.* 72:1926-1932.

Fry, F. J., Kossoff, G., Eggleton, R. C. and Dunn, F., 1970, Threshold Ultrasonic Dosage for Structural Changes in the Mammalian Brain, *J. Acoust. Soc. Am.* 48:1413-1417.

Galperin-Lemaitre, H., Kirsh-Volders, M. and Levi, S., 1975, Ultrasound and Mammalian DNA, *Lancet*, October 4, 1975, p. 662.

Gershoy, A., Miller, D. L. and Nyborg, W. L., 1976, Intercellular Gas: Its Role in Sonated Plant Tissue, *Ultrasound in Medicine* 2:501.

Gupta, A. and Wang, S., 1976, Effects of Low Intensity Ultrasound on Nucleic Acid Components," *in* "Ultrasonic Symposium Proc.", IEEE No. 76, CH1120-5SU, p. 92.

Harvey, E. N. and Loomis, A. L., 1928, High Frequency Sound Waves of Small Intensity and their Biological Effects, *Nature* 121:622-624.

Holmer, N. G., Johnson, A. and Josefsson, J. O., Effects of Ultrasonic Irradiation upon *Amoeba proteus, Z. Naturforsch.* 28c:607-609.

Henglein, A., 1985, Sonolysis of Carbon Dioxide, Nitrous Oxide and Methane in Aqueous Solution, *Z. Naturforsch.* 40b:100-107.

Law, W. K., Carstensen, E. L. and Miller, M. W., 1978, Effects of Localized Ultrasonic Irradiation on *Pisum sativum* Roots, *Env. Exp. Bot.* 18:207-218.

Lehamnn, J. and Herrick, J., 1953, Biologic Reactions to Cavitation. A Consideration for Ultrasonic Therapy, *Arch. Phys. Med. Rehab.* 34:85.

Lehmann, J. F. and Krusen, F. H., 1955, Biophysical Effects of Ultrasonic Energy on Carcinoma and their Possible Significance, *Arch. Phys. Med. Rehab.* 36:452-459.

McKee, J. R., Christman, C. L., O'Brien, W. and Wang, S., 1977, Effects of Ultrasound on Nucleic Acid Bases, *Biochem.* 16:4651.

Miller, D. L., 1977, The Effects of Ultrasonic Activation of Gas Bodies in *Elodea* Leaves During Continuous and Pulsed Irradiation at 1 MHz, *Ultrasound Med. Biol.* 3:221.

Miller, D. L., 1979a, A Cylindrical Bubble Model for the Response of Plant-Tissue Gas-Bodies to Ultrasound, *J. Acoust. Soc. Am.* 65:1313.

Miller, D. L., 1979b, Cell Death Thresholds in *Elodea* for 0.45- 10 MHz Ultrasound Compared to Gas-Body Resonance Theory, *Ultrasound Med. Biol.* 5:351.

Miller, D. L., Nyborg, W. L. and Whitcomb, C. C., 1979c, Platelet Aggregation Induced by Ultrasound under Specialized Conditions *in vitro, Science* 205:505-507.

Miller, D. L., 1985, Microstreaming as a Mechanism of Cell Death in *Elodea* Leaves Exposed to Ultrasound, *Ultrasound Med. Biol.* 11:285-292.

Reisz, P., Berndahl, D. and Christman, C. L., 1985, Free Radical Generation by Ultrasound in Aqueous and Non-Aqueous Solutions, *Environmental Health Perspectives*, in press.

Sacks, P. G., Miller, M. W. and Sutherland R. M., 1981, Influence on Growth Conditions and Cell-Cell Contact on Responses of Tumor Cells to Ultrasound, *Radiat. Res.* 87:175.

Sarvazyan, A. P., Beloussov, L. V., Petropovlovskaya, M. N. and Ostroumova, T. V., 1982, The Action of Low-Intensity Pulsed Ultrasound on Amphibian Embryonic Tissues, *Ultrasound Med. Biol.* 8:639-654.

Taylor, K. J. W. and Dyson, M., 1973, Toxicity Studies on the Interaction of Ultrasound on Embryonic and Adult Tissues, *Utrasonics in Medicine (Proc. 2nd World Congress Ultrasound in Medicine)* Excerpta Medica, Amsterdam, p.353-359.

ter Haar, G., Dyson, M. and Talbert, D., 1978, Ultrasound Induced Contractions in Mouse Uterine smooth Muscle *in vivo*, *Ultrasonics* 16:275-276.

ter Haar, G. R. and Daniels, S., 1981, Evidence for Ultrasonically Induced Cavitation *in vitro*, *Phys. Med. Biol.*, 26:1145-1149.

ter Haar, G., Daniels, S., Eastaugh, K. C. and Hill, C. R., 1982, Ultrasonically Induced Cavitation *in vivo*, *Br. J. Cancer* 45(Suppl V):151-155.

Thacker, J., 1973, The Possibility of Genetic Hazard from Ultrasonic Radiation, *Curr. Top. Radiat. Res. Quart.* 8:235.

Williams, A. R., Sykes, S. M. and O'Brien, Jr., W. D., 1976, Ultrasonic Exposure Modifies Platelet Morphology and Function *in vitro, Ultrasound Med. Biol.* 2:311.

Williams, A. R. and Miller, D. L., 1980, Photometric Detection of ATP Release from Human Erythrocytes Exposed to Ultrasonically Activated Gas-Filled Pores, *Ultrasound Med. Biol.* 6:251-256.

Williams, A. R., 1983, "Ultrasound: Biological Effects and Potential Hazards," Academic Press, New York.

INTERACTION MECHANISMS: NON-THERMAL, NON-CAVITATIONAL EFFECTS

Gail ter Haar

Physics Department, Institute of Cancer Research
Clifton Avenue
Sutton, Surrey, U.K.

INTRODUCTION

The way in which ultrasound interacts with tissue is con-
ventionally divided into three classes of mechanisms - thermal,
cavitational, and non-thermal, non-cavitational.   Heating and
cavitation are covered elsewhere in this volume (see chapters
by W.L. Nyborg and E. Carstensen in this volume).

The group of mechanisms carrying the umbrella name of
"non thermal, non cavitational effects" comprises a variety of
proposed physical mechanisms, the occurrence of many of which
has not been confirmed experimentally.   The problem of identification of these effects is shown diagrammatically in Figure
1.

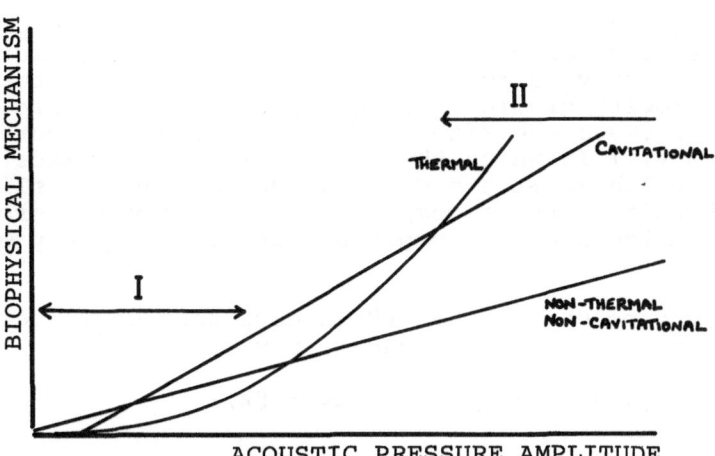

Fig. 1.   Graph demonstrating the inter-relationship between
thermal, cavitational and non thermal, non cavitational
effects.

On this figure, the vertical axis is labelled biophysical mechanism. This is meant to·represent a measurable biophysical effect. In the case of heating, for example, this may be temperature rise, or observed thermal damage. For cavitation, this may be subharmonic emission, or amount of vacuolation.

Acoustic pressure amplitude has been chosen as the parameter plotted on the abscissa, although intensity might also have been used. Pressure was chosen because cavitation and non-cavitational and non-thermal effects increase approximately linearly with pressure. Heating increases linearly with intensity (α(pressure)^2).

Two regions, I and II, have been marked on the graph. In region I there is no really dominant mechanism, thermal effects are small, and may be overshadowed by non-thermal effects. In region II, when biological endpoints are studied, thermal effects predominate and may mask the observation of any other effects produced. Thus, acoustic pressures in the range covered by region I may be considered as producing non-thermal effects, and acoustic pressures in region II may be thought of as producing thermal effects. At intermediate pressures, no one effect predominates. In region II, although the amount of cavitation or other effects may be greater than at lower pressure amplitudes, it can be difficult to detect their biological consequences, as the thermal disruption can be extreme. Also, the consequences of some of the mechanical effects may be altered by temperature, for example, shear stresses may be more disruptive to cell membranes at supra-normal temperatures (Dunn, 1985).

In summary, although different mechanisms can be detailed separately in terms of the physics involved, in reality they must interact, and cannot be observed in isolation. It is probably true to say that non-thermal, and cavitational effects always accompany thermal effects, but that non-thermal mechanisms can occur in the absence of significant heating.

Shear stresses

Under the action of an ultrasonic field, the particles in a fluid take up an oscillatory motion. If the fluid is near a rigid boundary, a non slip condition may exist that means that a velocity gradient is set up within the fluid. Nyborg (1978) discusses the situation for a cartesian coordinate system (x,y,z) in which the z direction is outwards from the boundary which is at z = 0. Because of the non slip condition at the boundary, the z component of velocity is zero at that point, and the x and y components increase rapidly with increasing z.

It can be shown, that the x component of velocity, u, at any distance z from the boundary may be written

$$u = u_0 (\cos \omega t - e^{-\beta z} \cos(\omega t - \beta z)) \qquad (1)$$

$$\beta^{-1} = \sqrt{\frac{2\eta}{\omega \rho_0}}$$

u_0 is a constant, ω is the angular frequency of the sound field, ρ_0 is the fluid density, and η is its shear viscosity.

Expression (1) has the value $u_o \cos \omega t$ for values of $z \gg \beta^{-1}$, and is zero for $z=0$. $u_o \cos \omega t$ is the "free field" velocity that would pertain in the liquid in the absence of the boundary. β^{-1} is the distance from the boundary in which the velocity essentially increases from zero to u_o and thus is the layer in which the velocity gradient is found. There is a shear stress associated with the velocity gradient, given by the product of the velocity gradient and the shear viscosity. Nyborg (1978) has calculated that for 1MHz ultrasound in water, the boundary layer is $0.56\mu m$ thick.

At the boundary, the velocity gradient is oscillatory, with amplitude

$$\left| \frac{du}{dz} \right| = \beta u_o \qquad (2)$$

Again, Nyborg (1978) calculated that for a 1MHz ultrasonic wave of intensity $1 W cm^{-2}$ grazing the boundary $z = 0$, $u_o = 11.5$ cm.s^{-1} and the velocity gradient, βu_o, is 2.10^5 s^{-1} at the boundary.

The viscous stress associated with this velocity gradient in water has an amplitude of 2040 dyne.cm^{-2}. This stress would be sufficient to cause biological damage if it were unidirectional, but it is oscillatory and reverses direction every half cycle.

Unidirectional velocity gradients are also set up in a fluid by acoustic microstreaming, which is a consequence of radiation pressure forces.

Acoustic microstreaming and radiation pressure

An ultrasonic wave exerts a force on any inhomogeneities in its path. In this case, an inhomogeneity is a region with acoustic properties that are different from those of the medium surrounding it. This force is in part oscillatory in nature, but also has a steady, unidirectional component that is known as the radiation force. The force on a perfectly reflecting target in the ultrasonic beam may be written

$$F = \frac{2IA}{C} \qquad (3)$$

where I is the intensity, C the sound velocity, and A the area presented by the target in a direction perpendicular to the beam.

The force on a large rigid sphere of radius a $(a \gg \lambda)$ is given by

$$F = \frac{\pi a^2 I}{C} \, Y_p \qquad (4)$$

where Y_p is a constant. For a small rigid sphere $(a \ll \lambda)$ equation 4 becomes

$$F = V_o \left[B \frac{\partial T}{\partial x} - \frac{\partial U}{\partial x} \right] + \Delta \qquad (5)$$

where V_o is the sphere volume, T and U are the second order approximations to the time averaged kinetic energy density (T) and potential energy density (U), and B is given by the term $3(\rho-\rho_o)/(2\rho+\rho_o)$ (ρ is the sphere density). (Nyborg 1967). Δ is a term that is only important when T and U are essentially uniform, as in plane progressive wave fields.

The force of a small compressible sphere is given by the sum of the force on a rigid sphere (equation 5) and a component due to the compressibility, F_C given by

$$F_C = - <V(t) \frac{dp}{dx} (x,t)> \qquad (6)$$

(< > denotes time average, $V(t)$ is the instantaneous volume of the sphere, and $p(x,t)$ is the acoustic pressure distribution along the x axis) (Crum, 1971; Eller, 1968).

Radiation pressure thus exerts a force on liquid drops, small particles and boundaries within a field and may cause them to move. This may be of particular interest where a blood vessel is irradiated in a standing wave field. This will be discussed later in this chapter. Local differences in radiation pressure will cause variations in force, and where one object is subject to these variations along its length, this may give rise to a torque, or to translational movement. A more detailed account of the physics of radiation pressure and acoustic streaming may be found in a specialist text (see, for example, Nyborg, 1965).

The fluid velocities induced by unidirectional acoustic streaming are spatially non-uniform, and so velocity gradients are set up within the field. Objects within the field are therefore subject to shear stresses. The non-slip condition discussed above means that at boundaries, the velocity is zero, and so velocity gradients tend to be highest in these regions. It can be shown that the steady stress (S_{steady}) exerted on a boundary due to the unidirectional streaming around a spherical object of radius b vibrating with amplitude ξ can be written

$$S_{steady} = (\frac{1}{2} \eta \omega^3 \rho \frac{\xi^2}{b})^{\frac{1}{2}} \qquad (7)$$

(Rooney, 1970).

This steady stress may be an order of magnitude less than the oscillatory stress, but it acts continuously, and therefore may be more significant in producing biological effect.

High shear stresses have been implicated in the damage to endothelium observed when blood vessels are irradiated in ultrasonic fields (Dyson et al, 1974; ter Haar et al, 1979). The damage was found on the luminal aspect of the plasma membrane, a site at which fluid is in contact with a membrane.

It should be noted that another, possibly more significant, source of microstreaming is the bubbles induced by cavitation. This topic is covered more fully in a chapter in this volume by Carstensen.

Inter particle forces

If two particles be close to each other in an ultrasonic field, there will be an interactive force between them resulting from the interaction of each oscillating body with the sound field re-radiated by the other.

When the line joining the centres of the two particles is parallel to the direction of propagation of a plane progressive wave field, the force is proportional to the product of the particle volumes, and increases with decreasing distance between the particles (Embleton, 1962). The theory has also been extended for the case when the line joining the centres is at an angle θ to the propagation direction (Gershoy and Nyborg, 1973). It was found that in this case there was a repulsive force along the direction of propagation, and an attractive force in the perpendicular direction. The form of the force is given by

$$F_\theta = F_O \sin 2\theta \tag{8}$$

$$F_r = F_O (3 \cos^2\theta - 1)$$

where
$$F_O = \frac{2\pi}{3} \left[\frac{(\rho - \rho_0)^2}{\rho_0} \right] \frac{a^3 b^3}{r^4} v_O^2$$

a,b are the particle radii, r is their separation, v_O is the velocity amplitude of the surrounding medium, ρ_0 is its density. For erythrocytes in plasma, this gives a maximum force (when they are touching) of 10^{-13}N in a $1Wcm^{-2}$, 3MHz field ($a = b = 4$ μm; $\rho/\rho_0 = 1.1/1.03$).

Standing wave effects

An ultrasonic wave will be reflected by an interface between two media of different acoustic impedance. Where the incident wave interacts with the reflected wave, a standing wave may be set up. In a standing wave, the points of maximum and minimum intensity remain fixed in space, the maxima (and the minima) being separated by half a wavelength.

The radiation forces that exist in a standing wave field are somewhat different from those in a progressive wave. For example, it can be shown that the force on a small rigid sphere (c.f. equation 5) may be written

$$F = V_O B \frac{\delta T}{\delta x} \tag{9}$$

(ter Haar and Wyard, 1978), and the force on a compressible sphere in a standing wave field may be expressed as

$$F = \frac{V_O P^2}{4\rho_0 C_0^2} k \sin 2kx . f(\rho/\rho_0) \tag{10}$$

where $f(\rho/\rho_0) = \left[\frac{\rho_0 C_0^2}{\rho C^2} - \left(\frac{5\rho - 2\rho_0}{3\rho + \rho_0} \right) \right]$

(ter Haar 1977).

This force is periodic in half a wavelength.

It has been observed that when blood vessels (either chick or mammalian) are exposed to an ultrasonic standing wave field, under the right conditions, circulating erythrocytes in small blood vessels clump into apparently static bands at the pressure nodes oriented normally to the field direction. (Dyson et al, 1974; ter Haar et al, 1979; Gould and Coakley, 1974). The plasma continues to flow through the vessel. The erythrocyte banding is in most cases reversible in the sense that the bands disappear when the ultrasound is switched off. Figure 2 shows the phenomenon in the blood vessels supplying the uterine horn of the mouse.   In this case, the reflector is presumed to be an air bubble in the gut.

It is thought that this phenomenon can occur whenever blood vessels overlie an ultrasonic reflector such as air or bone, and are irradiated with a continuous wave beam that is held still in relation to the reflector.   It is unlikely to occur when short pulses are used as standing wave fields are not created, and can be avoided under continuous wave conditions by movement of the ultrasonic transducer.

High shear stresses seem probable in the plasma filled spaces between bands.   This may lead to tissue damage. Another effect of this so called "blood cell stasis" is that, while the erythrocytes are trapped, tissues downstream are deprived of oxygen.

Non linear propagation

When a sinusoidal wave of sufficient amplitude propagates through a non linear medium, its shape will change, until it approximates to a sawtooth wave.   The crest of the wave travels faster than the trough.   The rate of change of momentum of a particle is much greater at the leading edge than at the trailing edge, and the force on it will therefore vary.   It has been shown that considerable distortion can occur in water for medical ultrasound beams.   If a shock front is formed, this may have considerable biological consequences.

Biological configurations for which effects may be significant

i.   Configuration 1

A liquid confined within fixed boundaries - for example, plasma within a blood vessel, or cytoplasm in a plant cell.

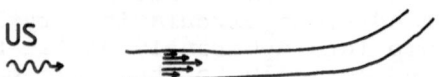

Fig. 3.   Configuration 1: A liquid confined within fixed
          boundaries.

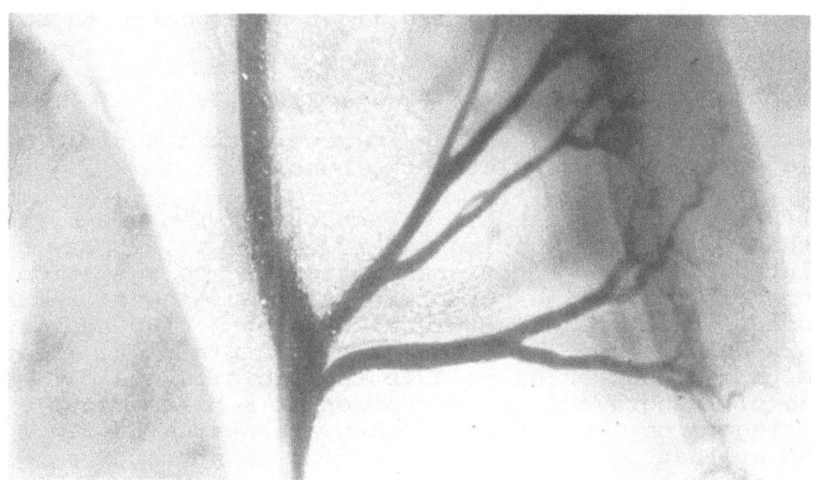

Fig. 2a.   Blood vessels supplying the uterine horn of the
           mouse.   A loop of gut can be seen on the left hand
           side.   Ultrasound off.

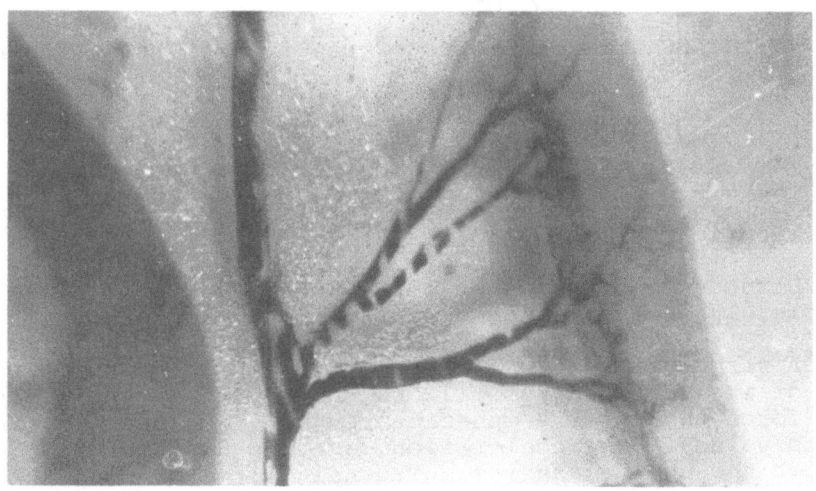

Fig. 2b.   Blood vessels supplying the uterine horn of the
           mouse.   A loop of gut can be seen on the left hand
           side.   Ultrasound on   (3MHz, 2Wcm^{-2}).   The bands
           are 0.25 mm apart.

When a fluid flows along a fixed boundary, a velocity gradient is set up, and shear stresses may be created. At sufficiently high acoustic pressures, acoustic streaming may occur which can increase the velocity gradient and thus alter the shearing forces. Biological damage may then be found at the vessel walls where shearing might be expected to be greatest.

ii.   Configuration 2

Where structures are free to move within a field - for example, erythrocytes, platelets, bubbles.

If a structure that has an acoustic impedance different from that of its surroundings is free to move, it may undergo translational and/or rotational motion due to radiation pressure effects. The most likely consequence of radiation pressure is that the structure will be pushed up against a boundary and trapped. In the case of a platelet, shear damage to a blood vessel wall in the vicinity could lead to release of factors and the formation of a blood clot. Particles may aggregate on a boundary if they are near a bubble that is trapped at that point, and is exerting an attractive force by virtue of its oscillations.

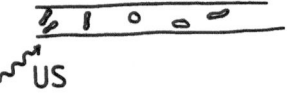

Fig. 4.   Configuration 2: structures free to move within the field.

iii.   Configuration 3

Structures constrained within their surroundings - for example, lysosomes, mitochondria within cell cytoplasm.

A structure that has an acoustic impedance different from that of its surroundings will be subject to a cyclic displacement force that, for a spherical object, is equal to the product of its volume, the acceleration, and the difference in density between the object and its surroundings. For most relevant biological systems, structural inclusions have much the same density as their surroundings and the effect will be small. If an "object" lies within a fluid, but is attached to a fluid/ solid interface in some way, it will be subject to the shear stresses created in the liquid, and may move within it, if it is sufficiently "floppily" bound.

iv. Configuration 4

Structures free to move within a field in the vicinity of an acoustic reflector - for example, erythrocytes in blood vessels overlying bone or gas.

The main acoustic reflectors to be found within the body are bone and gas (such as may be found in the lungs or gut). Where a continuous wave field exists, there is the possibility of standing wave formation when irradiating over sites containing these. If standing waves are set up, and the acoustic pressures involved are sufficient to overcome any normal flow that exists, small structures with density greater, and compressibility less, than that of the liquid in which they are suspended will move towards regions of velocity maxima. Gas bubbles smaller than resonant size move to pressure maxima, whereas those larger than resonant size move to pressure minima.

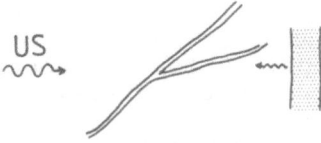

Fig. 5. Configuration 4: structures free to move within an ultrasonic field, in the vicinity of a reflector.

v. Configuration 5

Gaseous inclusions in tissue - for example, gas spaces in plant tissues.

If there is a small gaseous inclusion in tissue, then this may undergo volume resonances in a fashion similar to those of trapped cavitation bubbles, and streaming patterns with associated shear stresses may be set up in the vicinity. This has been most widely studied in plant tissues (Miller, 1983).

Relevance of effects discussed for medical ultrasound usage

There is no doubt that the effects discussed above can occur in an ultrasonic field when the exposure parameters are suitable. All the phenomena are well documented both theoretically and experimentally. The pertinent question that should be asked is whether or not they are relevant for medical ultrasound exposures, and whether they are beneficial or potentially hazardous.

Thermal and cavitational effects have been discussed in detail elsewhere in this book. They may occur to a significant degree in continuous and "tone burst" fields if the intensity is high enough. Theoretical calculations have shown that cavitation could occur as a result of diagnostic pulses at the acoustic pressure levels currently available in clinical machines. The relevance to medical ultrasound applications however, is hard to determine.

Although collapse cavitation is a potentially destructive phenomenon, stable cavitation and associated streaming patterns may be beneficial when "therapeutic" changes are sought. Induced fluid motion, for example, may cause an acceleration of normal diffusion processes occurring at extracellular membranes.

Radiation pressure will undoubtedly be a phenomenon that occurs in continuous wave or pulsed (tone burst) fields. It is unlikely to be important for diagnostic pulses. The situation is similar for acoustic streaming.

Standing waves can only form when an incident and a reflected wave coincide. In the complex geometry of the human body this is only probable when a continuously excited transducer is held stationary over an acoustic reflector.

All forms of ultrasonic beam whether continuous or pulsed have been shown to exhibit non linear propagation when the acoustic pressure in the beam is high enough. It is not known what the formation of a shock wave in, for example, amniotic fluid, may do in biological terms. It seems likely that the high frequency components would be attenuated rapidly. Further work is needed to investigate the occurrence of non linear wave propagation in tissues (Starrit et al, 1984) and its biological consequences.

SUMMARY

Non-thermal, non-cavitational effects occur in tissues. Their detection may be difficult if heating and cavitation mask the effects.

Table 1.   Relevance of effects for medical ultrasound exposures

EFFECT	CONTINUOUS WAVE	PULSED BEAMS	
		Tone Burst "therapy" pulses (ms duration)	Short pulses diagnosis (μs duration)
Significant thermal effects	√√	√	X
Cavitation	√	√	(√)
Radiation pressure	√√	√	X?
Streaming	√√	√	X?
Standing waves	√	X	X
Non linearity	√	√	√

115

REFERENCES

Crum, L.A., 1971, Acoustic force on a liquid droplet in an acoustic stationary wave. J. Acoust. Soc. Am. 50:157.

Dunn, F., 1985, Cellular inactivation by heat and shear. Radiat. Environ. Biophys. 24:131.

Dyson, M., Pond, J.B., Woodward, B., Broadbent, J., 1974, The production of blood cell stasis and endothelial damage in the blood vessels of chick embryos treated with ultrasound in a stationary wave field. Ultrasound Med. Biol. 1:133.

Eller, A.I., 1968, Force on a bubble in a standing acoustic wave. J. Acoust. Soc. Am. 43:170.

Embleton, T.F.W., 1962, Mutual interaction between two spheres in a plane sound field. J. Acoust. Soc. Am. 34:1714.

Gershoy, A., Nyborg, W.L., 1973, Microsonation of cells under near threshold conditions, in "Proc. Second World Congress on Ultrasonics in Medicine". Rotterdam 1973, (Int. Congress Series No. 309, ISBN 90 219 01870; Excerpta Medical Amsterdam 1974) pp. 360-365.

Gould, R.K. & Coakley, W.T., 1974, The effects of acoustic force on small particles in suspension. in Proc. Symp. Finite wave effects in fluids. IPC Science and Tech. Press, Lyngby, Denmark.

ter Haar, G.R., 1977, The effect of ultrasound standing wave fields on the flow of particles, with special reference to biological media. Ph.D. Thesis, University of London.

ter Haar, G.R., Dyson, M., Smith, S.P., 1979, Ultrastructural changes in the mouse uterus brought about by ultrasonic irradiation at therapeutic intensities in standing wave fields. Ultrasound Med. Biol. 5:167.

ter Haar, G.R., Wyard, S.J., 1978, Blood cell banding in ultrasonic standing wave fields: a physical analysis. Ultrasound Med. Biol. 4:111.

Miller, D.L., 1983, The botanical effects of ultrasound: a review. Env. & Exp. Botany, 23:1.

Nyborg, W.L., 1965, Acoustic streaming, in "Physical Acoustics" Vol. IIB Ch. 11. Ed. W.P. Mason, Academic Press, London/New York.

Nyborg, W.L., 1967, Radiation pressure on a small rigid sphere. J. Acoust. Soc. Am. 42:947.

Nyborg, W.L., 1978, Physical mechanisms for biological effects of ultrasound. HEW Publication (FDA) 78-8062.

Rooney, J.A., 1970, Hemolysis near an ultrasonically pulsating gas bubble. Science, 169:869.

Starrit, H.C., Perkins, M.A., Duck, F.A., Humphrey, V.F., 1985, Evidence for ultrasonic finit amplitude distortion in muscle using medical equipment. J. Acoust. Soc. Am. 77:302.

EXPERIMENTATION IN VITRO :

ULTRASOUND STUDIES AT THE MACROMOLECULAR LEVEL

Michael H. Repacholi

Chief Scientist
Royal Adelaide Hospital
Adelaide, South Australia 5000

INTRODUCTION

This paper describes what in vitro experiments are, their purpose, the various techniques used and what results have been found from exposing solutions of macromolecules to ultrasound. The following paper summarises the results of experiments performed on suspensions of cells.

In vitro experiments are performed with suspensions of macromolecules or with cells in culture medium or attached to the surface of a culture dish. Some investigations may involve ultrasound exposure of cells in the intact organism and subsequent examination of the cells in vitro.

IN VITRO EXPERIMENTATION

The purpose of in vitro experiments is generally two-fold. Using simple systems one is more likely to identify primary or direct effects that may occur from ultrasound exposure. In vitro experiments may be used to screen for effects, which, once identified, should then be persued to determine if they occur in an organism having a higher level of biological complexity. Secondly, the ability to study details of possible interaction mechanisms is greatly enhanced by in vitro experimentation. Subtle mechanisms may be studied without the potential complications of a system of higher complexity. For example, a multicellular organism exposed to ultrasound may exhibit an effect which masks, or may be an indirect consequence of a more subtle action of the beam.

Table 1 lists some of the end-points which may be studied by exposing suspensions of molecules to ultrasound.

TABLE 1. SOME END-POINTS OF MOLECULAR STUDIES

1. Identify mechanisms - cavitation, streaming, thermal, various forces

2. Determine thresholds for effects - degradation, cavitation, free radical production

3. Observe end-products of ultrasound induced chemical reactions

4. Compare relative damage from CW versus pulsed beams

5. Study molecular absorption characteristics - effects of molecular structure (proteins, DNA)

Bioeffects or interaction mechanisms identified from in vitro experimentation must be studied further to determine if they occur in higher organisms, because higher organisms may possess protective measures or other physical or chemical factors which do not make them susceptible to ultrasound in the same way. Thus the results of in vitro experimentation alone cannot be used to make a health risk assessment of ultrasound exposure in humans.

In vitro results need to be interpreted with care because, in many experiments, cell suspensions are in contact with foreign substances (culture dishes or test tubes made of plastic, rubber membranes etc.) during exposure to ultrasound. Complex acoustic fields may be reflected from these surfaces making it difficult to determine cell exposure levels and to compare results with studies having different experimental arrangements.

Experimental arrangements may take different forms as shown in figure 1. Figures 1a and 1b indicate that cells in culture dishes can be exposed by a transducer (T) from either above or below. Suspensions of cells in test tubes (TT) or special containers can be exposed in a water bath with ultrasound absorbing (ABS) material at one end to reduce the presence of standing waves (see figures 1b, 1c).

Cells exposed using experimental arrangements shown in figures 1a,b,c will be subjected not only to the direct beam but also to standing waves set up by reflections from the container walls. This may make the exposures to the cells difficult to interpret. The arrangement in figure 1d is designed to reduce standing waves to a minimum since using thin windows at either end will ensure that the beam incident on the front surface of the container (SC) does not significantly attenuate the beam. Further, the beam transmitted through the cell system will not be reflected by the rear surface. It is then possible to determine the free field beam intensity at the point in the water bath where the container will be located and assume, with reasonable certainty, that the cell suspension will be exposed to approximately the same beam intensity.

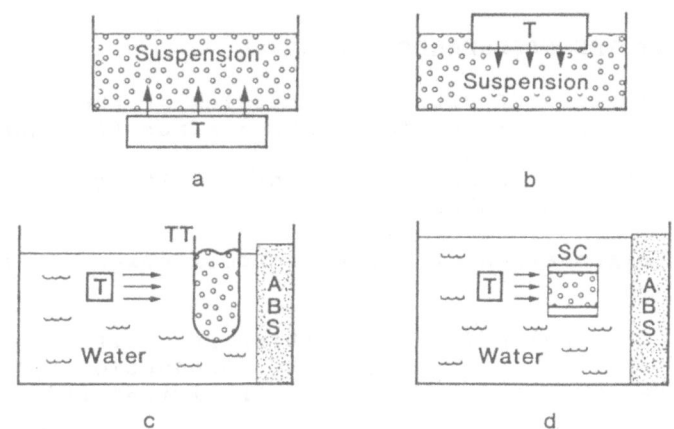

Figure 1. Various experimental arrangements for exposing molecules or cells to ultrasound (from NCRP, 1983).

TABLE 2. SOME FACTORS AFFECTING IN VITRO EXPERIMENTS

Factor	Variations
Cell Container	Size, shape, construction, composition, movement (rotating?)
Exposure parameters	Intensity, exposure duration, frequency, pulsed, focused, unfocused
Exposure position	Near field, far field
Ultrasound generator	Transducer, vibrating wire
Cell medium	Chemical composition, solid, liquid, dissolved gas
Environmental parameters	Temperature, pressure
Beam coupling medium	Degassed water, gel
Exposing arrangement	Traveling, stationary or standing waves

A variety of in vitro exposure conditions have been reported as tabulated in Table 2. It is therefore essential that the exact exposure conditions be noted so that interaction mechanisms or effects can be better compared with other experiments. Readers are referred to NCRP (1983) for a detailed discussion.

EFFECTS AT THE MACROMOLECULAR LEVEL

The results of ultrasound studies at the macromolecules level can be broadly divided into 3 kinds (Edmonds, 1972):

(i)   passive absorption of ultrasonic energy by macromolecules,

(ii)   degradation of large macromolecules in suspension, and

(iii)   chemical effects resulting from ultrasound induced cavitation causing the production of chemically active free radicals in the irradiated solution.

a) Absorption

There is reasonable evidence that the primary mechanism for the absorption of ultrasound by biological tissues is at the macromolecular level. Investigations have suggested that the absorption properties of blood are determined mainly by its protein content and that the absorption coefficient is directly proportional to the protein concentration (Carstensen, 1960; O'Brien & Dunn, 1972; Kremkau & Carstensen, 1972). The frequency dependence of ultrasound absorption by whole and homogenized liver tissue is very similar, however the absorption coefficients of whole liver are approximately 30 per cent higher than those of homogenized liver (Pauly & Schwan, 1971), suggesting that approximately two-thirds of the absorption occurs at the macromolecular level, with one-third due to the tissue structure (Carstensen, 1960; Pauly & Schwan, 1971).

Numerous studies have been conducted using solutions of proteins, polypeptides, and nucleic acids, but have not produced any clear-cut mechanism for the absorption of ultrasound in the neutral pH range. While proton transfer reactions between solute and solvent appear to be the mechanism for ultrasound absorption at pH values less than 5 and greater than 8, they are not significant near neutral pH. Changes to solvent-solute interactions, intramolecular hydrogen bonds, keto-enol equilibria, intramolecular proton transfer, or viscous processes have all been suggested as the mechanism for absorption at neutral pH (Lang et al., 1971; O'Brien & Dunn, 1972; Zana et al., 1972; Slutsky & White, 1972; Hussey, 1972). Proton exchange between phosphate ions and histidyl residues has been shown to occur around pH7 suggesting that perturbation of this equilibrium would be a mechanism for the absorption of ultrasound in the neutral pH range (Slutsky et al., 1980).

Kremkau & Carstensen, (1972) have suggested that intermolecular interactions appear to be important in ultrasound absorption since the specific absorption of haemoglobin solutions increases with increasing concentration of protein and the specific absorption of dextran and polyethylene glycol solutions increases with increasing polymerization up to about 100 monomer units (O'Brien & Dunn, 1972). Absorption of ultrasound by a solution of F-actin (polymer form) was shown (Sadykhova & El'Piner, 1970) to be much greater than that by a corresponding solution of G-actin (monomer form). Kremkau et al (1973) have reported that fixation of erythrocytes with acrolein or glutaraldehyde, which crosslinks macromolecular hydrophobic groups, resulted in as much as a fivefold increase in the specific absorption of ultrasound compared with unfixed samples.

There is evidence (Goss & Dunn, 1980) that the ultrasonic absorption characteristics of biopolymers in solution is affected by their molecular structure as well as by their concentration. For example, dilute solutions of collagen, which is a triple helix, and DNA, which is a double helix, exhibit a greater degree of ultrasonic absorption at 6MHz than do more concentrated solutions of less structured molecules such as haemoglobin and albumin. These studies have led to the conclusion that since the specific absorption increases as the level of organization increases, interactions between macromolecules may be affected by ultrasound.

b) Degradation

Exposure of degassed solutions of DNA to 0.98MHz ultrasound at intensities of 25 to 31W/cm^2 resulted in a decrease in molecular weight from 2.2 x 10^7 to 4 x 10^6 (Hawley et al. 1963). This degradation occurred within the first 15 seconds of exposure and little further degradation for up to 2-minutes, suggesting that a limiting molecular weight had been reached. No cavitation (as evidenced by visible bubbles) or heating could be detected and the authors suggested that the degradation was due to viscous stresses in the molecule resulting from the density difference between DNA and water. This study appears to be one of only a few suggesting a mechanism of action other than cavitation.

Studies on calf thymus DNA exposed in vitro with 1MHz focused ultrasound caused degradation of the DNA at 200W/cm^2 with exposures of 10 minutes or longer (Coakley & Dunn, 1971, 1972). Transient cavitation seemed insufficient to account for the breakage observed and the authors suggested that the mechanism involved microstreaming (probably from stable cavitation). Greater degradation occurred with the 200W/cm^2 intensity (apparently in the absence of cavitation) than with an intensity of 515W/cm^2, where transient or collapse cavitation was suspected to occur.

Degradation of calf thymus or salmon sperm DNA was reported after exposure to 1MHz ultrasound radiation for 3 minutes at intensities greater than 0.4W/cm^2 (Hill et al., 1969). The molecular weight decreased with increasing ultrasound intensity up to 3W/cm^2 and no further decrease occurred with intensities up to 8W/cm^2 indicating that a limiting molecular weight had been reached. This terminal molecular weight was also obtained with a 5-minute exposure at 2.5W/cm^2; longer times (up to 20 minutes) caused no further DNA degradation. These results with low intensity ultrasound could only be obtained if the exposure vessel were rotated during the experiment. The authors concluded that the mechanism for the ultrasound-induced DNA degradation probably involved stable cavitation in which the microbubbles were induced to move in a circular path by rotation of the vessel thus increasing their effective lifetimes.

Irradiation of calf thymus DNA with 1MHz ultrasound resulted in considerable damage as evidenced when the lengths of sonicated and control DNA samples were examined by electron microscopy after exposure to as little as 20mW/cm^2 (Galperin-Lemaitre et al., 1975).

c) Free radicals

Studies performed on components of DNA and RNA such as nucleotide bases, nucleosides and nucleotides (Gupta & Wang, 1976; Wang, 1977; Wang & Gupta, 1977) have yielded interesting results. Exposure of the bases to intensities of 3 and 5W/cm^2 resulted in the production of sonoproducts with the order of reactivity being: thymine>uracil>cytosine>guanine>adenine. In the case of thymine, 50 percent had reacted after an exposure duration of 20 minutes at 5W/cm^2. The same sequence of reactivity of nucleic acid bases is obtained whether the bases are in solution alone or as an integral part of the nucleic acid molecule (Braginskaya and Dunn, 1981). No sonolysis products were observed when nitrous oxide (a free radical scavenger) was present. This suggests strongly that free radicals mediate the sonoreaction of the nucleic acid components.

The production of free radicals in aqueous suspensions of cells or nucleosides appears to be mediated by transient cavitation (Clarke and Hill, 1970; Fu et al, 1979; Weissler et al, 1980; Ciaravino, 1982). Nucleosides (base + sugar) and nucleotides (base + sugar + phosphate) were found to be less reactive than their corresponding bases suggesting that the additional sugar or phosphate group affords some protection from sonolysis. Analysis of the sonoproducts obtained indicated that they were mainly glycols which the authors suggested were formed by reaction of the nucleotide bases with OH free radicals produced in water as a result of cavitation (Gupta & Wang, 1976). Similar results were obtained with pulsed ultrasound at a time average intensity of 3W/cm^2 (Wang & Gupta, 1977). It was found that the extent of sonolysis was greater with the pulsed ultrasound (pulse durations of 20 usec to 10 msec) than with continuous wave and that a greater effect was observed with the longer pulse widths.

The mechanisms by which free-radical mediated thymine-base damage is caused by ionizing radiation and ultrasound must be different. With ionizing radiation, free radicals will be produced very near the intracellular site of interaction whereas with ultrasound, free radicals are most likely produced outside the cell and must diffuse into the cell to interact with the DNA (NCRP, 1983). The cell outer membrane is a very complex organ and highly

selective in what can diffuse across. It is not clear how ultrasound induced free radicals would diffuse across the plasma membrane.

d) Enzyme activity

The effect of ultrasound on the activity of various
enzymes has been extensively studied (see review in
Repacholi, 1981) but producing conflicting results. An
analysis and comparison of exposure parameters indicate
that, in general, where the irradiation conditions could
produce cavitation, and hence highly reactive free
radicals, enzyme inactivation was found. This was well
demonstrated by Klibanov et al, (1974) who added chloroform
(an efficient donor of free radicals) to the enzymes
solution and found that the rate of enzyme inactivation
increased sharply. Further, in the presence of ethanol,
the ultrasound had little effect on the enzymatic activity
of the solution. Klibanov et al, (1974) also demonstrated
a threshold of enzyme inactivation which coincided with the
threshold of cavitation production. The threshold value at
880kHz frequency was approximately $1W/cm^2$.

Enzyme activity has been shown (Young and Smithwick,
1976; Muhfeld and Sachs, 1975; Belewa-Staikowa et al, 1970)
to increase in cells fragmented or extensively disrupted by
ultrasound. Young and Smithwick (1976) suggested that the
ultrasound caused more rapid solubilization of the enzyme,
presumably increasing the reaction rates. In the case of
increased antibody activity (Muhfeld and Sachs, 1975),
ultrasound may increase the accessibility of hidden cell
surface antigens.

Ultrasound effects on enzymes and on enzyme-catalayzed
reactions in vitro have been performed on achymotrypsin,
trypsin, aldolase, lactic dehydrogenase, and ribonuclease.
The solutions were exposed from 0.12 seconds to 10 minutes
to ultrasound having frequencies of 1 to 27MHz and
intensities as high as $10^4W/cm^2$ (Coakley & Dunn,
1972). The investigators concluded that cavitation was
necessary for enzyme degradation and that if these studies
could be extrapolated to in vivo conditions it appears that
proteins would be damaged only with very intense fields.
Degassed solutions of catalase and malate dehydrogenase
were sonicated for 15-90 min with a vibrating wire driven
at 20kHz (tip displacement amplitudes varied from 15-26 um)
(Kashkoolie et al, 1980). While catalase appeared to be
unaffected by the ultrasound treatment, the enzyme activity
of malate dehydrogenase decreased exponentially with
increasing time of sonication. The authors concluded that
the enzyme inactivation was due to acoustic microstreaming
and was not a result of collapse cavitation or temperature
elevation. Although these results suggest that enzymes can
be damaged by a nonthermal and noncavitational mechanism,
the low frequency used and the lack of conventional
intensity values makes it difficult to evaluate this study
with respect to medical ultrasound exposure. However,
since interactions between macromolecules such as proteins
appear to be affected by ultrasound, it is possible that
subcellular structures could be more sensitive to damage
from low intensity ultrasound (Edmonds, 1972) than their
component biomolecules.

CONCLUSIONS

A selected summary of results is given in Table 3 to provide an overview of ultrasound induced effects on macromolecular solutions. Solutions of macromolecules such as proteins and nucleic acids are capable of absorbing ultrasound in the megahertz frequency range. There is evidence suggesting that approximately two-thirds of the absorption occurs at the macromolecular level and about one-third occurs at the level of the tissue structure. Proton transfer reactions appear to be involved in this absorption process along with intermolecular interactions and relaxation of the tissue lattice.

Damage of macromolecules in suspension exposed to ultrasound is generally as a result of cavitation, although some evidence exists for non-thermal, non-cavitational mechanisms occurring. One report has indicated that DNA can be degraded in solution with low intensity ($200mW/cm^2$) ultrasound (Galperin- Lemaitre et al. 1975). It is unlikely that this data can be extrapolated to the in vivo situation since the structure of DNA in solution bears little resemblance to its structure in vivo. DNA in vitro may be less sensitive to destruction by ultrasound since it is complexed with proteins which could protect the DNA from damage.

The role of free radicals in producing damage in molecules exposed to ultrasound has been shown from various experiments. When free radicals scavengers are used, the molecular damage is greatly reduced.

TABLE 3
SELECTED EFFECTS OF ULTRASOUND ON SUSPENSIONS
OF MACROMOLECULES

SATA INTENSITY	EXPOSURE TIME	WAVE FROM	EFFECT OBSERVED	REFERENCE
200	30	cw	DNA Molecular weight reduced	Galperin- Lemaitre et al (1975)
250	-	cw	Threshold for production of free radicals in aqueous solution	Carmichael et al (1984)
500	2	cw	Threshold for release for iodine from K1 solution	Hill et al (1969)
510	-	cw	Threshold for DNA base lysis	McKee et al (1977)
6600 (SPTA)	15	cw	Free radical production in biological media	Edmonds and Sancier (1983)

Transient or collapse cavitation appears to be responsible for almost all effects produced on macromolecular solutions by ultrasound. Unless similar mechanisms are found to occur in vivo, valid questions could be raised concerning the value of continuing research on macromolecules to identify possible biological effects of ultrasound exposure.

REFERENCES

Braginskaya, F.I. and Dunn, F. (1981). Some aspects of the effect of ultrasound on biological structures, Biophysics 26: 550.

Campbell, P.N. and Kernot, B.A. (1962). The incorporation of (C^{14}) leucine into serum albumin by the isolated microsome fraction from rat liver. Biochem. J. 82: 262-266.

Carstensen, E.L. (1960). The mechanism of the absorption of ultrasound in biological materials. IRE Trans. Med. Electron. 7: 158-162.

Ciaravino, V. (1982). Effects of 1MHz ultrasound on Chinese hamster V-79 cells: cavitation mechanisms and effects on proliferation. Doctoral Thesis, University of Rochester, New York.

Clarke, P.R. and Hill, C.R. (1970). Physical and chemical agents of ultrasonic disruption of cells. J. Acoust. Soc. Am. 47: 649.

Coakley, W.T. and Dunn, F. (1971). Degradation of DNA in high-intensity focused ultrasonic fields at 1MHz. J. Acoust. Soc. Am. 50: 1539-1454.

Coakley, W.T. and Dunn, F. (1972). Interaction of megahertz ultrasound and biological polymers. In: Interaction of Ultrasound and Biological Tissues. J.M. Reid and M.R. Sikov (Eds.). HEW Publication (FDA) 73-8008, pp. 43-45.

Edmonds, P.D. (1972). Effects on macromolecules. In: Interaction of Ultrasound and Biological Tissues. J.M. Reid and M.R. Sikov (Eds.). HEW Publication (FDA) 73-8008, pp. 5-11.

Fu, Y.K., Miller, M.W., Lange, C.S., Griffiths, T.D. and Kaufman, G.E. (1980). Ultrasound lethality to synchronous and asynchonous Chinese hamster V-79 cells. Ultrasound Med. Biol. 6: 39.

Galperin-Lemaitre, H., Kirsch-Volders, M. and Levi, S. (1975). Ultrasound and mammalian DNA. Lancet 1: 662.

Goss, S.A. and Dunn, F. (1980). Ultrasonic propagation properties of collagen. Phys. Med. Biol. 25(5): 827-837.

Gupta, A.B. and Wang, S.Y. (1976). Effect of low
    intensity ultrasound on nucleic acid components.
    Ultrasonics Symposium Proceedings. IEEE 76 CH1120-5SU:
    92-96.

Hawley, S.A., Macleod, R.M. and Dunn, F. (1963).
    Degradation of DNA by intense, noncavitating
    ultrasound. J. Acoust. Soc. Am. 35(8): 1285-1287.

Hill, C.R., Clarke, P.R., Crowe, M.R. and Hammick,
    J.W. (1969). Biophysical effects of cavitation in a
    1MHz ultrasonic beam. In: Ultrasonics for Industry
    Conference Papers. Iliffe and Sons, Ltd., London, pp.
    26-30.

Hill, C.R. (1972). Ultrasonic exposure thresholds for
    changes in cells and tissues, J. Acoust. Soc. Am. 52:
    666-672.

Hughes, D.E. (1972). The interaction of ultrasound
    with cells. In: Interaction of Ultrasound and
    Biological Tissues. J.M. Reid and M.R. Sikov (Eds.).
    U.S. Dept. of HEW Publication (FDA) 73-8008, pp. 61-63.

Hussey, M. (1972). Proton transfer processes: One of
    the modes of interaction of ultrasound with proteins
    and DNA. In: Interaction of Ultrasound and Biological
    Tissues, J.M. Reid and M.R. Sikov (Eds.). U.S. Dept.
    of HEW Publication (FDA) 73-8008, pp. 31-35.

Kashkooli, H.A., Rooney, J.A. and Roxby, R. (1980).
    Effects of ultrasound on catalase and malate
    dehydrogenase. J. Acoust. Soc. Am. 67(5): 1798-1801.

Kremkau, F.W. and Carstensen, E.L. (1972).
    Macromolecular interaction in sound absorption. In:
    Interaction of Ultrasound and Biological Tissues. J.M.
    Reid and M.R. Sikov (Eds.). U.S. Dept. of HEW
    Publication (FDA) 73-8008 pp. 37-42.

Kremkau, J.W., Carstensen, E.L. and Aldridge, W.G.
    (1973). Macromolecular interaction in the absorption
    of ultrasound in fixed erythrocytes. J. Acoust. Soc.
    Am. 53(5): 1448-1451.

Lang, J., Tondre, C. and Zana, R. (1971). Effect of
    urea and other organic substances on the ultrasonic
    absorption of protein solutions. J. Phys. Chem. 75(3):
    374-379.

NCRP (1983). Biological effects of ultrasound:
    Mechanisms and clinical implications, National Council
    on Radiation Protection and Measurements Report No 74,
    NCRP, 7910 Woodmont Ave, Bethesda, MD 20814.

O'Brien, W.D. and Dunn, F. (1972). Ultrasonic
    absorption by biomacromolecules. In: Interaction of
    Ultrasound and Biological Tissues. J.M. Reid and M.R.
    Sikov (Eds.). U.S. Dept. of HEW Publication (FDA)
    73-8008, pp. 13-19.

Pauly, H. and Schwan, H.P. (1971). Mechanism of absorption of ultrasound in liver tissue. J. Acoust. Soc. Am. 50(2): 692-699.

Peacock, A.R. and Pritchard, N.H. (1969). Some biological aspects of ultrasound. Progress in Biophysics, 18: 185-208.

Sadykhova, S. Kh. and El'Piner, I.E. (1970). Absorption of ultrasonic waves in aqueous solutions of biopolymers. Soviet Physics - Acoustics 16(1): 101-107.

Slutsky, L.J. and White, R.D. (1972). Proton transfer and acoustic absorption in protein solutions. In: Interaction of Ultrasound and Biological Tissues. J.M. Reid and M.R. Sikov (Eds.). U.S. Dept. of HEW Publication (FDA) 73-8008, pp. 27-29.

Slutsky, L.J., Madsen, L., White, R.D. and Harkness, J. (1980). Kinetics of the exchange of protons between hydrogen phosphate ions and a histidyl residue. J. Phys. Chem. 84: 1325-1329.

Von der Decken, A. and Campbell, P.N. (1964). The effect of ultrasonic vibrations on the protein synthesizing activity of microsome preparations from rat liver. Biochem. J. 91(1): 195-201.

Wang, S.Y. (1977). Ultrasonic radiation of nucleic acids and compondnets. In: Symposium on Biological Effects and Characterizations of Ultrasound Sources. D.G Hazard and M.L. Litz (Eds.). U.S. Dept. of HEW Publication (FDA) 78-8048, pp. 196-205.

Wang, S.Y. and Gupta, A.B. (1977). Effect of pulse ultrasound on nucleic acid components. Ultrasonics Symposium Proceedings. IEEE 77 CH 1264-ISU.

Weissler, A., Cooper, H.W. and Snydner, S. (1980). Chemical effect of ultrasonic waves: Oxidation of potassium iodide solution of carbontetra chloride. J. Amer. Chem. Soc., 72: 1769.

Zana, R., Lang, R., Tondre, C. and Sturm, J. (1972). Interactions of ultrasound with proteins and nucleic acids in solutions. In: Interactions of Ultrasound and Biological Tissues. J.M. Reid and M.R. Sikov (Eds.). U.S. Dept. of HEW Publication (FDA) 73-8008, pp. 21-26.

EXPERIMENTATION IN VITRO :

EFFECTS OF ULTRASOUND ON CELL SUSPENSIONS

Michael H. Repacholi
Chief Scientist, Royal Adelaide Hospital
Adelaide, South Australia 5000

INTRODUCTION

Elucidating the mechanisms of action of a particular agent is usually more readily performed and analysed using cell suspensions instead of the whole animal because of the absence of numerous uncontrollable variables. In vitro experiments are also important for suggesting new endpoints to study in vivo. Effects that have been observed in mammalian cells exposed to ultrasound include: modification of macromolecular synthetic pathways and cellular ultrastructure; cell lysis, inactivation, and altered growth properties; and chromosomal alterations.

Since proteins and DNA are key macromolecules in cells, many studies have been performed to determine if ultrasound can alter their rate of synthesis. Increases or decreases in protein or DNA synthesis would suggest that ultrasound may be inducing direct damage which is being repaired. Alterations in synthesis could be due to changes in the complicated intracellular processes leading to the production of protein or DNA. This paper summarizes some of the more important experimental data and conclusions are made on their significance.

PROTEIN SYNTHESIS

Protein synthesis was observed to be stimulated in human fibroblasts 4 days after exposure to 3MHz ultrasound for 5 min at intensities of $0.5-2.0W/cm^2$ (Harvey et al., 1975). Continuous wave (cw) exposure at $0.5W/cm^2$ caused the total protein synthesis in fibroblasts to increase by 20%, while exposure to pulsed ultrasound (pulse duration, 2ms; duty factor, 0.2) at the same average intensity resulted in a 30% increase compared with control values (Harvey et al., 1975; Webster et al., 1978). The stimulation which appeared to be inversely related to the ultrasound frequency in the range 1-5MHz, did not occur when the cells were pretreated with cortisol. This suggested that the increased protein synthesis observed was due to damage to the lysosomal and plasma membranes (possibly by cavitation), since no ultrastructural changes occurred if the cells were exposed at elevated pressures.

An increase in protein synthesis in hepatic, renal, and myocardial tissue treated with a single, 5min exposure to a therapy transducer at intensities of both 0.2 and 0.6W/cm^2 was observed by Belewa-Staikowa & Kraschkowa (1967). However, protein synthesis was retarded at 1W/cm^2. A similar effect was observed by Repacholi (1980) who found that stimulation of protein synthesis occurred in suspensions of human lymphocytes exposed to low cw therapeutic (SATA) intensities (870kHz, 1.1W/cm^2, 30 min), and retardation at higher intensities (3-4W/cm^2).

A summary of selected data on induced changes in protein synthesis resulting from exposure to ultrasound is shown in Table 1. These data generally support the hypothesis that exposure to low intensity ultrasound is simulatory while high ultrasound reduces protein synthesis.

Table 1

Selected Results on Ultrasound -
Induced Changes in Protein Synthesis

SATA INTENSITY mW/cm^2	WAVE FORM	EXPOSURE TIME MIN	OBSERVED EFFECT	REFERENCE
200	cw	5	enhanced	Beleva-Staikowa & Kraschkowa (1967)
500	cw	5	enhanced (20%)	Harvey et al (1975)
500	pulsed	5	enhanced (30%)	Webster et al (1978)
600	cw	5	enhanced	Ross & Edmonds (1983)
1000	cw	5	retarded	Beleva-Staikowa & Kraschkowa (1967)
1100	cw	30	enhanced	Repacholi (1980)
1700	cw	5	induced	Ross & Edmonds (1983)
3000	cw	30	retarded	Repacholi (1980)
3600	cw	5	retarded	Ross & Edmonds (1983)

It has been suggested (NCRP, 1983) that because the exposed cultures contain fewer cells and the two populations (exposed and control) may not be confluent (synchronised or acting in the same manner), and altered uptake of precursor may result. This is possible, but it is normal experimental procedure to ensure the same cell concentration exists in both samples. Further, the cells are not normally synchronised prior to exposure and it would be expected that the same degree of asynchrony existed post-exposure.

DNA

Increased DNA synthesis in vitro was observed 1, 2, and 3 days after exposure of excised neonatal mouse tibiae to cw 1MHz ultrasound at $1.8W/cm^2$ (Elmer & Fleischer, 1974). However, no statistically significant differences were observed in either protein accumulation or in bone elongation compared with the controls.

Levels of (^3H) thymidine and (^3H) deoxyuridine incorporated into DNA decreased to 54% and 42% of control values, respectively, following exposure of mouse leukaemia 1210 cells to 2.22MHz ultrasound for 10 min, at a mean spatial intensity of $10W/cm^2$ (Kaufman & Kremkau, 1978). Ultrasound caused reversible injury in the cell, which was not readily reversed in the presence of cytotoxic drugs, and this resulted in a significant decrease in the lethal potential of the leukaemia cells.

A significant immediate inhibition in the incorporation of (^3H) thymidine was also found by Repacholi et al. (1979) and Repacholi (1980), when Concanavalin A (Con-A) stimulated human lymphocytes were exposed in vitro to therapeutic ultrasound (cw, near-field, 870kHz, $4W/cm^2$, for 30 min) 24 to 48 hours post stimulation. The uptake of the radioactive precursors returned to control levels, 2-3 days after exposure (Repacholi, 1980, 1981). This result was confirmed by Vivino et al (1985) after exposing Con-A stimulated murine spleen cells at lower intensities (spatial peak values from 16 to $300mW/cm^2$) of 1.6MHz ultrasound in the presence of a Nuclepore membrane that contained stabilised gas bubbles. Stable cavitation not only reduced the uptake of (^3H) thymidine but induced cell lysis at spatial peak intensities above $75mW/cm^2$ (SATA intensity of $15mW/cm^2$).

Fung et al (1978) exposed activated human lymphocytes to cw ultrasound for 0-30 min using a commercial fetal Doppler unit. The uptake of (^3H) thymidine over an 18-h period, 1 day after ultrasound exposure, was found to be biphasic. There were lymphocytes that showed significant stimulation in uptake at short exposure times (3-12 min exposure) with a return to control values at longer exposure times (15-30-min exposure), and lymphocytes that did not exhibit any stimulatory effect at short exposures times, but showed a significant reduction in uptake with 12- and 30-min exposures.

Liebeskind et al (1979) exposed synchronized HeLa cells in culture to pulsed 2.5MHz ultrasound at a SATA intensity of 17mW/cm^2 (35.4W/cm^2 SPTP intensity) and induced unscheduled, non-S-phase (repair) DNA synthesis. This result suggested that the DNA had been damaged by the ultrasonic exposure. A similar effect was reported by Repacholi & Kaplan (1980), who found non-S-phase unscheduled DNA synthesis in human peripheral blood lympocytes exposed to cw near-field, 870kHz ultrasound at 4W/cm^2 for 30 min.

A summary of selected results of induced changes in DNA synthesis by MHz ultrasound is given in Table 2. As in the previous section, it appears that low intensity ultrasound has a stimulatory effect and high intensity and repressive effect on DNA synthesis. The data on changes in DNA and protein synthesis in cells exposed to ultrasound suggest that one or more of the following may be the cause:

a) Release of hydrolytic enzymes from damaged lysosomes could lead to a derepression of DNA and induction of protein synthesis as well as to increased DNA synthesis (Stewart and Stratmeyer, 1982).

b) Repair synthesis would show as an increase in protein synthesis and in non-S-phase DNA synthesis.

c) At higher intensities where ultrasound could damage cell membranes, a decreased DNA synthesis could result from a decrease in the transport of nucleotide precursors from damaged plasma membrane. Similarly, disruption of the endoplasmic reticulum could cause a decrease in protein synthesis.

Table 2

Selected Results on MHz Ultrasound – Induced Changes in DNA Synthesis

SATA INTENSITY mW/cm^2	WAVE FORM	EXPOSURE TIME min	OBSERVED EFFECT	REFERENCE
5	cw	3,6	stimulated	Fung et al (1978)
5	cw	30	suppressed	Fung et al (1978)
17	pulsed		increased (non-s-phase)	Liebeskind et al (1979)
1800	cw		increased	Elmer and Fleisher (1974)
4000	cw	30	increased (non-s-phase)	Repacholi & Kaplan (1980)

Table 2 continued

4000	cw	30	decreased (stimula- ted cells)	Repacholi (1980)
10000	cw	10	decreased	Kaufman & Kremkau (1978)

d) Cavitation seems the most likely mechanism to produce the above results (Vivino et al, 1985), although non-cavitational stresses and streaming could play a role.

SISTER CHROMATID EXCHANGES (SCE)

The significance of SCE in relation to biological hazard is not understood, though the phenomenon is generally held to be undesirable. For some other types of insults, sister chromatid assay has been suggested to be a sensitive measure of genetic damage, because the frequency of exchanges increases after exposure of cells to known mutagens and carcinogens (Stetka & Wolff, 1977). The SCE method has been advocated as a direct test of mutagenic or carcinogenic agents (Latt & Schreck, 1980; Shiraishi & Sandberg, 1980). The data on production of SCEs by ultrasound exposure will be reviewed in a separate paper in this volume.

CELL MEMBRANE

A number of investigators have reported ultrasonically-induced functional alterations in the plasma membrane. These include increased permeability, decreased active transport, decreased non-mediated transport, and decreased electrophoretic mobility.

A 5% decrease in the non-mediated transport of leucine in avian erythrocytes following a 30-min, 1MHz ultrasound exposure at an intensity of $0.6W/cm^2$ was reported by Bundy et al (1978). However, no change was observed in the active transport of (^{3}H) thymidine in human lymphocytes exposed to cw 870kHz ultrasound at intensities up to $4W/cm^2$, for 30 min (Repacholi, 1980).

A reduction in the electrophoretic mobility of Ehrlich ascites tumour cells observed by Repacholi (1970) and Repacholi et al (1971) was found to be directly proportional to the square root of the ultrasonic frequency used in the range of 0.5-3.2MHz (Taylor & Newman, 1972). This reduction in mobility was reported to be independent of the pulse length over the range of 20us-10ms (peak intensity was $10W/cm^2$; duty factor, 0.1; exposure time, 5 min). The change in mobility was presumably a result of alteration of the surface charge of the cells. This effect was also reported by Joshi et al (1973) to be due to cavitation and later reported to be reversible and non-lethal by Hill and ter Haar (1981).

An increase in the permeability of human erythrocyte membranes to potassium ions was observed following ultrasound exposure _in vitro_ for 5-30 min (1MHz, 0.5-3.0W/cm^2) (Lota & Darling, 1955). A decrease in potassium content was reported to occur following sonication of rat thymocytes for 40 min, using an ultrasonic therapy unit operated at 3MHz and 2W/cm^2 (Chapman et al., 1980). These changes appeared to be a result of both a decreased influx and an increased efflux of potassium. Changes in membrane permeability to sodium and calcium ions have also been shown for similar exposures (Dyson 1985).

Changes in the concentrations of membrane-associated cAMP and cGMP have profound effects on a wide variety of cellular processes. However, no alterations in the amount of cAMP and cGMP could be detected following exposure of human amniotic cells or mouse peritoneal cells to cw 1MHz ultrasound at 1W/cm^2 for 33 min (Glick et al., 1979).

Dispersed, cultured human cells seeded in plastic Petri dishes were reported (Siegel et al, 1979) to show significantly reduced cellular attachment after 0.5 min of exposure to a pulsed, 2.25MHz clinical diagnostic ultrasound source (approximate SATA intensity, 10mW/cm^2). The authors suggested that, if cellular attachment were to be altered _in vivo_, it could affect implantation, morphogenesis, and development. These results may be related to findings described by Liebeskind et al (1981a) on morphological changes in cell surface characteristics observed after pulsed diagnostic ultrasound exposure. Mouse 3T3 cells examined for up to 37 days after a single exposure showed abnormally large numbers of microvilli and cell projections. Thirty-seven days represents 50 generations for this cell line and suggests that the altered cell surface characteristics were a result of a hereditary change. However, Mummery (1978) had not previously observed these changes following exposure of fibroblasts to either pulsed or cw therapeutic ultrasound.

Martins (1971) reported that scanning electron micrographs of M3-1 cells exposed to 1MHz ultrasound at 1.0 and 0.25W/cm^2 showed a characteristic bumpy outer surface, compared with the smooth outer surface of unexposed cells.

The motility _in vitro_ of sparse populations of human embryo lung fibroblasts was found to increase after exposure to 3MHz ultrasound at SPTP intensities of 0.5-2.0W/cm^2, pulsed 2ms on, 8ms off for 20 min. This was the result of an increase in mean speed (Mummery, 1978). The author suggested that this effect could be implicated in the beneficial therapeutic action of ultrasound on wound healing.

An increase in the calcium ion content of human embryonic lung fibroblasts resulted from _in vitro_ exposure to 3MHz ultrasound, at SPTP intensities of 2 and 4W/cm^2 pulsed 2ms on, 8ms off, for 20 min. The effect was still observed when the cells were washed with ethylene diamine tetraacetic acid (EDTA) after treatment, but was suppressed by doubling the ambient pressure during sonication. This strongly implicates acoustic cavitation as the dominant mechanism (Mummery, 1978).

Table 3 gives a summary of results found on membranes of cells exposed to ultrasound. In summary, there are several reports indicating that diagnostic levels of pulsed ultrasound can cause structural and functional changes in cell surface characteristics. Because of the importance of the cell surface in immune determination, receptor topography carrier systems, and cell-cell recognition, these changes could have quite important ramifications in vivo. However, the interpretation of the results of cell culture experiments in terms of an in vivo situation is speculative, because of the difficulty in bridging the gap between experimental in vitro work and effects that may occur in the patient. The mechanism of these effects appears to be cavitation and it has yet to be shown that cavitation can occur in vivo.

ULTRASTRUCTURAL CHANGES

Electron microscopic examination of human fibroblasts, irradiated with pulsed, 3MHz ultrasound at an SATP intensity of $0.5W/cm^2$ (duty factor 0.2), revealed: more free ribosomes; increased dilation of the rough endoplasmic reticulum; increased damage to mitochondria and to lysosmal membranes; and more cytoplasmic vacuolation (Harvey et al., 1975). Exposure of HeLa cells to 0.75MHz ultrasound at an intensity of $0.9W/cm^2$ for 20-120 min a caused: slits in the cells; holes in the nuclear membranes; separation of the inner and outer nuclear membranes; increases in cell debris; exploded mitochondria; and lesions in the endoplasmic reticulum (Watmough et al., 1977). The results suggested that some of the damage, such as rupture of the nuclear and plasma membranes, may have been due to shear stresses resulting from microstreaming around oscillating microbubbles (stable cavitation).

Microtubule systems of Heliozoan were studied using a commercial pulsed diagnostic device emitting $2.5mW/cm^2$ for 10-20s at 5MHz (Cachon et al 1981). Ultrasound exposure caused the microtubules to become disorganised within their axopods. Subsequently the organisms stopped moving and died rapidly. Electron microscopic examination of Con-A stimulated human blood lymphocytes exposed for 30 min to 870kHz cw ultrasound at $4W/cm^2$ also revealed disruption of microtubule formation (Repacholi, 1980). Results of studies on human lymphocytes and Erlich ascites carcinoma cells suggested a possible disturbance of the mitotic spindle at metaphase following ultrasound exposure (Schnitzler, 1972). Clarke & Hill (1970) reported that, in L51784 cells, susceptibility to ultrasonic disintegration increased during mitosis. It was suggested that cells are particularly susceptible to damage by ultrasound during mitosis, because major changes in the cell membrane and in the internal structure during this phase of the cell cycle.

Table 3 Selected Studies on Ultrasound - Induced Changes to Cell Membrane

SATA INTENSITY mW/cm^2	WAVE FORM	EXPOSURE TIME min	OBSERVED EFFECT	REFERENCE
10	Pulsed	0.5	Decreased attachment	Siegel et al (1979)
17	Pulsed	-	Altered surface character-istics	Liebeskind et al (1981a)
250	cw	0.5	Altered topography	Martins (1971)
500-2000 SPTP	Pulsed	20	Increased Motility - no surface character change	Mummery (1978)
500	cw	5	Increased K$^+$ permeab.	Lota & Darling (1955)
600	cw	30	Decreased non-mediat. transport	Bundy et al (1978)
700	cw		imperfect. morphology	Rozeboro (1977)
1000	Pulsed	5	Reduced electro-phoretic mobility	Repacholi (1970) Taylor & Newman (1972) Joshi et al (1973)
1000	cw	10	Detachment of multi-cellular spheroids	Conger et al (1981)
2000	cw	40	Decreased potassium content	Chapman et al (1980)
4000	cw	30	No active transport change	Repacholi (1980)

Changes were observed when a 3T3 fibroblast and normal rat peritoneal fluid cells were exposed to pulsed 2MHz ultrasound at 15mW/cm^2 for 30 min post-sonication ultrastructural (Liebeskind et al., 1981b). The authors suggested that low-intensity, pulsed ultrasound could alter both cellular ultrastructure and metabolism and that the persistence of disturbance in cell motility, many generations after sonication in vitro, is especially important. It can be speculated that, if fetal cells were to be sustain subtle damaged, it might affect cell migration during organogenesis.

Mitochondria appear to be some of the most sensitive intracellular organelles to ultrasound exposure, exhibiting swelling, loss of cristae, and eventual disruption of the outer membrane. The endoplasmic reticulum seems to be less sensitive to ultrasound exposure than mitochondria, but, with increasing exposure times, dilation of the cisternae, loss of surface ribosomes, and vesiculation occurs. Most cell damage from sublethal exposures appears to be reparable within four days; however, changes in the mitochondria persist for longer periods of time and may be irreversible (Stephens et al., 1978).

A summary of studies on ultrastructural changes observed in cells exposed to ultrasound in vitro is given in Table 4. These data provide evidence that pulsed ultrasound may be more detrimental in terms of producing an effect than the equivalent SATA intensity in the cw mode. However, as seen in Table 5, Dooley et al (1983) found quite the opposite effect on cell survival.

Table 4.
Selected Studies on Ultrasound –
Induced Ultrastructural Changes
in Cells Suspensions

SATA INTENSITY mW/cm^2	WAVE FORM	EXPOSURE TIME min	OBSERVED	REFERENCE
2.5	pulsed	0.2	disorganised microtubules	Cachon et al (1981)
15	pulsed	30	altered internal structure, increased microvilli	Liebeskind et al (1981a,b)
200	cw	2	rupture to myofibrils	Samosodova & El'Piner (1966)
500	pulsed	5	damage to mitochondria, etc	Harvey et al (1975)
800	cw	5	increased platelet aggregation holes in nuclear membranes	Chater & Williams (1977)
900	cw	0.3	increased cell debris, etc	Watmough et al (1977)
4000	cw	30	disorganised microtubules	Repacholi (1980)

MAMMALIAN CELL SURVIVAL AND PROLIFERATION

From the mid-1970's investigators began to focus their attention on quantifiable biological variables such as cell survival and proliferative capacity. Lysis of mouse lymphoma cells in suspension, at ultrasound frequencies and intensities used in clinical medicine, has been documented and correlated with acoustic cavitation (Coakley et al., 1971). Maeda & Murao (1977) found significant growth suppression in human amniotic cells in cultures exposed to 2MHz cw ultrasound at intensities higher than $0.8W/cm^2$ for 1h. Maeda & Tsuzaki (1981) also observed growth suppression in cultured human amniotic cells exposed to pulsed, 2MHz ultrasound at SATA intensities higher than $60mW/cm^2$ (1kHz pulse repetition rate, 3-us duration, $80W/cm^2$ SPTP intensity).

The importance of peak pulse intensities and other parameters, such as pulse duration and pulse repetition frequency, has been reported by other investigators (Barnett, 1979; Saravazyan et al., 1980). It has been suggested that intact cells surviving ultrasound exposure remain unaffected, in terms of subsequent growth and proliferation rates (Clarke & Hill, 1969). However, other studies have shown that many of the intact nonlysed cells in suspension remaining after ultrasound exposure are non-viable, as determined by both vital dye exclusion and colony-forming ability (Kaufman et al., 1977).

Exposure of HeLa and CHO cells for 2-5 min to 1MHz cw ultrasound resulted in a threshold for cell lysis at an intensity of approximately $1W/cm^2$, with the maximum effects occurring at an intensity of $10W/cm^2$ (Kaufman et al., 1977). Colonies formed from sonicated cells contained fewer cells and a higher frequency of giant cells than colonies formed from appropriate controls (Miller et al., 1977).

Table 5 gives a summary of data on effects of ultrasound on cell survival and proliferation.

Ultrasound exposure to cells in suspension can lead to cell death by disintegration (lysis) and cavitation is an important mechanism in the process. What remains in some doubt is whether ultrasound at low megahertz frequencies causes cell death either by disintegration or otherwise, in the absence of cavitation at normal physiological temperatures. A number of reports in the literature indicate that this may be so but, in view of the technical difficulty of monitoring cavitation activity, these must be treated with some reservations. Where such investigations

Table 5

Selected Studies on Cell Survival
and Proliferaton

SATA INTENSITY mW/cm^2	WAVE FORM	EXPOSURE TIME min	OBSERVED EFFECT	REFERENCE
60	pulsed	-	growth suppress.	Maeda & Tsuzaki (1981)
500	cw		growth suppress.	Clarke et al (1970)
800	cw	60	growth suppress.	Maeda & Murao (1977)
1000	cw	2-5	lysis	Kaufman et al (1977)
2000 (SPTA)	cw	10	decreased cell surv.	Dooley et al (1983)
2000 (SPTA)	pulsed	10	no decrease survival	Dooley et al (1983)

have been carried out systematically (Coakley et al 1971; Hill 1972; Morton et al 1983) a clear correlation between cell death and cavitation has generally been found.

Although Hill and ter Haar (1981) suggest there is no evidence for a time lag after exposure before cell death occurs, studies on cells in suspension have shown ultrasound exposure can induce both immediate and delayed effects (Kaufman & Miller, 1978). Studies performed at elevated temperatures showed that immediate cell lysis was independent of temperature (up to 43°C), whereas cellular inactivation (as measured by a reduction in plating efficiency) was temperature dependent (Li et al., 1977). These studies indicate that immediate cell death may be caused by large-scale cellular damage (probably resulting from some form of cavitation activity), whereas the delayed effects depend on the cell's ability to repair sublethal damage. These repair mechanisms are less efficient at elevated temperatures

There is quite a wide range of "threshold intensities" for the lysis of isolated cells in suspension. Variables contributing to this wide variation include: the gas content of the medium; exposure geometry; ultrasound exposure parameters; and the number and availability of cavitation nuclei. In any given medium, the last of these factors depends critically on the treatment of the medium immediately prior to exposure and the degree of agitation during exposure (Williams, 1982). Similarly Armour and Corry (1982) found that cell killing depended on the amount of gas dissolved in the treatment medium.

CONCLUSIONS

Exposure to ultrasound can cause changes in the ultrastructure of cells in culture, which lead to disruptions on macromolecular synthetic pathways. Various cell components may be susceptible to damage; these include the nuclear, lysosomal, and plasma membrane, microtubules, the mitotic spindle, and the endoplasmic reticulum. Both ultrastructural and functional changes in the plasma membrane have been reported following exposure to relatively low-intensity pulsed ultrasound. Because of the importance of the cell surface in such functions as immune determination, receptor topography carrier systems, and cell-cell recognition, these changes could have quite important ramifications in vivo.

Cavitation appears to be the dominant mechanism responsible for many of the ultrasonically-induced structural changes. Church and Miller (1983), using classical radiation target theory, have proposed that non-trapped bubbles tunnel into cells while undergoing stable cavitation and produce cell lysis by one or more transient events inside the cell. This theory adds a new dimension for study since it is believed that forces produced by stable cavitation should be strong enough in themselves to lyse plasma membranes from outside the cell.

Ultrasound exposure alters both cellular ultrastructure and metabolism. Cells exposed in vitro to ultrasound appear to be more prone to cell death during mitosis. Suppression of cellular growth has been reported under cw and pulsed exposure conditions.

It is quite difficult to make any quantitive determination of in vitro since they depend so much on the experimental arrangement. For example, Williams (1982) found threshold intensities for the in vitro lysis of human erythrocytes in the range from about 100 to 700mW/cm^2 within the same apparatus. The only change in the experimental arrangement was the speed of rotation of the erythrocyte container during ultrasound exposure. Similarly Armour and Corry (1982) found ultrasound induced all killing depended on the frequency of the beam, free radical scavengers and attachement to membranes.

REFERENCES

Armour, E.P. and Corry, P.M. (1982). Cytotoxic effects of ultrasound in vitro dependence on gas content frequency, radical scavengers and attachment. <u>Rad. Research</u>, <u>89</u>: 369-380.

Barnett, S.B. (1979). Bioeffects of pulsed ultrasound. <u>Austral. Phys. Sci. Med.</u>, <u>2-7</u>: 397-403.

Belewa-Staikowa, R. & Kraschkowa, A.M. (1967). Effects of bio-physical factors on the redox processes and biological oxidation. Effect of ultrasonics on the protein content and transaminase activity of organs. <u>Radiobiol. Radiother.</u>, <u>8</u>: 655-662.

Bundy, M.L., Lerner, J., Messier, D.L., & Rooney, J.A. (1978). Effects of ultrasound on transport in avian erythrocytes. <u>Ultrasound Med. Biol.</u>, <u>4</u>: 259-262.

Cachon, J., Cachon., & Bruneton, J.H. (1981). An ultrastructural study of the effect of very high frequency ultrasound on a microtubular system. <u>Biol. Cell</u>, <u>40</u>: 69.

Chapman, I.V., Macnally, N.A., & Tucker, S. (1980). Ultrasound-induced changes in rates of influx and efflux of potassium ions in rat thymocytes <u>in vitro</u>. <u>Ultrasound Med. Biol.</u>, <u>6</u>: 47-58.

Chater, B.V. and Williams, A.R. (1977). Platelet aggregation induced <u>in vitro</u> by therapeutic ultrasound. Thomb. Haemos. 38: 640-651.

Church, C.C. and Miller, M.W. (1983). The kinetics and mechanisms of ultrasonically - induced cell lysis produced by non-trapped bubbles in a rotating culture tube. Ultrasound Med. Biol. 9(4): 385-393.

Clarke, P.R. & Hill, C.R. (1969). Biological action of ultrasound in relation to the cell cycle. <u>Exp. Cell Res.</u>, <u>58</u>: 443-444.

Clarke, P.R. & Hill, C.R. (1970). Physical and chemical aspects of ultrasonic disruption of cells. <u>J. Acoust. Soc. Am.</u>, <u>50</u>: 649-653.

Coakley, W.T., Hampton, D., & Dunn, F. (1971). Quantitative relationships between ultrasonic cavitation and effects upon amoebae at 1MHz. <u>J. Acoust. Soc. Am.</u>, <u>50</u>: 1546-1553.

Conger, A.D.; Ziskin, M.C. and Wittels, H. (1981). Ultrasound effects on mammalian multicellular spheroids. J. Clinical Ultrasound 9: 167-174.

Dooley, D.A., Child, S.Z., Carstensen, E.L. and Miller, M.W. (1983). The effect of continuous wave and pulsed ultrasound on rat thymocytes in vitro. <u>Med. Biol.</u> 9: 379-384.

Dyson, M. (1985). Therapeutic applications of ultrasound.
In: Biological effects of ultrasound. W.C. Nyborg and
M.C. Ziskin eds. Churchill Livingston, New York,
p121-133.

Elmer, W.A. & Fleischer, A.C. (1974). Enhancement of DNA
synthesis in neonatal mouse tibial epiphyses after
exposure to therapeutic ultrasound. J. Clin.
Ultrasound, 2: 191-195.

Fung, H.K., Cheung, K., Lyons, E.A., & Kay, N.E. (1978).
The effects of low-dose ultrasound on human peripheral
lymphocyte function in vitro. In: White, D. & Lyons,
E.A., ed. Ultrasound in medicine, New York, Plenum
Press, Vol. 4, pp. 583-586.

Glick, D., Adamovics, A. Edmonds, P.D., & Taenzer, J.C.
(1979). Search for biochemical effects in cells and
tissues of ultrasonic irradiation of mice and of the in
vitro irradiation of mouse peritoneal and human
amniotic cells. Ultrasound Med. Biol., 5: 23-33.

Harvey, W., Dyson, M., Pond, J.B., & Grahame, R. (1975).
The in vitro stimulation of protein synthesis in human
fibroblasts by therapeutic levels of ultrasound. In:
Kazner, E. et al., ed. Proceedings of the 2nd European
Congress on Ultrasonics in Medicine, Munich 12-16 May
1975, Amsterdam, Excerpta Medica, pp. 10-21. (Excerpta
Medica International Congress Series No. 363).

Hill, C.R. (1972). Ultrasonic exposure thresholds for
changes in cells and tissues. J. Acoust. Soc. Am. 52:
667-672.

Hill, C.R. & ter Haar, G. (1981). Ultrasound. In: Suess,
M.J., ed. Nonionising radiation protection, Copenhagen,
World Health Organisation Regional Office for Europe
(WHO Regional Publications, European Series No. 10).

Joshi, G.P., Hill, C.R., & Forrester, J.A. (1973). Mode of
action of ultrasound on the surface change of mammalian
cells in vitro. Ultrasound Med. Biol., 1: 45-48.

Kaufman, G.E. & Miller, M.W. (1978). Growth retardation in
Chinese hamster V-79 cells exposed to 1MHz ultrasound.
Ultrasound Med. Biol., 4: 139-144.

Kaufman, G.E., Miller, M.W., Griffiths, T.D., Ciaravino,
V., & Carstensen, E.L. (1977). Lysis and viability of
cultured mammalian cells exposed to 1MHz ultrasound.
Ultrasound Med. Biol., 3: 21-25.

Kaufman, J.S. & Kremkau, F.W. (1978). Influence of
ultrasound on mouse leukaemia cell DNA synthesis,
membrane integrity, and uptake of anticancer drugs in
vitro. In: White, D. and Lyons, E.A. ed. Ultrasound in
medicine, New York, Plenum Press, Vol 4, 589-590.

Latt, S.A. & Schreck, R.R. (1980). Sister chromatid
exchange analysis. Am. J. Hum. Genet., 32 (3):
297-313.

Li, G.C., Hahn, G.M., & Tolmach, L.J. (1977). Cellular inactivation by ultrasound. Nature (Lond), 267: 163-165.

Liebeskind, D., Bases, R., Elequin, F., Neubort, S., Leifer, R., Goldberg, R., & Koenigsber, M. (1979a). Diagnostic ultrasound: effects on the DNA and growth patterns of animal cells. Radiology, 131: 177-184.

Liebeskind, D., Bases, R., Koenigsberg, M., Koss, L., & Raventos, C. (1981a). Morphological changes in the surface characteristics of cultured cells after exposure to diagnostic ultrasound. Radiology, 138: 419-423.

Liebeskind, D., Padawer, J., Wolley, R., & Bases, R. (1981b). Diagnostic ultrasound: Time-lapse and transmission electron microscopic studies of cells insonated in vitro. Presented at the L.H. Gray Conference in Oxford, England, July 13-16. New York, Albert Einstein College of Medicine.

Lota, M.J. & Darling, R.C. (1955). Changes in permeability of red blood cell membrane in a homogeneous ultrasonic field. Arch. phys. Med. Rehabil., 36: 282-287.

Maeda, K. & Murao, F. (1977). Studies on the influence of ultrasound irradiation on the growth of cultured cell in vitro. In: White, D. & Brown, R.E., ed. Ultrasound in medicine, New York, Plenum Press, Vol 3B, pp. 2045-2049.

Maeda, K. & Tsuzaki, T. (1981). The effect of pulsed ultrasound on cultured mammalian cells in vitro. Jpn. J. Med. Ultrason. 8: 276-278.

Martins, B.I. (1971). A study of the effects of ultrasonic waves on reproductive integrity of mammalian cells cultures in vitro: PhD Thesis, University of California (AEC Contract No. W-7405-ang-48 Publ. LBL-37).

Miller, M.W., Ciaravino, V., & Kaufman, G.E. (1977). Colony size and giant cell formation from mammalian cells exposed to 1MHz ultrasound radiation. Radiat. Res., 71: 628-634.

Morton, K.I., ter Haar, G.R., Stratford, I.J. et al. (1983). Subharmonic emission as an indicator of ultrasonically induced biological damage. Ultrasound Med. Biol. 9(6): 629-633.

Mummery, C.L. (1978). Effect of ultrasound on fibroblasts in vitro. PhD Thesis, University of London.

NCRP (1983). Biological effects of ultrasound: Mechanisms and clinical implications. National Council on Radiation Protection and Measurements, Report 74, NCRP, 1710 Woodmont Ave. Bethesda, Maryland 20814.

Repacholi, M.H. (1970). Electrophoretic mobility of tumour cells exposed to ultrasound and ionizing radiation. Nature (Lond), 277: 166-167.

Repacholi, M.H. (1980). The effect of ultrasound on human lymphocytes: a search for dominant mechanisms of ultrasound action. PhD Thesis, University of Ottawa.

Repacholi, M.H. (1981). Ultrasound: Characteristics and biological action, National Research Council of Canada, Ottawa, pp. 284, (Pub. NRCC 19244).

Repacholi, M.H., & Kaplan, J.C. (1980). DNA repair synthesis observed in human lymphocytes exposed in vitro to therapeutic ultrasound. In: Proceedings of the American Institute of Ultrasound in Medicine Convention, New Orleans, Sept. 15-19, p.42.

Repacholi, M.H., Woodcock, J.P., Newman, D.L., & Taylor, K.J.W. (1971). Interaction of low intensity ultrasound and ionising radiation with the tumour cell surface. Phys. Med. Biol., 16: 221-226.

Repacholi, M.H., Kaplan, J.G., & Little, J. (1979). The effect of therapeutic ultrasound on the DNA of human lymphocytes. In: Kaplan, J.G., ed. The molecular basis of immune cell function, Amsterdam, Elsevier/North Holland Biomedical Press, 443-446.

Ross, P. & Edmonds, P.D. (1983). Ultrasound induced protein synthesis as a result of membrane damage. Supp. to J. Ultrasound in Medicine 2(10): 47.

Rozeboro, J.A. (1977). Ultrastructure of HeLa cells and thoracic duct lymphocytes: pre and post ultrasonic irradiation. In: White, D. and Lyons, E.A. eds: Ultrasound in Medicine 3B, Plenum Press, New York, p 2036.

Sarvazyan, A.P., Belousov, L.V. Petroipavlovskaya, M.N., & Ostroumova, T.V. (1980). The interaction of low intensity ultrasound with developing embryos. In: Ultrasound Interaction in Biology and Medicine, International Symposium, Nov. 10-14. Castle-Reinhardsbrunn GDR, p. C-18.

Samosudova, N.Y. & El'Piner, I.Y. (1966). Ultrastructure of myofibrils exposed to ultrasonic waves. Biofizyka 11(4): 713-715.

Schnitzler, R.M. (1972). Ultrasonic effects on mitosis - a review. In: Reid, J.W. & Sikov, M.R., ed. Interaction of ultrasound and biological tissues, Washington, DC, US DHEW, pp. 69-72 (US Dept HEW Pub. (FDA) 73-8008).

Shiraishi, Y. & Sandberg, A.A. (1980). Sister chromatid exchange in human chromosomes, including observations in neoplasia. Canc. Genet. Cytogenet., 1: 363-380.

Siegel, E., Goddard, J., James, A.E. & Siegel, M.S. (1979). Cellular attachment as a sensitive indicator of the effects of diagnostic ultrasound on cultured human cells. _Radiology_, _133_: 175-179.

Stephens, R.H., Torbit, C.A., Groth, D.G., Taenzer, J.C., & Edmonds, P.D. (1978). Mitochondrial changes resulting from ultrasound irradiation. In: White, D. & Lyons, E.A. ed. _Ultrasound in medicine_, New York, Plenum Press, Vol. 4, pp. 591-594.

Stetka, D.G. & Wolff, S. (1977). Sister chromatid exchanges as an assay for genetic damage induced by mutagen-carcinogens. I. _In vivo_ test for compounds requiring metabolic activation. _Mutation Res._, _41_: 333-342.

Stewart, H.F. & Stratmeyer, M.E. (1982). An overview of ultrasound: Theory measurement medical applications and biological effects. U.S. Dept. Health, Education and Welfare. FDA 82-8190, Washington, D.C. pp 134.

Taylor, K.J.W. & Newman, D.L. (1972). Electrophoretic mobility of Ehrlich cell suspensions exposed to ultrasound of varying parameters. _Phys. Med. Biol._, _17_: 270-276.

Vivino, A.A., Boraker, D.K., Miller, D. and Nyborg, W. (1985). Stable cavitation at low ultrasonic intensities induces cell death and inhibits ^{3}H-TdR incorporation by Con-A stimulated murine lymphocytes in vitro. Ultrasound Med. Biol. 11(5): 751-759.

Watmough, D.J., Dendy, P.P., Eastwood, L.M., Gregory, D.W., Gordon, F.C.A., & Wheatley, D.N. (1977). The biophysical effects of therapeutic ultrasound on HeLa cells. _Ultrasound Med. Biol._, _3_: 205-219.

Webster, D.F., Pond, J.B., Dyson, M., & Harvey, W. (1978). The role of cavitation on the _in vitro_ stimulation of protein synthesis in human fibroblasts by ultrasound. _Ultrasound Med. Biol._, _4_: 343-351.

Williams, A.R. (1982). Absence of meaningful thresholds for bioeffect studies on cell suspensions _in vitro_. _Br. J. Cancer_, _45_ (Supp. 5): 192-195.

EFFECTS ON SOFT TISSUES WITH SPECIAL REFERENCE TO THE CENTRAL NERVOUS SYSTEM

A. R. Williams

Dept. of Medical Biophysics
University of Manchester Medical School
Oxford Road, Manchester M13 9PT

INTRODUCTION

One of the earliest proposed applications of ultrasound in medicine was to produce trackless lesions at specific sites within the brain for the treatment of certain types of discrete and localised cerebral tumours. While this application was superseeded by cryosurgical techniques before it had been accepted as a routine clinical procedure, it still resulted in the generation of a large body of reliable experimental data on the effects of high intensity ultrasound first on the mammalian brain and later on other soft tissues.

The histological detection systems used as the end points for the above studies are relatively insensitive in that they usually rely on large scale protein denaturation or the autolytic changes which occur following the death of the cells to provide the contrast betwen normal and damaged tissue. Functional endpoints are more sensitive and can demonstrate interactions of nervous tissue with ultrasound fields at much lower intensities than are observed using histological endpoints. It would be expected that stimulating endpoints (where the sensory structures at the afferent nerve endings are stimulated directly by the ultrasound field) or developmental endpoints (i.e. where embryonic or rapidly proliferating nervous tissue is being irradiated) would be even more sensitive and should yield the lowest "threshold" values for an ultrasound bioeffect. However, the experimental complexities and the random variability inherent in any measuring system increase as the sensitivity of that system to an external stimulus is increased. Thus, while a developmental endpoint may intuitively be expected to reveal an interaction with ultrasound at the lowest possible power levels, in practice it is very difficult to ascribe a high level of confidence to any single study.

Heating within Focal Lesions in vivo

As has been described earlier, the rate at which heat is deposited within a tissue is a function of the product of the acoustic intensity at that site and the absorption coefficient of the tissue. The temperature rise caused by this heat will depend upon the shape and volume of the heated region, its density and specific heat and the rate at which the heat is being removed by conduction and convention via the blood which is perfusing the heated volume. For tissue such as the cornea or the lens of the eye which have virtually no blood flow and a moderately high absorption coefficient, it is found that thermal lesions can be produced at relatively low acoustic intensities. However, as the vascularity of the tissue increases, and especially if the rate of blood perfusion through the tissue is increased in response to a small local increase in temperature (i.e. the hyperaemic reflex) then greater acoustic intensities are required to produce a thermal lesion even though the absorption coefficient of that tissue may be higher than that of a tissue which is poorly vascularised (e.g. the white matter of the brain).

Johnston and Dunn (1976) observed that the "threshold" condition for the production of focal lesions appeared to be essentially independent of the applied frequency. At first sight this is surprising because the absorption coefficient of all tissues increases with increasing frequency and so we would expect more heat to be deposited at the same intensity at the higher ultrasonic frequencies. This is indeed the case, but it is offset by the fact that for any given geometry the dimensions of the focal volume decrease as the frequency is increased so that the rate of heat loss by conduction is increased. These two factors tend to balance each other maintaining a relatively constant lesion volume which is independent of frequency (Lerner et al., 1973).

(a)   Histological Endpoints

There is remarkable agreement between the data obtained by different groups of workers on the relationship between the peak acoustic intensity at the focus of a bowl or lens and the duration of a single pulse of ultrasound necessary to produce a "threshold" lesion in mammalian brain in vivo (Fry et al., 1970; Robinson and Lele, 1972). This data essentially falls on a single line characterised by $It^{\frac{1}{2}} = 200 \; Ws^{\frac{1}{2}}/cm^2$ where I is the spatial peak temporal average acoustic intensity within the focal volume. For short duration pulses (which have the highest intensity) the histological appearance of the lesion is characterised by "holes" in the sections and disrupted cells characteristic of cavitational activity. Conversely, the longer duration pulses at lower intensity (less than about 700 W/cm^2) produce lesions which are indistinguishable from thermal lesions produced by non-acoustic means. At intermediate pulse lengths both mechanisms may co-exist and it has even been proposed that other unconfirmed mechanisms may occur.

Histological studies at the level of the light microscope have shown that the white matter of the brain exhibits a lower "threshold" than grey matter, possibly reflecting its reduced vascular perfusion. At the level of the electron microscope Borrelli et al. (1981) have shown that changes in the terminal synapses are amongst the earliest signs of morphological damage to nervous tissue.

The moderately high attenuation coefficient of nervous tissue means that it is one of the most susceptible of the soft tissues to the damaging effects of ultrasonic irradiation. For example, Herrick (1953) and Anderson et al. (1951) report that they were able to destroy the sciatic nerves of experimental animals using high therapeutic intensities of ultrasound without affecting the histological structure of the surrounding muscular tissue. The spinal cord is particularly at risk because of the intimate association between the spinal nerves and the sympathetic nerve ganglia and the highly absorbing bony vertebral column. Consequently, the exposure conditions commonly used to irradiate the foeti of pregnant mice (e.g. 80-200 sec exposure of 2 MHz continuous wave ultrasound using a broad beam transducer at an average intensity of 1 W/cm^2)·frequently results in maternal hind limb paralysis which is associated with grossly distended urine-filled bladders and impacted masses of _faecal material within the flaccid intestines indicative of inactivation of the autonomic system (Stolzenberg et al, 1980).

(b) Functional Endpoints

Less attention has been paid to the functional effects of low-intensity ultrasound on the nervous system. Stuhlfauth (1952) demonstrated that the temperature within the sciatic nerve of a rabbit irradiated with MHz ultrasound was higher than that of the surrounding tissues. Studies on the peripheral nerves of frogs and cats have shown that focused ultrasound can reversibly block axonal conduction with the small fibres being more susceptible than the large fibres (Young and Henneman, 1961). Interruption of nervous conduction has also been reported by Herrick (1953) and Tippe (1979). Takagi et al. (1960) reported that reflex discharges were stimulated and that spontaneous discharges appeared on the ventral root of the spinal cord at an intensity of 3.2 W/cm^2. Doubling the intensity resulted in additional spontaneous discharges but a decrease in reflex discharges. Madsen and Gersten (1961) and Esmat (1975) also report ultrasound-induced changes in the conduction velocities of peripheral nerves whereas other laboratories (including my own) have been unable to demonstrate any changes at therapeutic intensities and frequencies (unpublished observations).

Hu and Ulrich (1976) applied pulsed 2.25 to 5 MHz ultrasound (SATA intensity 3 mW/cm^2; SATP intensity 1.5 W/cm^2) to the brains of anaesthetized squirrel monkeys and were able to detect the presence of additional electronic discharges (evoked potentials). These signals appeared immediately after the ultrasound was switched on and disappeared after 2 or 3 min even though the ultrasound remained on. The authors attempted to eliminate sources of artifact resulting from direct electrical pickup, but all electroencephalographic measurements are so extremely sensitive to electrical interference that artifactual effects have not been ruled out. These observations should be repeated in an independent laboratory.

Tsutsumi et al. (1964) reported that the levels of the enzymes glutamate oxaloacetate transaminase (GOT) and glutamate pyruvate transaminase (GPT) in the serum and cerebrospinal fluid of dogs were increased after the animals had been exposed to 2 MHz ultrasound (average intensity 1.5mW/cm^2, pulsed 4 μs on and 15 ms off, peak intensity 5.8 W/cm^2) for 6-10 hours. The animal's brain was irradiated through the intact skull and so the intensity of the incident ultrasonic beam was attenuated by reflection at the tissue-bone interfaces and by absorption within the bone itself. Their results show that despite a marked variation from animal to animal, there appeared to be a statistically significant increase in the levels of these enzymes which reached a peak about 6 hours after irradiation before returning to normal. It is difficult to extract details of the experimental arrangement from this article, but the dogs were apparently anaesthetized and then immobilized in gypsum so that they could be awake but restrained during the long exposure period. In view of the psychological trauma associated with immobilizing active animals such as dogs for long periods (over 9 hours for 7 of them) it is not surprising that there were changes in the level of these (and presumably many other) enzymes and that these levels returned to normal a few days after the animals had been released from the gypsum. The authors did not include adequate control series (i.e. animals which had been immobilized for similar periods under the same conditions but not exposed to ultrasound) and so the results obtained by Tsutsumi et al. (1964) should be viewed with some scepticism. If this work should be repeated, it would be more humane, and the results more interpretable, if the animals were to be kept anaesthetized throughout the sonication period. A better alternative would be to attach a less cumbersome version of the transducer to a more docile animal which could be conscious and unrestrained during the exposure period.   Ideally informed human volunteers could be used even though it would not be advisable to sample the cerebrospinal fluid in this case.

(c)   Sensory Endpoints

It is known that moderately high intensities of pulsed ultrasound can stimulate the frog cochlea to generate trains of impulses at the pulse repetition rate of the acoustic source (Gavrilov et al., 1975).   It has also been reported that about 10 mW/cm^2 of 6-150 kHz ultrasound provoked modifications of the bioelectric potentials recorded from in vitro frog neuromuscular preparations (Nagy and Mihalas, 1974).   It is therefore possible that some signals may have been generated at the diagnostic intensities used by Hu and Ulrich (1976) even though they were not deliberately irradiating the internal ear (a structure which is designed for the conversion of acoustic waves into nervous impulses).   Providing that the acoustic intensities employed are not high enough to damage the sensory or neural tissues, the reversible elicitation of trains of impulses should not constitute a potential hazard to the wellbeing of adult animals.

In 1975 David et al. reported the novel observation that pregnant women were able to detect an increased number of foetal movements during the period that their foeti were being subjected to ultrasound from either of two common doppler foetal heart monitors.   Each patient was studied for 30 min with the ultrasonic transducer taped to her abdomen, but it was only energized (without the patient's knowledge) for the second half of the observation period.   A mean increase of 90% in the number of foetal movements was recorded.   Attempts to duplicate these observations in other laboratories using a more stringent experimental protocol have yielded one positive (Sheldon, 1978) and three negative results (Docker and Petoussi, 1982; Hertz et al. 1979; Powell-Phillips and Towell, 1979).   If this effect is real then it may reflect a direct stimulation of the foetal CNS by the ultrasound. One possible mechanism which could result in a direct nervous stimulation by pulsed ultrasound would be if each pulse of the ultrasound caused a small displacement of a sensory structure within the cochlea or else slightly warmed the sensory cells.   Either of these perturbations could result in trains of nervous impulses at the pulse repitition frequency which could be interpreted by the brain as audible sound.

(d)   Developmental Endpoints

Murai et al. (1975a) exposed the shaved abdomen of pregnant rats to the acoustic field emitted by a commercial doppler device (2.3 MHz, SATA intensity 20 mW/cm^2) for 5 hours.   Seven types of reflex neuromotor response were evaluated in the subsequent offspring during the first 21 days after birth; these were the righting reflex, cliff-top aversion, negative geotaxis, grasp reflex, vibrissa placing response and acceleration righting reflex.   Only the grasp reflex showed a statistically significant (though not large) difference between the irradiated and the sham-irradiated animals.   A complication of these experiments is that the pregnant animals had to be immobilized for the duration of the 5 hour treatment and there were even more significant differences between the offspring of the restrained but mock-irradiated animals and those of the unrestrained controls.   Another criticism of these investigations is that they were not performed double-blind. This is important because many of the reflexes measured involved an element of subjective assessment and were thus open to unconscious bias in the case of an ambiguous response.

In a subsequent paper, Murai et al. (1975b) reported on the results of four "emotional reactions" in the three groups of animals who had been irradiated in utero as described above (i.e. their mothers had either been restrained and irradiated, restrained but not irradiated, or unrestrained and unirradiated). The animals were evaluated at 120 days of age and the parameters evaluated were ambulation in an open field, defecation and urination responses in an open field, vocalization response in reaction to being handled by humans and their escape response from electric shock. The vocalization as a result of handling and response to electric shock both showed significant differences between the irradiated and mock-irradiated groups, even though these results are subject to the same criticisms as those of their first article. Two tests for cognitive (learning) response made at the age of 150 days showed negative results.

Brown et al. (1981) have performed an extensive series of well-devised studies to measure the effects of low levels of continuous wave ultrasound on reflex development and the acquisition of conditioned reflexes in the offspring of ICR mice which had been irradiated in utero. The pregnant animals were shaved and immersed in a water bath and exposed to 1 MHz c.w. ultrasound for 3 min at intensities of 0, 50 or 500 mW/cm^2. Their offspring were evaluated for the number of days required to develop a conditioned food cup response to a compound stimulus (light plus a 2800 Hz tone) as well as the time taken to attain five developmental reflexes (pivoting, walking, forelimb grip, accelerated righting, and the ability to stay on a rotating rod). Neither of the two groups of offspring exposed to ultrasound differed significantly from their mock-exposed controls for any of the measured parameters.

The positive bioeffect observations reported by Murai et al. (1975a,b) give cause for concern but, even if proved to be reproducible, do not necessarily indicate that diagnostic intensities of ultrasound are hazardous. The experimental problems inherent in restraining conscious animals throughout long irradiation periods cause many psychological and physiological changes which may mask or accentuate any effects caused by ultrasound (Brodie and Hanson, 1960). For example, it is well known that psychological stress during pregnancy produces detectable effects upon the behavioural development of the offspring (Thompson, 1957).

REFERENCES

Anderson, T. P., Wakin, K. G., Herrick, J. F., Bennett, W. A. and Krusen, F. H., 1951, An experimental study of the effects of ultrasonic energy on the lower part of the spinal cord and peripheral nerves, Arch. Phys. Med., 32:71.

Borrelli, M. J., Bailey, K. I. and Dunn, F., 1981, Early ultrasonic effects upon mammalian CNS structures (chemical synapses), J. Acoust. Soc. Amer., 69: 1514.

Brodie, D. A., and Hanson, H.M., 1960, A study of the factors involved in the production of gastric ulcers by the restraint technique, Gastroenterology, 38: 353.

Brown, N. T., Galloway, W. D. and Henton, W. W., 1981, Reflex development following in utero exposure to ultrasound, Proc. Aug. AIUM Meeting, San Francisco, 1301: 119.

David, H., Weaver, J. B. and Pearson, J. F., 1975, Doppler ultrasound and fetal activity, Brit. Med. J., 2: 62.

Docker, M. F. and Petoussi, N., 1982, Does pulsed ultrasound stimulate the foetus?, Ultrasound Med. Biol., 8:45.

Esmat, N., 1975, Investigations of the effects of different doses of ultrasonic waves on the human nerve conduction velocity. J. Egypt. Med. Assoc., 58:395.

Fry, F. J., Kossoff, G., Eggleton, R. C. and Dunn, F., 1970, Threshold ultrasonic dosages for structural changes in the mammalian brain, J. Acoust. Soc. Amer., 48: 1413.

Gavrilov, L. R., Tsirulnikov, E. M. and Shchekanov, E. E., 1975, Responses of the auditory centers of the frog midbrain to the labyrinth stimulation by focussed ultrasound, Fiziol. Zh. SSSR, 61: 213.

Herrick, J. F., 1953, Temperatures produced in tissues by ultrasound: experimental study using various techniques, J. Acoust. Soc. Amer., 25: 12.

Hertz, R. H., Timor-Tritsch, I., Dierker, L. J., Chik, L. and Rosen, M. C., 1979, Continuous ultrasound and fetal movement, Amer. J. Obstet. Gynecol., 135: 152.

Hu, J. H. and Ulrich, W. D., 1976, Effects of low-intensity ultrasound on the central nervous system of primates, Aviat. Space and Environ. Med. June: 640.

Johnston, R. L. and Dunn, F., 1976, Ultrasonic absorbed dose, dose rate and produced lesion volume, Ultrasonics, July: 153.

Lerner, R. M., Carstensen, E. L. and Dunn, F., 1973, Frequency dependence of thresholds for ultrasonic production of thermal lesions in tissue, J. Acoust. Soc. Amer., 54: 504.

Madsen, P. W., and Gersten, J. W., 1961, The effects of ultrasound on conduction velocity of peripheral nerves, Arch. Phys. Med. Rehab., 42: 645.

Murai, N., Hoshi, K. and Nakamura, T., 1975a, Effects of diagnostic ultrasound irradiated during fetal stage on development of orienting behaviour and reflex ontogeny in rats, Tohoku J. Exp. Med., 116: 17

Murai, N., Hoshi, K., Kang, C-H. and Suzuki, M., 1975b, Effects of diagnostic ultrasound irradiated during fetal stage on emotional and cognitive behaviour in rats. Tohoku J. Exp. Med., 117: 223.

Nagy, I. I. and Mihalas, G. I., 1974, Bioelectric potential modification under low intensity ultrasonic field, Proc. 8th Intern. Congr. Acoustics, Lond., 363.

Powell-Phillips, W. D. and Towell, M. E., 1977, Doppler ultrasound and subjective assessment of fetal activity, Brit. Med. J., 2: 101.

Robinson, T. C. and Lele, P. P., 1972, An analysis of lesion development in the brain and in plastics by high-intensity focused ultrasound at low-megahertz frequencies, J. Acoust. Soc. Amer., 51: 1333.

Stolzenberg, S. J., Edmonds, P. D., Torbit, C. A. and Sadmore, D. P., 1980, Toxic effects of ultrasound in mice: damage to central and autonomic nervous systems, Toxicol. Appl. Pharmacol., 53: 432.

Stuhlfauth, K., 1952, Neural effects of ultrasonic waves, Brit. J. Phys. Med., 15: 10.

Takagi, S. F., Higashino, S., Shihuya, A. and Osawa, N., 1960, The action of ultrasound on the myelinated nerve, the spinal cord and the brain, <u>Jap. J. Physiol.</u>, 10: 183.

Thompson, W. R., 1957, Influence of prenatal maternal anxiety on emotionality in young rats. <u>Science</u>, 125: 698.

Tippe, A. 1979, Sound field effects on the electrophysiological functions of myelinated nerves, <u>Proc. 4th Ultrasound Med. Biol. Symp.</u>, 1: 106.

Tsutsumi, Y., Sano, K., Kuwabara, T., Takakura, K., Hayakawa, I., Suzuki, T. and Katanuma, M., 1964, A new portable echo-encephalograph, using ultrasonic transducers; and its clinical applications, <u>Med. Electron. Biol. Eng.</u>, 2: 21.

Young, R. R. and Henneman, E., 1961, Reversible block of nerve conduction by ultrasound, <u>Arch. Neurol.</u>, 4: 83.

OCULAR EFFECTS

Vincenzina Mazzeo

University Eye Clinic
Ferrara, Italy

INTRODUCTION

The use of ultrasound in ophthalmology involves three fields: diagnosis, therapy and surgery. Diagnosis, wich includes biometry (i.e. the measurement of the thickness of eye components), is the most widely used. The first paper on diagnostic ultrasound was published by Mundt and Hughes in 1956. In little less than 30 years development has occurred to the extent that nowadays computerized techniques of ultrasound tissue characterization seem to have reached the point of performing "acoustic biopsy in vivo" (Coleman et al., 1983). This 30 year development has led to an increase in the number of devices manufactured, but their number is still relatively small in comparison with the technological advances which have characterized other fields of diagnostic ultrasound. Since the very beginning the problem of safety of diagnostic procedures has been of great concern in clinical field. However, after only a few studies this problem was put aside.

Surgical tools have been in everyday practice since 1973. The use of ultrasound to remove cataracts has become very popular even though complications were reported soon after its introduction.

THERAPEUTIC ULTRASOUND

The first paper describing an ultrasound effect on the eye was published by Zeiss in 1938. Early papers from Eastern European Countries were only available in their original languages, so their experimental conditions are described as quoted by others or in reviews. The description of the effects encountered will be subdivided following the anatomy of the eye: anterior segment, excluding the (namely cornea, aqueous, iris, and ciliary body), lens, vitreous body, retino-choroidal layer including retinal circulation and sclera.

Bioeffect experiments were performed with two major end-points:
1. to discover at what levels anatomical damage would occur to the target,
2. to find subtle physiological changes which would explain the beneficial effect of ultrasound delivered to the eye especially for those tissues which have repair capabilities.
It is obvious that ultrasound intensity levels used to produce histological damage to eye tissue are much higher than those producing submicroscopic and physiological effects. A thermal effect is generally considered to be the dominant mechanism of action of ultrasound energy. Most papers on biological effects refer to experimental situations which are vastly different from the clinical one, making it difficult to compare results. Rabbit eyes were used in the majority of in vivo experiments since they simulate those of humans quite well. Particular emphasis is given to clinical papers because in some countries ultrasound therapy is widely used. In general the benefits obtained are evaluated subjectively by the patients

a) Cornea, aqueous humor, iris and ciliar body

While Ricci and Buonsanto (1953) did not find any histological changes in rabbit eyes exposed to ultrasound ($6W/cm^2$ 1-3 MHz), in clinical trials they found that ultrasound seemed to be absorbed by blood and exudates from the anterior chamber. The dilatation of conjunctival and anterior uvea vessels seem to be the cause of this beneficial effect (Hápten and Palmer, 1954).

Extensive experimental research to determine safe exposure levels was made by Baum (1956). He demonstrated that no damage occurred in the anterior segment from a 5 minute single exposure to $0.25\,W/cm^2$ at 1 MHz of pulsed ultrasound (duty cycle from 1:5 to 1:20) for 3 minutes at $1\,W/cm$. Reversible and irreversible damage was found at $1.5 - 2\,W/cm^2$ and at $2.5 - 3\,W/cm^2$ respectively using the same exposure conditions. He stated that a linear relation existed between the acoustic power and the temperature and that all effects were due to temperature increase. All pathological changes occurred in the anterior part of the eye.

The group at Brno University showed that a 2 minute exposure of cw at 800 MHz with a SATA intensity greater than $0.5\,W/cm^2$ did not produce any temperature increase while pulsed diagnostic ultrasound lasting up to 8 minutes caused an increase in the temperature of the aqueous humour of 0.75°C (Preisová et al.,1965). Although no temperature increase was found using $1\,W/cm^2$ of pulsed ultrasound, they noticed some histopathological changes in the corneal epithelium and stroma, and hyperemia

of the iris and ciliary body vessels. Histological changes occurred more in the pulsed mode than in the continuous one
(Hrazdira et al., 1967).

Experimental and clinical studies conducted by Tsok (1963)
suggested that no histological changes occurred in ocular tissues with 0.5 W/cm^2 ultrasound at 1.625 MHz with 3 or 5 minutes
single or multiple exposure, while the same exposure produced
an increased resorption of blood and exudates in clinical trials.
A 10 minute exposure produced corneal oedema and congestion of
iris and ciliary body vessels in rabbits. When the ultrasound
intensity was increased from 1 to 4 W/cm^2 and exposure times from
3 to 10 minutes, dystrophic changes were found in the cornea
(cellular proliferation, stromal oedema). Also haemorrage was
observed around overfilled iris vessels and the ciliary body
was swollen. Having determined levels of safe exposure the author
(Tsok, 1963) went on with patient treatment. He produced clinical papers on inflammation reduction in the anterior segment
and augmented clearing of corneal opacities in conjunction with
a drug introduced into the cornea by electrophoresis(Tsok, 1967).
Intensity levels used were 0.2 - 0.3 W/cm^2.

The Daisonic NSY-02 ultrasound therapeutic equipment for
myopia treatment appeared on the market in 1964. It had an acoustic output of 100 mW/cm and a working frequency of 1.4 MHz.
Clinical results reported by Lacaillon-Thibon in 1967 on anterior segment inflammation are very confusing and contracditory.
It seems that this treatment had an effect or some diseases and
not on others, the evaluation of the results being left to clinical judgement of the user only.

Russian researchers investigated subtle effects such as
cytochemical (Marmur and Pleviskis, 1973) and biochemical changes while studying major effects on the lens at higher intensities (Narbut, 1974). Marmur and Pleviskis (1973) studied the
concentration of RNA and aminogroups in the cytoplasm of basal
layer cells of corneal epithelium of the rabbit (0.5, 1, 2 hours
and 10 days) after exposure to 0.2 - 1 W/cm^2. Cytochemical changes were found to be related to the intensity of ultrasound. A
temporary increase in the concentration of aminogroups lasted
for longer times at higher exposures. Since they did not find
any change in the DNA of the epithelial cells they concluded
that no mutagenic effect is to be expected. An increase in albumin and hexosamine content in the aqueous humor of rabbit was
found at the threshold intensity to produce cataract e.g. 400 W
/cm^2 after 10 minute exposure (Narbut, 1974). An increased permeability of the cornea and an alteration of the epithelial
layer were found at low levels 0.2 - 0.4 W/cm^2 at 880 kHz cw or
pulsed ultrasound (pulse duration 10 ns) (Aristarkova and Nuritdov, 1974). The former phenomenon was utilized to introduce
drugs into the eye and was named "phonophoresis", while the
latter developed earlier using pulsed ultrasound.

The last paper in this period dealing with a physiological endpoint was published by Greguss (1975) who studied the pupillary response at $0.1 - 1 \, W/cm^2$ at 0.8 and 2.4 MHz. No further study on the cornea was published till 1982 when Mark and Bennerman (1982) produced evidence of intraparenchimal lesions in rabbit using a special transducer at very high ultrasonic intensities. These very small lesions due to hyperthermia closely resemble those lesiones produced by hyperthermia in other tissues.

b) Lens

The lens is a structure which is very sensitive to many physical and chemical agents. It has no repair capability, being completely avascular and having only a single layer of cells before the posterior capsule. The opacification of part or all of the lens is called a cataract and is due to the precipitation of the proteins which form the submicroscopic structure of lens fibres. It is not known how ageing produces the alteration of these proteins but it is well known that many agents influence their chemical state. Physical agents known to produce cataracts of different types are heat, ionizing radiations and microwaves. For this reason the lens was the first part of the eye studied to see if it was sensitive to ultrasound.

In 1938 Zeiss produced a reversible cataract in bovine lens in vitro with $100 \, W/cm^2$ at 250 kHz cw exposure. The cataract became irreversible with increasing exposure times. He also produced a cataract using focused ultrasound at $10 \, W/cm^2$. Kawamoto reproduced these results in 1947.

Lavine and co. (1952) using pulsed ultrasound at 3.25 MHz found a partial irreversible cataract with a single exposure lasting 1 minute at an intensity of $150 \, W/cm^2$. When the exposure time was 5 minutes, a total, irreversible cataract was produced. No effect occurred when the ratio of pulse length to pulse interval was kept less than 1:1. This suggested a thermal mechanism in which a certain amount of time was needed to dissipate the heat delivered to the lens from each pulse.

Purnell (1967) and Sokollu (1969) reproduced the Lavine type cataract (i.e. a fulciform cataract occurring deep in the lens substance and along the axis of the beam). These cataracts are irreversible and non progressive. Using cw ultrasound at 3.5 MHz, an intensity of $25 \, W/cm^2$ is enough to produce a cataract in 40 seconds. With pulsed ultrasound exposure a series of thresholds curves were drawn. It was demonstrated that, with a constant pulse duration of 1.2 msec at $45 \, W/cm^2$, the number of pulsed necessary to produce the cataract increases from 0.5 to almost 2 seconds. At intensities up to $135 \, W/cm^2$ in steps of $15 \, W/cm^2$, the number of pulses remained constant at different levels. At $75 \, W/cm^2$ the number of pulses required to produce a cataract goes to infinity when the pulse interval is increased

from 2 to 5 sec. At higher intensities the number of pulses
remains constant even if the pulse interval is increased. The
term cataract producing unit (CPU) was used for describing effects on other ocular tissues. The value of the CPU was 135 W/
cm (cw and 0.5 sec exposure at 3.5 MHz). The safe level determined with pulsed ultrasound refers to the intensities to produce a cataract and depends on the pulse length and duty cycle.
In their experiment with a pulse length of 1.2 msec and a duty
cycle of around 19 %, not enough energy could be generated to
produce a cataract. A lower intensity level was found to produce
a cataract (Fukunaga and co, 1969). After a 1 minute exposure
at 30 W/cm^2 and 3 MHz, a reversible haze cataract was found in
rabbits eyes, while after 3 and 5 minutes exposure, small and
large snow-balls cataracts were found.

A clinical report of prophylaxis of secondary cataracts
appeared in 1968 by Sokolenko. He used a Soviet made therapeutic
device at 830 kHZ, pulsed mode with pulse length of 4 msec, 0.4
W/cm^2 and multiple exposure (10-12) of 5 minute each.

The use of ultrasound to produce a soft cataract suitable
for needle aspiration was tested by Coleman and colleagues (1972).
The lenses of rabbit eyes were exposed to focused ultrasound
for periods from 2 seconds to one minute at intensities of 100-
500 W/cm^2 and at a frequency of 4.2 MHz. The radiation was pulsed
at 10Hz and had a 50 % duty cycle. The histological results 60
days after the exposure showed very hard cataracts. The lenti-
cular substance underwent softening only in the peripheral sections of the induced cataracts where low intensity levels were
encountered.

A clear demonstration of thermally induced cataract was
produced by Coleman et al. (1978 a,b) with ultrasound at 9.8MHz,
focused at intensities from 200 to 2000 W/cm^2. The type of cataract produced went from "haze" to complete cataract with increasing exposure times. The type of cataract also varied with
acoustic intensity. In their recent review Coleman et al.(1985a)
reported: "The effects of thermal conduction were evident in
lesion geometry. For short high-intensity exposure thermal conduction is not important because lesions form before significant
conduction occurs. When the beam is focused on the anterior lens
surface a small cataract can be formed where the beam is focused.
For lower intensities longer exposures are required to produce
minimal cataract and there is a sufficient time for significant
thermal condition both in the lateral and axial directions under
these conditions, minimal cataracts are broader and situated
deeper into the lens". The threshold curve of acoustic intensities versus exposure time is consistent with a thermal mechanism.
An exposure duration of 0.1 sec is enough to produce a minimal
cataract. Over the threshold limit the relationship of intensity
levels and exposure time is constant, under the threshold for
exposure shorter than 0.1 sec higher intensity levels are neces-

sary but not in linear fashion (Coleman et al., 1985b). Lizzi et al. (1985) conclude that the production of minimal cataracts can be used in sealing anterior traumatic ruptures and it is also useful to understand treatment of avascular tumours.

c) Vitreous body

The vitreous body has been widely studied alone or in conjunction with other parts of the eye such as the lens. The vitreous structure is quite peculiar and degeneration or as a consequence of vitreous inflammation or haemorrhage. Since vitreous opacities from degeneration do not clear spontaneously, while inflammatory or haemorragic opacities do or clear with use of drugs, it is very difficult to evaluate the clinical papers on ultrasound therapy of this disorder. Only a few experimental works have been carried out on rabbits with sham exposed animals and controls.

Kleifeld (1953) found contradictory results in a clinical trial on vitreous haemorrage clearing. His subjects were exposed to a single exposure of pulsed ultrasound lasting 30 minutes with a duty cycle of 50 % (pulse duration 1/6 second) to an intensity of 6-8 W/cm^2. Moore and coll. (1955) found an increased temperature in the vitreous body when exposing rabbit eyes to 10 W/cm^2. Donn (1955) studied the effect of 900 W/cm^2 on the vitreous body in vitro and in vivo. He found no effect till air bubbles were added to the vitreous body. In another clinical paper Hudelo and coll. (1957) found decreased vitreous opacities in subjects exposed to cw ultrasound at 960 kHz at 5-6 W/cm^2 for multiple sessions (10 to 12) of 5 minute each. Similar results were found by Marek (1958) and by Astrakhovic (1973), but at lower intensities (less than 1 W/cm^2). Gilbert Baum (1956, 1957) found only a slight increase in vitreous haemorrage resorption in rabbit eyes at 1 MHz and intensity levels considered safe for the anterior segment i.e. 0.25 W/cm^2 for 5 minutes (duty cycle 50 %, prf 20 Hz) and 1 W/cm for 3 minutes. A reduction in viscosity of fluids separated from the vitreous after in vitro exposures was found by Balint and co. (1962). They thought this was due to depolymerization.

An increased resorption of experimental haemophthalmos in rabbits was described by Tsok (1963). This increase was produced only when the insonification of the vitreous was made through the scleral route instead of the anterior segment. The ultrasound exposure parameters were: 0.5 W/cm^2, 1.625 MHz, 3-5 minutes.

Daisonic ultrasound therapy equipment was used by Lecaillon-Thibon (1967) to clear vitreous opacities of patients with haemophthalmos. Clinical results did not show a clearly favourable influence on outcome. The acoustic intensity delivered was not considered strong enough to produce an effect on vitreous haematomes.

Coleman and co. (1969) studied the effect of ultrasound on dye dispersion in the vitreous _in vitro_. The dye dispersion in the vitreous contained in a glass cuvette was obtained at 100 W/cm^2 of cw ultrasound at 1.27 MHz and exposure times varying from 2 up to 20 minutes. Under the same conditions with pulsed ultrasound (prf from 10Hz to 1 kHZ) _in vivo_, the dye bubble was clearly seen to move in the vitreous of living rabbits. Each movement corresponded to a single pulse at prf below 20 Hz. The pulsed system appeared to aid diffusion and lessen danger to surrounding tissues provided that the focal core of the ultrasonic beam was correctly positioned on the eye.

Narbut (1974) demonstrated in rabbit eyes that if an intensity level strong enough to produce cataract (400 W/cm^2) was maintained for 10 minutes several changes occurred in the vitreous body, namely, an increase in vitreous viscosity and increase in protein content (albumines and hexosamines).

A very extensive study was made by Coleman and coll.(1978a) to test the utility of ultrasound therapy in the resorption rates of experimentally produced membranes in rabbit eyes. In this study cw exposures were compared with the pulsed ones at different prf (1kHz and 10Hz); delivering different ultrasound intensities for a total exposure time of 5 sec (single exposure of 1 second each were delivered at 5 different points 1mm apart of each membrane). Sham exposed animals and control animals were also considered. Pulsed ultrasound with SATA intensities from 410 to 562 W/cm^2 at a prf of 10 Hz decreased the resorption time by 58 %. No effect was found using the same pulse conditions under 167 W/cm^2. Since histological examination of treated membranes in those animals sacrificed before resorption showed no structural abnormalities in their structure and since the membranes showed higher displacement at each pulse at 10 Hz prf, a mechanical action was supposed. Unfortunately in treating membranes near the ocular walls many cases of chorio-retinal lesions were produced even if the ultrasound beam was focused on the membrane. For these reasons this kind of treatment is no longer considered valid. In fact, the authors concluded that the risk to benefit ratio was too low to introduce it into clinical practice.

d) Retino-choroidal layer (including retinal circulation) and optic nerve

No anatomical or functional effects of ultrasound have been reported using the exposure conditions: 0.5 to 10 W/cm^2 and 2.5 minutes up to a total exposure time of 72 minutes (Moore et al., 1955; Hudelo et al., 1957; Ricci and Buonsanto, 1953; Tsok, 1963). Donn (1955) had previously reported that while performing his experiments on vitreous liquefaction in rabbit eyes, he found a displacement of the nuclear layer of the retina. This phenomenon was not found by Baum (1956).

The first evidence of an ultrasound effect on the posterior part of the eye was given by Purnell et al (1964).Chorio-retinal adhesions were produced both through the anterior segment and the conjunctival route to seal retinal tears. The focal point had to be placed on the retina. The ultrasound effects varied from a transitory oedema to perforation of the globe. The dimensions of the submicroscopic lesion did not excedd 1.4 mm and the major focal lesion, 2 mm. When starting cw exposure at a relatively low energy level, blanching of the choroidal circulation occurs at the focal point. Histological examination of different specimens suggests that in some cases the retina was still intact even if herniated or pulled out through the hole produced in the choroid and sclera. This phenomenon suggests different sensitivities in the different layers.

Trier (1967), using a Daisonic unit, attempted to repeat the experiments of Yamamoto et al (1963): to verify whether the treatment produced an increase in arterial blood pressure in retinal arteries and a change in vessels diameter. No difference was found in either parameters among patients exposed to ultrasound and to sham sonication.

Amelioraration of subjective symptoms and evolution were described in tapeto-retinal degenerations by Tanev and Todorov (1971), Lutker and Nurieva (1973), Sigaeva et al (1973) at cw exposure at 880 kHz. Acoustic intensities were between 0.2-0.3 W/cm^2. Multiple exposures of 5 minutes each (from 10 up to 12) were used. To produce experimental evidence of the way ultrasound therapy was acting on the retina, Marmur and co-workers (1973a,b) and Marmur and Saldan (1973) studied the histological changes produced by ultrasound on the photoreceptors and on the retinal vessels. 82 rabbits were subjected to ultrasound therapy at 880 kHz and intensities of 0.2 and 1 W/cm^2. An exposure time of 5 minutes was kept constant. The authors stated: "E.M. and histochemical studies revealed high ultrasonic sensitivity of photoreceptors and a stimulating influence of therapeutically admissible intensities of ultrasound on mitochondrial activity and synthetic processes". A harmful action of increased doses of ultrasound was found on photoreceptors. A vasodilating effect was demonstrated at the same intensities by photographing the retinal vessels of rabbit eyes and then calculating the difference in their caliper. The amelioration of optic nerve atrophies at 0.2-0.4 W/cm^2 for a total exposure time of 60-72 minutes (12-14 single exposures of 5 minute each) was thought to be the consequence of this phenomenon (Marmur et al., 1973a,b).

No damage in retinal structure of cats was found by Barnett and Kossoff (1977) with their system aiming at reproducing the exposure condition of their diagnostic equipment. After 30 minutes of irradiation of pulsed ultrasound focused on the retina (frequency 7.5 MHz and prf 16 kHz) no histological changes were found at 100 W/cm^2 (SPPA).

An intensity versus time threshold damage curve was published by Lizzi et al. (1977). It clearly shows the same shape for both ultrasound and light damage, suggesting a similar thermal mechanism. A retino-choroidal lesion was produced at an exposure time of 0.1 sec and intensity level of 2000 W/cm² of cw ultrasound at 9.8 MHz. With a single exposure lasting 20 sec the intensity necessary to produce the same lesion decreased to less than 200 W/cm². The histological examination of the eyes treated showed that the retina, choroid, sclera all had some damage at different rates with the different exposure levels. They concluded that: "The clinical implications of the histopathological findings indicate that therapeutically controlled, mild suprathresholds are feasible because the ocular tunics remain intact in such lesions without significant and lasting ultrasonic destruction of the choroid and sclera. Furthermore, the retinal tissue does not melt during the treatments, but survives in healed lesions in an inverse relationship to the energy level used".

Further studies were made to find out if pulsed regimens were more active in producing chorio retinal lesions suitable for treating retinal ruptures (Lizzi et al., 1984a). The intensity levels necessary to produce minimal irreversible effects were 60, 75-100 and 120-140 W/cm² for a single exposure of 10 seconds of ultrasound at 9.7 MHz, pulse duration of 0.1 sec, duty factor 50 % and PRF from 2 to 8 Hz. Short pulses (e.g. 400 μsec) delivered at high repetition frequency (e.g. 3 kHz) produced the same average intensity threshold values as those found for cw conditions. The increased effect with low prf values was explained with the reduction of blood flow which occurs at each pulse and lasts virtually the whole duration of the pulse thus increasing the thermal effect. Purnell et al. (1964) suggested "The most likely mechanism responsible for choroidal blanching is related to radiation force". A very precise theoretical model of lesions produced by hyperthermia has been found to predict lesion dimensions taking in account also the possible cooling effect of blood circulation (Lizzi et al. 1984b).

Blanching of detached choroids was observed by Tanev et al. (1984) on the fifth day of treating choroidal detachments by therapeutic ultrasound (800 kHz, daily sessions of 5 minutes each and acoustic intensity of 0.2-0.3 W/cm²).

e) Sclera and Intra ocular pressure (IOP)

Very few studies have been performed on glaucoma patients. Experiments on rabbit eyes (Purnell, 1967), while showing a significant drop of pressure of 5 % in treated animals were not able to determine the anatomical reason for this. in fact 30 % of animal eyes with pressure reduction showed no microscopic evidence of ciliary body injuries or break down of the blood-aqueous barrier. No attempt at treatment was made on patients since the dosage needed to obtain a pressure reduction was very painful.

A clinical trial was conducted by Astrakhovic (1973) who found that after therapeutic ultrasound delivered in multiple sessions (15-20), a decrease in the tonographic indices in patients with high grade complicated myopia occurred.

While studying chorio-retinal lesions it was found that a scleral thinning could be obtained, leaving intact a thin layer of retina (Coleman et al., 1978). The scleral thinning was produced by coagulating and weakening the collagen of the sclera in order to enhance aqueous outflow. The decrease of IOP can also be achieved by disrupting the ciliary epithelium in order to reduce aqueous production as in cyclodiathermy. A special transducer was constructed which included a central light surrounded by a diagnostic transducer, and in turn was surrounded by the therapeutic one whose basic frequence was 1.46 MHz (Lizzi et al., 1984). The focal zone dimensions can be varied by selecting an appropriate operating frequency. The intensity of sound at the focal zone has been calculated using a thermal model. No side effects were to be expected outside the focal zone. Average intensities as high as 2000 W/cm^2 were employed at a frequency of 4.6 MHz (SPTA intensity at -3 dB beam width). Histological changes in rabbit eyes three months after insonification showed a marked but highly localized thinning of the sclera. Over this thinning, where tha aqueous humour goes out of the bulbus, a "conjunctival bleb" was formed. These experiments were reproduced in pigs whose sclera better resemble the thickness of the human sclera. The first results on patients followed (Coleman et al., 1985a,b) and further encouraging results were presented by Lizzi et al. (1985).

SAFETY OF DIAGNOSTIC ULTRASOUND

The safety of diagnostic ultrasound has always been of great concern to all users. Arvo Oksala (1967), a pioneer in diagnostic ultrasonography, reported: "Right at the beginning of ultrasonic diagnosis Mundt and Hughes, Oksala and Lehtinen, as well as Baum and Greenwood among others came to the conclusion in their estimations that the intensity in diagnostic ultrasound equipment is so low that it cannot do any harm to the eye. Another factor which reduces danger is the pulsive form of ultrasound, in which case the duration of impulses is a fraction of the whole examination time. As early as in 1956, when examining the effect of pulsive ultrasound on the eye, Baum estimated that both at an intensity of 0.25 W/cm^2/5 min and 1 W/cm^2/3 min would be safe and harmless. Oksala and Lentinen figured out that the intensity of their equipment was about 2-3 mW/cm^2 and the duration of the examination a few minutes. In 1960 Baum and Greenwood announced that the average intensity of their equipment was approximately 0.07 W/cm^2. Jansson wrote that the maximum intensity of the Krautkramer equipment he used was 1-1.5 W/cm^2 and the average one 0.1-0.15 mW/cm^2. Stalkamp and Nover examined more than 100 patients with Krautkamer equipment with an intensity of about

5 mW/cm^2 without any harm at all. According to Freeman the maximum intensity of the usual ultrasonic equipment is approximately 3-5 W/cm^2, the average being much less. In 1965 Nover and Glanschneider wrote that the average sound intensity in diagnosis is about 5-50 mW/cm^2. Gersterner has studied this question of safety and mentions that for a normal examination, the proportion of the on-time of the off-time is approximately 1:1000. The intensity of the equipment cannot be measured directly, as it is very low, but it can be estimated e.g. from voltage and capacitance in the crystal. Gerstner calculated that an examination would raise the temperature only about 0.0008°C. All studies of ultrasound published so far have shown that the method is quite harmless to the eye". This last sentence can be repeated today. The equipment mentioned in Prof. Oksala lecture is no longer in use, being substituted by more sophisticated machines, especially in the field of contact B-scan.

The safety of diagnostic ophthalmology was evaluated by Ziskin and colleagues (1974). They found no effects after a four hour sonification at diagnostic intensities. Further, no effects were found by Barnett and Kossoff (1977). The characteristics of their diagnostic equipment are summarized below: Transducer, 3 cm diameter, frequency 7.5 MHz, energy per pulse 0.1 µJoules; peak pulse intensity at focus 90 W/cm^2; 20 dB beam width at focus, 1.2 mm ; PRF 1.1 kHz; duration of irradiation per pulse, 38 µsec.; total number of pulses, 42; time average power, 110 µW; total exposure energy for single pulse, 7 µJoules. They were very accurate in describing these characteristics and very few diagnostic devices have been described so carefully.

Problems related to acoustic output measurement are beyond the purpose of this paper and are discussed in other parts of this text. The difficulties of measuring acoustic intensities in the mW and µW range are well known. Recently a series of very precise miniature hydrophones were manufactured and used for measuring the acoustic output of equipment in common use. Unfortunately their response is very good only for frequencies generally lower than those used in ophthalmology (up to 20 MHz). More highly focused transducers are used for biometry and pachimetry but the necessity for resolving thin layers such as the cornea (0.5 mm thickness) involves shorter pulse lengths so that the actual ultrasound exposure time remains very low.

SURGICAL DEVICES

Ultrasonic devices to remove cataracts were introduced by Kelman in 1967. The device breaks up the cataract into small pieces and washes them out through the same instrument. The instrument consists of a titanium tip vibrating at an ultrasonic frequency of about 40 kHz. Vibrations are mostly longitudinal but in some instruments transverse oscillations occur. Fluid is introduced into the instrument both for cooling and washing out the cataractuous pieces through the needle itself. Sucking out lens particles and fluid occurs through a silicon sleeve surrounding the tip. Vibrations are obtained by connecting the vibrating tip to a magneto strictive transducer.

Trier (1985) published a very extensive review paper to which I'll refer. The first clinical results published by Kelman (1969) were not very favourable. However, complications were lower after surgeons become more familiar with this technique. Early results were disappointing enough to promote a number of studies to understand why these complications occurred. Because most of the damage was to the cornea (i.e. corneal endothelium), experimental and clinical studies were undertaken to decide whether or not these effects were a consequence of the direct action of ultrasound.

Several factors might be involved in damaging corneal endothelium during this kind of intervention. They are:
a) air bubble presence in the anterior chamber – the importance of this factor was suggested by Leibovitz and Lang (1974), but rejected by Olson and coll. (1978a,b).
b) irrigation and aspiration of fluids – the use of saline balanced solution in the irrigation and aspiration does not produce alterations (Polak, 1978; McCarey et al. 1976).
c) temperature increase – this was the principal cause of the early disastrous results and is still present at any failure of the irrigation system. Appropriate quantities of irrigation fluids are necessary for cooling (Benolken et al., 1974).
d) the mechanical effect on the lens nucleus – this factor exists in all type of extracapsular cataract surgery. The mechanical damage due to the small pieces of lens cannot be demonstrated or denied because it only exixts together with the ultrasonic field and cannot be created by different methods.
e) effects of the ultrasonic field, especially cavitation and microstreaming – the damage to the corneal endothelium created by the ultrasonic field has been demonstrated by several authors (Olson et al., 1978a,b; Panzica and Amasio, 1979; Talbot et al., 1981). Cavitation, if it occurs, does not extend far from the tip, approximately 1 mm (Kuwahara, 1972).

REFERENCES

Aristarkhova,A.A. and Nuritdov, V.A., 1974, The effect of ultrasound on the corneal permeability. Vest. Oftal., 3:46.
Astrakhovic, Z.A., 1973, Action of ultrasonic therapy on the changes in tonographic indices in patients with high grade complicated myopia. Oftalmol. ZH, 28: 410.
Bálint, A., Együd, K., and Sallai, A., 1962, Alterations in the viscosity of the vitreous humor of eyes exposed to ultrasound and sound complex containing ultrasonic impulses. Ophthalmologica (Basel), 140: 645.

Barnett, S.B., and Kossoff, G., 1977: Negative effects of long duration pulsed ultrasound on the retina of cats. In "Ultrasound in Med.", 3/B, White D. ed. Plenum Press, N.Y.,N.Y,2025.

Baum, G., 1956: The effect of ultrasonic radiation upon the eye and ocular adnexa. Am. J. Ophthalmol. 42: 696.

Baum, G., 1957: The effect of ultrasonic radiation upon the rate of absorption of blood from vitreous. Am. J. Ophthalmol. 44: 150.

Benolken, R.M., Emery, J.M. and Landis, D.J., 1974: Temperature profiles in the anterior chamber during phacoemulsification. Inv. Ophthalmol. 13: 71.

Coleman, D.J., Konig, W.F., Lizzi, F.L., Weininger, R.B., and Burt, W.J., 1969: Vitreous liquefaction by ultrasound. In "Ultrasonics in Ophthalmology" K.A. Gitter, A.H.Keeney, L. K. Sarin, D. Meyer edts. C.V. Mosby St. Louis, 337.

Coleman, D.J., Lizzi, F.L., 1983: Computerized ultrasonic tissue characterization of ocular tumors. Am. J. Ophthal. 96: 488.

Coleman, D.J., Lizzi, F.L., Burt, W., and Wen, H., 1972: Properties observed in cataracts produced experimentally with ultrasound. Am. J. Ophthalmol. 71: 1284.

Coleman, D.J., Lizzi, F.L., Driller, J., Rosado, A.L., Burgess, S.E.P., Torpey, J.H., Smith, M.E., Chang, S., and Rondeau, M.J., 1985b: Therapeutic Ultrasound in the treatment of glaucoma. II Clinical Applications. Ophthalmology, 92: 347.

Coleman, D.J., Lizzi, F.L., Driller, J., Rosado, A.L., Chang, S., Iwamoto, T., Rosenthal, D., 1985a: Therapeutic ultrasound in the treatment of glaucoma: I - Experimental Model. Ophthalmology, 92: 339.

Coleman, D.J., Lizzi, F.L., El-Mofty, A.A.M., Driller, J., and Franzen, L.A., 1978a: Ultrasonic accelerated resorption of vitreous membranes. Am. J. Ophthalmol., 89: 490.

Coleman, D.J., Lizzi, F.L., and Jakobiec, F.A., 1978b: Therapeutic ultrasound in the production of ocular lesions. Am. J. Ophthalmol. 86: 185.

Donn, A., 1955: Ultrasonic wawe liquefaction of the vitreous humour in living rabbits. Arch. Ophthal. 53: 223.

Fukunaga, K., Watanaba, T., Karimoto, S., and Yamamoto, T.,1968: Ultrasonic cataract preliminary report. Folia Ophthalmol. Jap. 20: 915.

Haptén, K., and Palmer, E., 1954: The effect of ultrasonic vibration on the living rabbit eye. Acta Ophthalmol., 32: 227.

Hrazdira, I., Preisová, J., and Anton, M., 1967: The temperature in the interior of the eye after ultrasound application. Albrecht v. Graefes Erch. Ophthal. 171: 300.

Hudelo, A., Hamery, A., and Perlmutter, B., 1957: Les ultrasons en ophtalmologie. Ann. Oculist. 190: 684.

Kawamoto, I., 1947: Experimental studies on the effects of ultrasonic waves on the eyeball. Nippon Gankwa Gakukway Zasshi 51: 12.

Kleinfeld, O., 1953: Beobachtungen bei der Beandlung des menschlishen Auges mitt ultraschall. Klin. Mbl. Augenheik. 123:743.

Kuwahara, Y. 1972: Aspiration method of a hard cataract. Ultrasonic vibration. Igaku Shoin, Tokyo.

Lavine, O., Langerstran, K.H., Bawyth, C.M., Fox, F.E., Griffin, V., and Thaler, H., 1952: Effects of ultrasonic waves on the refractive media of the eye. Arch. Ophthal. 47: 204.

Lecaillon-Thibon, B., 1967: Resultat du vibreur de Yamamoto ("Daisonic") en therapeutique ophthalmologie. In "Ultrasonic in ophthalmology, A. Oksala and H. Gernet edts. Karger, Basel-New York, 37.

Leibowitz, H.M., and Lang, R.A., 1974: Corneal endothelium: the effect of air in the anterior chamber. Arch. Ophthal. 92:227.

Lizzi, F.L., Coleman, D.J., Driller, J., Yablonski, M., Greenall, P., Smith, M., and Rosado, A. 1985: Therapeutic ultrasound in clinical treatment of medically refractive glaucoma. In: "WFUMB 85", R. Gill and M.J. Dadd edts. Pergamon Press, Sydney, 432.

Lizzi, F.L., Coleman, D.J., Driller, J., Ostromogilsky, M., Chang, S., and Greenal, P., 1984a: Ultrasonic hyperthermia for ophthalmic therapy. IEEE Transactions on sonic and ultrasonics, SU 31: 473.

Lizzi, F.L., Driller, J., Ostromogilsky, M., and Coleman, D.J.? 1984b: Thermal model for ultrasonic treatment of glaucoma. Ultrasound Med. Biol. 10: 289.

Lizzi, F.L., Franzen, L.A., Driller, J., and Coleman, D.J., 1977: Ultrasonically induced lesions in the retina, choroid and sclera. In "Ultrasound in Med." 3A, White, D. edt., Plenum Press, N.Y., N.Y., 1081.

Lutker, L.S., and Nurieva, S.M. 1973: Microwave and ultrasonic therapy of tapetoretinal degeneration of the retina. Vest. Oftalmol. 5: 69.

Marek, P., 1958: Ultrasound treatment in ophthalmology. Szememetz, 95: 104.

Mark, D.B., and Benermann, R., 1982: Intracorneal lesions produced with focused ultrasound. Curr. Eye Res., 2: 323.

Marmur, R.K., Dumbrova, N.E., and Plevnskis, V.P., 1973b: Submicroscopic and cytochemical change in photoreceptors of the retina induced by ultrasound. Oftalmol. Zh., 28: 589.

Marmur, R.K., and Plevinskis, V.P., 1973a: Effects of ultrasound on nucleic acids and aminogroups of corneal proteins. Oftalmol. Zh., 28: 383.

Marmur, R.K., and Saldan, I.R., 1973a: Study of effect of ultrasonic energy on the retinal circulation. Oftalmol. Zh., 28: 47.

Marmur, R.K., Shpak, N.I., and Elashkn, N.I., 1973b: Effectivity of ultrasonic therapy in patients with partial atrophy of the optic nerve depending on etiology and duration of the process. Oftalmol. Zh., 28: 403.

McCarey, B.E., Polack, F.M., and Marshall, W., 1976: The phacoemulsification procedure: I: The effect of irrigating solutions on the corneal endothelium. Inv. Ophthalmol., 15: 449.

Moore, C.H., Herrick, J.F., and Martens, T.G., 1955: Some effects of ultrasonic energy on the rabbit eye. Arch. Ophthal., 54:922.

Mundt, G.H., and Hughes, W.E., 1956: Ultrasonics in ocular diagnosis. Am. J. Ophthal., 42: 488.

Narbut, N.P., 1974: Experimental simulation of cataract by means of focused ultrasound. Vest. Oftal., 2: 47.

Narbut, N.P., Vasilieva, U.S., and Gavrilov, L.R., 1974: Change in content of albumins and hexosaming in the aqueous and vitreous after irradiation with focused ultrasound. Oftalmol. Zh., 29: 277.

Olson, L.E., Marshall, J., Rice, N.S.C., and Andrews, R., 1978a: Effect of ultrasound on the corneal endothelium: I-The acute lesion. Br. J. Ophthalmol., 62: 134.

Olson, L.E., Marshall, J., Rice, N.S.C., and Andrews, R., 1978b: Effect of ultrasound on the corneal endothelium: II-The endothelial repair process. Br. J. Ophthalmol., 62: 145.

Panzica, G.C., and Amasio, E., 1969: Note ultrastrutturali sugli effetti determinati della facoemulsificazione sull'endotelio corneale del coniglio. Boll. Oculist., 58: 315.

Polack, F.M., 1978: Damage to endothelium in phacoemulsification. In "Highlights of Ophthalmology" B.F. Boyd, edt., 15: 130.

Preisova, J., Hrazdira, I., and Dolemek, A., 1965: The influence of ultrasound on the surface temperature of the eye. Ser.Med. (Fac. Med. Brun.) 38, 215 as quoted in WHO, 1982.

Purnell, E.W., Sokollu, A., and Holasek, E., 1964: The production of focal chorioretinitis by ultrasound. Am. J. Ophthal., 58: 953.

Purnell, E.W., 1967: Therapeutic use of ultrasound. In: "Ophthalmic ultrasonography", R.E. Goldberg and L.K. Sarin edts. Saunders, Philadelphia, 145.

Ricci, A., and Buonsanto, M., 1953: Tentativi di ultrasonoterapia in oculistica (ricerche sperimentali e cliniche). Boll. Oculist., 32: 107.

Schwab, F., 1954: Impulschallversuche am Auge. (I. Impulsversuche am der Linse). V. Graefes Arch. Ophthal., 115: 97.

Sigaeva, O.L., Kazakova, M.A., and Mozherenkov, V.P., 1973: Ultrasonic therapy in certain eye diseases. Vest. Ophthalmol., 4: 76.

Sokolenko, O.M., 1968: Ultrasound in the prophylaxis of secondary cataract. Vest. Oftal., 4: 48.

Sokollu, A., 1969: Ultrasonic therapeutics. In: "Ophthalmic Ultrasound, K.A. Gitter, A.H., Keeney, Sarin, D.Meyer edts. CV Mosby, St. Louis, 321.

Talbot, J.F., Marshall, J., Sherraid, E., Kohner, E.M., and McLeod, D., 1981: Experimental phacoemulsification: effects on the corneal endothelium. In "The cornea in health and disease", P.D. Trevor Roper ed. Royal Soc. of Medicine and Academic Press, London, 805.

Tanev, V., Goleminova, E., and Starov, N., 1984: Ultrasonic treatment of choroidal detachment. SIDUO X. Abstract book, 42.

Tanev, V., and Todorov, N., 1971: Personal experience with ultrasound therapy in some eye diseases. Ophthalmologia (Sofia), 19: 27.

Trier, H.G., 1967: Erste Erfahrungen mit einen japanischen sogenamiten Ultraschall. Behandlungsgerat (Daisonic NSY-62). In "Ultrasonic in ophthalmology", A. Oksala and H. Gernet edts. S. Karger, 45.

Trier, H.G., 1985: Ultrasonics devices for surgery (cataract removal and vitrectomy) in ophthalmology. J.E.M.U., 6: 17.

Tsok, R.M., 1963: The effects of ultrasound on the normal tissues of the eyes and on the course of experimental haemophthalmos. Vest. Oftalm., 4: 65.

Tsok, R.M., 1967: Simultaneous ultrasound and electrophoresis treatment of long-standing corneal opacifications. Vest. Oftal., 6: 70.

W.H.O., 1982: Ultrasound. Environmental Health Criteria, 22, World Health Organisation, Geneve.

Yamamoto, Y., Kitukawa, H., Kato, M., and Hilkawa, T., 1963: Studies on penetration into aqueous humor of colymicin and the effect of ultrasonic waves. J. Clin. Ophthal., 17: 875.

Zatulina, N.I., and Aristarkhowa, A.A., 1974: Ultrasound produced cytological changes in the corneal epithelium. Vest. Oftalmol., 4: 47, as quoted in WHO, 1982.

Zeiss, E., 1938: Ueber Linsenueranderung und herausgenommen Rindherhinsen durk Ultraschalleinwirkung. Arch. Ophthal., 139: 301.

Ziskin, M., Romayandanda, N., and Harris, K., 1974: Ophthalmologic effect of ultrasound at diagnostic intensities. J. Clin. Ultrasound, 2: 119.

HAEMATOLOGICAL EFFECTS

A.R. Williams

Dept. of Medical Biophysics
University of Manchester Medical School
Oxford Road, Manchester, England

INTRODUCTION

The role of blood perfusion in the maintenance of tissue viability
is so vital that it is not possible to administer any diagnostic or
therapeutic ultrasound exposure without also irradiating blood and the
vessels which contain it. If ultrasound produces a relatively small
change in the functional properties of the blood (e.g. an effect on
leucocytes and their role in the immunological protection of the animal)
or in the ability of blood to flow through small vessels (i.e. any
tendency to induce the blood to clot), it can exert a disproportionately
large effect on the well-being of that animal.

Most of the experimental investigations of the bioeffects of
ultrasound on blood performed to date have concentrated on one of four
major topics. These are (a) The mechanical lysis of red blood cells in
vitro, (b) Effects on platelets and their role in the coagulation of
blood, (c) Functional effects on leucocytes, and (d) Vascular effects.
Each of these topics will be reviewed separately after a brief discussion
of some of the mechanisms by which the energy of the ultrasonic wave can
be transformed into forces which can damge blood cells or otherwise
change their behaviour. This is particularly important in the case of
ultrasound interacting with blood because the choice of the experimental
system or the limitations imposed by the measuring technique frequently
change the order of dominance of the various reaction mechanisms so that
a bioeffect which is readily demonstrable with a dilute suspension of
blood cells in the laboratory may not necessarily occur in vivo under
realistic exposure conditions.

INTERACTION MECHANISMS

The dominant mechanisms whereby ultrasound is able to irreversibly
change cellular structure or function are presumed to be either thermal
(where the temperature rise has to be high enough to denature some
proteins) or cavitational (where cells may be mechanically disrupted
without experiencing a significant rise in temperature). Blood cells
suspended in a relatively non-absorbing medium like plasma are less
likely to be affected by temperature rise than cells in compact or
"solid" tissues because the absorbed heat can flow out of the small

171

cells and into the cooler suspending medium (Love and Kremkau, 1980). This effect is accentuated if the cells are suspended in saline media in vitro. However this cooling effect cannot happen if the cells are packed tightly together (i.e. at very high haematocrits); in this case thermal effects may once again dominate as they appear to do in many soft tissue interactions. Bearing in mind the fact that blood is constantly in motion and so the residence time of any given volume element of blood in the ultrasound beam is short, it is unlikely that the blood cells will experience a damaging temperature rise except perhaps when they are traversing the microvasculature of a heated tissue.

Cavitational activity, on the other hand, involves the pulsation of gas and vapour filled bubbles and is dependent upon the acoustic pressure amplitude of the incident ultrasonic field, the number, size and availability of the gas bubbles or micronuclei from which they can grow, the geometry of the acoustic exposure situation as well as many other factors including the composition and partial pressures of the various gasses within the irradiated medium, its temperature, ambient pressure, etc. In general, it is the availability of the micronuclei which determines whether or not cavitational activity is going to occur at a given therapeutic or perhaps even diagnostic intensity level. The elevated pressure produced inside a small gas bubble by the effects of surface tension result in the progressive shrinkage of that bubble which will cause it to dissolve completely unless it is protected by some form of surface coat or skin, or it is embedded within an irregularity on the surface of a solid body such as a dust particle (Crum, 1979). It is presumed that the rate of occurrence of these nuclei within the well-filtered densely packed cell interior is less than that in the more fluid extracellular environment. Micronuclei are easy generated within liquid samples in vitro by mechanical handling, contact with solid surfaces (especially if scratched or hydrophobic), by being stirred (Williams, 1982) or exposed to ionizing radiation (Messino et al., 1963).

Thus, the exposure of blood cells to ultrasound in vitro can significantly change the exposure conditions for those cells, particularly if they have been resuspended in a saline medium at low haematocrit. Thermal effects will have been minimised even though the duration of the exposure of any given cell has been increased, whereas cavitational effects will have been maximised. This is especially true if some form of stirring or agitation system has been employed to maintain the cells as a homogenous suspension.

Other less obvious changes in the exposure situation include the recent observation by Miller and Williams that cavitation in a medium of low haematocrit disrupts the adjacent cells whereas in a medium of high haematocrit the radiation pressure force attracts so many cells towards the oscillating bubble that it is damped and the cells are not disrupted. Great care must therefore be exercised in the extrapolation of a bioeffect observed using isolated blood cells in vitro to the prediction of a potential hazard in vivo.

(a) Lysis of red blood cells in vitro

Erythrocytes are readily obtained as a homogenous suspension of cells consisting almost entirely of a membrane enclosing a solution of haemoglobin. The ease of assay for free haemoglobin together with the established clinical use of osmotic fragility tests has resulted in several attempts to devise mechanical fragility tests using cavitating ultrasound as the destructive agent (Tarssanen, 1976; Akopyan and Abuladze, 1982). The basis of a mechanical fragility test should be that all the cells are subjected to the same constant force for an indefinite period and the rate at which the cells are disrupted by that force is measured — the weakest cells being the first to break. However, in the present case, cavitation events are occurring randomly within the cell suspension and disrupting the cells adjacent to that event. Thus, while the overall shape of the haemolysis/rate curve is the same as that of the osmotic fragility curve, it is entirely due to statistical chance whether or not any given erythrocyte will be disrupted at the beginning or near the end of the sonication period. These techniques are not therefore likely to yield much useful clinical information even though there is an apparent correlation between haemolysis rate and erythrocyte diameter.

Ultrasonic bioeffects due to cavitational activity would be expected to occur at the lowest intensities in media containing pre-formed gas bubbles of a size close to the resonant dimensions for that particular driving frequency. In early work at kilohertz frequencies this was accomplished by drilling holes having diameters of the order of millimetres in the polished face of a metal velocity transformer (Hughes and Nyborg, 1962). More recently stabilised gas bubbles having diameters of the order of microns (i.e resonant at megahertz frequencies) have been used, the bubbles being trapped in the pores of hydrophobic Nuclepore membranes (Miller et al., 1979). If the use of these stabilised gas bubbles is combined with a sensitive technique capable of detecting the rupture of a small number of cells (e.g. a photometric technique employing firefly Luciferin/Luciferase for the detection of free ATP) then ultrasound-induced haemolysis can be observed at spatial peak intensities as low as 20 to 30 mW/cm^2 at 1.6 MHz, c.w. (Williams and Miller, 1980).

It requires more acoustic energy to cause a micronucleus to grow into a bubble than is needed to drive that bubble into oscillation so that it can generate the streaming forces which modify or destroy biological tissues (Nyborg, 1978). Consequently, any factor which generates micronuclei and/or assists the ultrasonic field in the initial stages of bubble growth will greatly enhance the amount of cavitational activity generated by any given "supra threshold" ultrasonic intensity. Williams (1982) showed that the number of erythrocytes lysed by the same intensity of ultrasound (0.6 or 1.0 W/cm^2 SATA, c.w., 0.75 MHz) increased as the rotational speed of a magnetic stirring bar contained within the sample chamber was increased. A similar enhancement of ultrasound-induced cavitational activity was also observed if the stirring bar was removed and the entire sample chamber oscillated at 50 Hz or repeatedly struck by the corners of a rotating hexagonal metal bar. It is presumed that the enhancement of cavitational activity by stirring results from both the generation of micronuclei (i.e. hydrodynamic nucleation and possibly also jet-edge nucleation from the moving solid interface) and the enhancement of bubble growth within the pressure gradients developed by the stirrer. If a stirred erythrocyte suspension is irradiated with pulsed ultrasound (0.75 MHz, 2 ms on and 8 ms off for 5 min) then cell lysis attributable to cavitational activity can be obtained at SATA intensities as low as about 2 mW/cm^2 (A.R. Williams, unpublished observations).

(b) <u>Effects on platelets and their role in the coagulation of blood</u>

Platelets are blood-borne anucleate cell fragments which can be stimulated by a wide range of chemical and physical factors including collagen, adenosine diphosphate (ADP), electrical current, mechanical trauma and hydrodynamic shear stress. Their first response to a supra-threshold stimulus is to undergo a shape change (a disc to echinocyte transition) and become "sticky" so that they attach themselves to any available solid surface (adhesion) or to each other (aggregation). This shape change is usually followed by the "release reaction" which involves the active expulsion of the contents of the platelet's secretory granules and vacuoles. These contents can be roughly divided into three classes of chemicals, these are :- (1) vasoactive substances such as histamine and serotonin which result in a transient vasoconstriction; (2) platelet aggregating factors including ADP which cause more platelets to attach themselves to the growing platelet thrombus; and (3) coagulation factors (including platelet factor 3) which initiate and accelerate the plasma coagulation system resulting in the rapid conversion of fibrinogen to fibrin and the eventual formation of a true red blood clot (Thomas, 1977).

Numerous diverse techniques have been employed to investigate the effects of ultrasonic energy on platelets and their physiological role both in vitro and in vivo. For the sake of simplicity, this topic has been sub-divided into three broad sections, these are:- (1) The effects of acoustic microstreaming fields on platelets (i.e. the use of models simulating the small-scale streaming fields developed around oscillating gas bubbles). The object of these studies is to see if cavitation-induced forces could initiate blood coagulation in vitro and in vivo. (2) Effects of ultrasound on platelets and the blood coagulation system in vitro; and (3) The effects of ultrasound on blood in vivo.

(1) The effects of acoustic microstreaming fields on platelets

Small gas bubbles are difficult to work with in acoustics (unless they are stabilised within holes in solid bodies) because they tend to spontaneously dissolve and/or be driven out of the region of interest by radiation pressure forces. However, the acoustic microstreaming fields generated around the hemispherical tips of small metal wires or probes oscillating at ultrasonic frequencies while immersed in a liquid (Williams et al, 1970) are similar to those generated by gas bubbles oscillating in a stable manner (especially if the bubbles are in contact with a solid surface) (Rooney, 1970). These metal models of stable cavitational activity are less prone to artefact and more amenable to quantification than most gas bubble-induced acoustic microstreaming fields.

Nyborg (1975) developed an approximate linear theory which predicted that the magnitude of the hydrodynamic shear stresses generated within these acoustic microstreaming fields should increase as the square of the displacement amplitude of the oscillating body. Williams (1974) exposed functionally inert human platelets containing radioactively labelled serotonin to the acoustic microstreaming field generated around a 250 μm diameter steel or tungsten wire oscillating in a transverse mode at 20 kHz and observed that (as predicted) the amount of serotonin released increased in a linear manner when plotted against the square of the wire displacement amplitude. These platelets were unable to undergo their release reaction because they had been anticoagulated with EDTA, and so the serotonin could only have been liberated by mechanical disruption of the platelets. These experiments therefore strongly indicate that it is the acoustic microstreaming field generated around wires or gas bubbles which disrupts platelets and that the mechanical fragility of platelets is about one tenth that of erythrocytes.

If a small blood vessel is exposed in an anaesthetised animal, these metal wires or probes can be pressed against the outside of the vessel wall so as to make an indentation similar to that made by pushing a finger into an air or water-filled balloon. The mechanical coupling between the wire and the vessel wall is so efficient that the indented portion of the vessel wall can be driven to oscillate at the same ultrasonic frequency and at the same displacement amplitude as the metal wire (Williams, 1977). When transilluminated and viewed under the microscope it can be seen that the oscillating portion of the vessel wall generates an acoustic microstreaming field within the intact blood vessel and that a variety of displacement amplitude dependent biological effects can be observed. These effects are qualitatively similar whether the wire is oscillating in a transverse mode at 20 kHz or in a longitudinal mode at 85 kHz but the absolute values of displacement amplitude are different because of the different boundary layer thicknesses at the two frequencies as well as the frequency dependence of the shear stress generated at any given displacement amplitude (Nyborg, 1965).

At the lowest displacement amplitudes used, the flowing blood could be seen to be deflected from its normal streamlines and to form twin vortices at the point of contact with the wire tip. No damage to the blood cells or the endothelium could be detected although slightly higher displacement amplitudes resulted in the adhesion of platelets having partially disrupted membranes to the apparently normal endothelium (Williams, 1981). At higher displacement amplitudes the twin vortices grow to fill the lumen of the small vesels and gelatinous aggregates of platelets are observed to form in the centre of the vortices and to embolise downstream where they adhere to the vessel wall if they touch it. At even higher displacement amplitudes the platelet thrombus emerges as a continuous stream from the microstreaming vortices and solidifies downstream (due to the formation of fibrin) where it may occlude the blood vessel.

Thus, platelets are easily disrupted and/or stimulated to participate in the formation of thrombus both in vitro and in vivo by acoustic microstreaming fields. These observations suggest that similar fields generated around oscillating gas bubbles (if they were to occur in blood during ultrasound exposure in vivo) could pose a potential thrombogenic hazard.

(2) Effects of ultrasound on platelets and the blood coagulation system
     in vitro

Platelets in anticoagulated whole blood or in platelet rich plasma (PRP, i.e. anti-coagulated blood where the erythrocytes and most of the leucocytes have been removed by centrifugation) are usually exposed to ultrasound in vitro under free field exposure conditions. Williams et al. (1976a) demonstrated that 5 min exposures of citrated PRP to one M Hz ultrasound resulted in a time dependent decrease in the recalcification time (i.e. the time taken to form macroscopic strands of fibrin following the addition of enough calcium ions to overcome the effects of the anticoagulant). This increased tendency of the blood to clot was associated with numerous morphological changes in the structure of the clot as seen by electron microscopy. Sonicated PRP gave larger, less rigid clots containing multivacuolated cells and numerous platelet fragments which were not present in control samples. These changes in recalcification time and clot morphology could be duplicated by incubating control PRP with small quantities of homogenised PRP prior to recalcification (Williams et al., 1976b).

The large number of small platelets in a sample of PRP efficiently scatter a beam of visible light. However, if the platelets are induced to aggregate to form a smaller number of larger particles, then the transmissivity of the light beam through the sample is greatly increased.

Thus, time-dependent changes in the optical density of a PRP suspension are a sensitive measure of the rate and extent of platelet aggregation (this is the basis of optical aggregometry). Activated platelets must collide with each other before they can aggregate and so the samples must be stirred throughout the aggregation process. Chater and Williams (1977) devised an ultrasound exposure apparatus whereby the rate and extent of platelet aggregation could be measured while the samples were being exposure to MHz ultrasound under free field conditions.

It was found that ultrasound exposure alone could induce human platelets in citrated PRP to aggregate. At any given ultrasonic frequency there was an apparent "threshold" intensity below which the sample did not aggregate (this was typically about $0.6 - 0.8$ W/cm^2 SATA for c.w. 0.75 MHz ultrasound). At any given supra-threshold intensity, the extent of aggregation decreased as the ultrasonic frequency was increased. For any one human donor the amount of aggregation produced by a given supra-threshold intensity was remarkably constant. However, PRP from different donors sometimes exhibited wide variations in the rate and extent of aggregation induced by the same intensity of ultrasound. This variability was traced to the different inherent sensitivities of the different platelets to physiologically-induced aggregation. Those samples which required low concentrations of ADP to induce aggregation required a lower "threshold" intensity of ultrasound whereas those samples requiring high concentrations of ADP before aggregating had higher "threshold" intensity values (Chater and Williams, 1977).

These ultrasound induced aggregation measurements together with the recalcification time data outlined above strongly suggested that ultrasound was exerting its effects by disrupting a small proportion of the platelet population (possibly via a cavitational mechanism) and it is the materials released from the disrupted platelets which was responsible for the observed changes. This hypothesis is supported by the observation that PRP samples irradiated with "sub-threshold" intensities of ultrasound (i.e. intensities less than the value required to induce spontaneous aggregation) were refactory (i.e. less sensitive to low concentrations of an aggregating agent) when challenged with more ADP. This is analogous to the observation that two sub-threshold doses of ADP given about 10 min apart do not result in platelet aggregation even though the final ADP concentration is greater than the threshold value for a single administration of ADP.

Additional information supporting this hypothesis came from measurements of the rate of liberation of β-Thromboglobulin (β-TG) a platelet-specific protein of unknown function which is contained within the platelet α-granules and is liberated when they undergo the release reaction or are disrupted (Ludlam et al., 1975). The concentration of β-TG in blood plasma can be measured with an accuracy of about $\pm$ 3ng/ml by means of a specific radioimmunoassay and normal plasma values range from 20 to 40 ng/ml rising to more than 5,000 ng/ml in serum where all of the platelets have undergone the release reaction.

Williams et al. (1978) exposed anticoagulated whole blood from human donors to 0.75 mHz c.w. ultrasound in both the presence and absence of a mixture of EDTA and theophylline which effectively prevents platelets from undergoing their release reaction. At any supra-threshold intensity it was found that the presence of these release inhibitors decreased the amount of β-TG liberated by ultrasound to about 30% of the value obtained in their absence. The only plausible mechanism for liberating β-TG from these functionally inert platelets is by mechanically disrupting them as would occur if the damaging mechanism was some form of acoustically-induced cavitational activity. This argument in favour of cavitation is supported by the fact that high levels of β-TG release were always accompanied by a corresponding increase in the level of free plasma haemoglobin from disrupted erythrocytes.

All of the above results indicate that some form of cavitational activity is being generated at "suprathreshold" intensities of ultrasound which subsequently disrupts a small proportion of the platelet population (and also some of the erythrocyte population if they are also present). When enough cells have been disrupted, the materials liberated from these cells (especially ADP) will induce other undamaged functional platelets to undergo their normal release reaction (liberating β -TG and more ADP) and to aggregate, thus initiating a self-perpetuating cycle which continues as long as there are normal platelets present.

As in the case of erythrocytes, the ultrasonic intensity needed to initiate platelet aggregation is greatly reduced if the irradiated medium is stirred or agitated or supplied with pre-formed gas bubbles of resonant size stabilised within the pores of Nuclepore membranes. Miller et al. (1978) showed that human platelets in citrated PRP formed aggregates in the vicinity of the gas-filled pores at spatial peak intensities of only 16 to 32 mW/cm^2 (c.w., 2.1 MHz). These platelets could also be induced to aggregate by the ultrasonic field emitted by a common doppler diagnostic instrument used for the detection of the foetal heart. Some of these platelets have been disrupted or induced to undergo the release reaction because the inclusion of the Luciferase/Luciferin enzyme system for the detection of free ATP results in the emission of light shortly after the ultrasound has been switched on (Miller et al., 1979).

(3) The effects of ultrasound on blood in vivo.

The investigations outlined above indicate that platelets are primarily damaged in vitro as a result of some form of cavitational activity and so it is reasonable to presume that similar effects would occur if cavitational activity were to be induced within the intact vascular system in vivo. This was confirmed by Chater and Williams (1982) who drove a 25 k Hz cell disintegrator (Rapidis 50, Ultrasonics Ltd) off resonance until it could be pressed against the wall of an exposed blood vessel in a rabbit without puncturing it, and yet could still produce transient cavitation in freshly-drawn blood. The plasma levels of histamine (a normal intracellular constituent of rabbit platelets) and free haemoglobin downstream of the sonication site were elevated while the transducer was activated indicating that cavitation was occuring within the following blood and disrupting both platelets and erythrocytes.

Preliminary in vivo investigations using megahertz frequencies of ultrasound were inconclusive in that Zarod and Williams (1977) found occasional small aggregates of platelets trapped within the mirocirculation of the external ear of a guinea pig after its main blood supply vessel (the central ear artery) had been subjected to 1 W/cm^2 of pulsed 0.75 MHz and c.w. 3MHz ultrasound. However, subsequent investigations demonstrated significant temperature elevations under these exposure conditions and so the platelet aggregates may have been initiated by tissue thromboplastins released from thermally damaged endothelium.

In a subsequent series of investigations, butterfly cannulae were inserted into the anticubital veins of healthy adult human volunteers and a 0.75 MHz transducer positioned about one inch upstream of the puncture site (Williams et al., 1981). Blood samples were collected before, during and after the transducer had been activated at the highest intensity that the volunteers would tolerate (typically 0.35 to 0.5 W/cm^2 SATA, c.w.) and anticoagulated with EDTA and theophylline which also rendered the platelets functionally inert. There was no detectable elevation in the plasma levels of β -TG in the samples collected while the ultrasound was being administered. In an attempt to subject blood in vivo to higher intensities of ultrasound we used the rabbit model described above. Rabbit platelets do not contain a β-TG like material that we could measure, but they are loaded with histamine which is liberated when they undergo the release reaction or are disrupted. Rabbit blood vessels were exposed to the highest intensities emitted by a commercially available therapeutic device (2.4 W/cm^2 SATA, 0.75 MHz, c.w.) but no increase in the level of plasma histamine or free haemoglobin could be detected. A water-filled thin metal cone was attached to the transducer housing resulting in a maximum SATA intensity of 17.4 W/cm^2, but this also resulted in no significant change in plasma histamine or free haemoglobin levels (Chater and Williams, 1981).

Contradictory results were reported by Wong and Watmough (1980) who found evidence of intravascular haemolysis after they irradiated the beating hearts of anaesthetised mice for 5 min with 0.7 to 2 W/cm^2 (SATA, c.w.) of 0.75 MHz ultrasound. One of the major differences between this exposure situation and the ones employed above are that here the blood is being violently agitated within the heart while it is being exposed to the ultrasound. It is possible that these turbulent rheological conditions could generate nucleation sites and/or assist the growth of nuclei to form bubbles so that cavitational activity could occur in vivo at ultrasonic intensities which are known to be ineffective in non-turbulent blood. This possibility is currently under investigation in several laboratories but preliminary results apparently indicate that intravascular cavitation does not occur at therapeutic intensities of ultrasound in rabbits or dogs even when the beating heart is irradiated (Gross et al., 1985).

Lunan et al,(1979) exposed anaesthetised mice to whole body ultrasonic irradiation for 5 min at 2 MHz at a spatial average intensity of 1 W/cm^2 in a 37°C water bath. They found that platelets from animals sonicated four hours previously aggregated less efficiently than those from control animals. It is not known if this reflects a direct effect of ultrasound on the platelets (i.e. a possible refractory phase following a "sub-threshold" stimulation) or a general systemic effect resulting from the release of substances such as prostaglandins into the animal's blood stream.

Somewhat more controversial results were reported by Sanada et al. (1977) who investigated changes in the morphology of human platelets obtained from patients whose hearts were being exposed to ultrasound from a commercially available diagnostic cardiac apparatus (2.25 MHz, SATA intensity 0.5 mW/cm^2). They found that the number of circulating platelets having pseudopodia (one of the earliest detectable changes in "stimulated" platelets) increased with time of exposure and tended to a plateau value after about 15 min. The number of platelets with pseudopodia gradually decreased with time after the ultrasound was switched off, and the authors claim (but do not provide any statistical evidence or even raw data) that the patients platelet count was found to have been "significantly" reduced. The magnitude of the effects reported here are surprisingly large, especially in view of the results of Lunan et al. (1979) who found no significant difference between the platelet numbers in the blood of control mice and those exposed to 1 W/cm^2 of 2 MHz ultrasound. One possible source of artefact which was not eliminated by Sanada et al (1977) was the progressive time - dependent activation of platelets by the needle of the indwelling catheter system which remained in position for the duration of each measurement series (40 or 60 min).

Equally controversial results were reported by Yaroniene (1978) who
subjected the hearts of rabbits for 2 weeks or 1 month to 2 MHz ultrasound
(either c.w. at 10_2mW/cm^2 or pulsed 4 μs on, PRF of 1k Hz and SATA
intensity 0.4 mW/cm^2) from a portable ultrasonic device which was
strapped to the animals body. Histological investigation showed changes
in the chest muscles, myocardium and liver: the reported changes included
capillary expansion, microthrombus formation and erythrocyte aggregation.

One potential health hazard involving the possible interaction
between ultrasound and platelets which has not yet been investigated in
detail concerns the role of ultrasonic contrast agents. Most of these
agents function by introducing large numbers of micron-sized gas bubbles
into the blood stream so as to efficiently scatter the interrogating
ultrasound beam and so generate strong echoes (Roelandt, 1982). However,
these bubbles are efficient scatterers because they are close to the
resonant dimensions for the ultrasound frequencies being employed. Thus,
the use of ultrasonic contrast agents simulates the in vitro experiments
using gas bubbles of resonant dimensions stabilised within the pores of
hydrophobic Nuclepore membranes. These in vitro gas bubbles can induce
platelet aggregation at diagnostic intensity levels and so it is not
unreasonable to presume that the gas bubbles introduced during contrast
echocardiography may be capable of producing similar effects. This topic
is currently under investigation.

Apart from a few unconfirmed and poorly described articles, it can be
concluded that diagnostic and low therapeutic intensities of ultrasound do
not appear to damage platelets in vivo or initiate blood coagulation
(provided that excessive temperature elevations are avoided). There are
several exceptions to this statement; one is that the effects of
turbulent blood flow on the induction of acoustically-driven cavitation
have not been fully explored. It would therefore be prudent not to expose
the beating heart of the adult or foetus to high therapeutic intensities of
ultrasound. Another exception is that the potential thrombogenic effects
of ultrasonic contrast agents have not been adequately investigated,
especially in combination with other factors which might enhance their
potentially destructive effects such as turbulent flow fields and/or the
development of standing waves.

(c) Functional effects on leucocytes

Crowell et al. (1977) subjected white cell enriched canine plasma to
the acoustic microstreaming field generated around a tungstem wire
oscillating transversely at 20 k Hz. They observed cell lysis at wire
displacement amplitudes greater than 8 μm but also measured changes in
phagocytic and bacteriocidal indices and metabolic activities at amplitudes
significantly less than the value required to disrupt the cells. Visual
observation of the number of bacteria engulfed by (and/or adhering to the
surface of) the polymorphonuclear neutrophilic leucocytes showed that the
average cell's phagocytic index increased with increasing displacement
amplitude up to about 7 μm and therafter decreased with increasing
displacement amplitude. Conversely, the number of bacteria killed by each
leucocyte (i.e. its relative bacteriocial capacity) declined progressively
with increasing displacement amplitude suggesting that more bacteria may be
attached to the outside of sheared cells rather than being engulfed by
them. The authors suggest that this increased adhesion could be the result
of changes in the distribution of charges on the cell surface resulting
from exposure to the microstreaming field as has been shown for human
erythrocytes exposed to MHz ultrasound.

(d) Vascular effects

The ultrasonic exposure conditions are markedly different for a tissue or organ subjected to an acoustic field having a strong standing wave component as compared with that same organ subjected to the same incident intensity beam in the absence of the reflected wave. Dyson et al. (1974) have shown that the standing wave results in the reversible accumulation of the blood cells in discrete bands spaced one half wavelength of the compressional wave (i.e. blood cell stasis). There is no single "threshold" intensity for the production of this effect since it depends upon the ultrasonic frequency, the magnitude of the standing wave component, the animal's blood pressure, the velocity of blood flow within that vessel, the dimensions and orientation of the vessel relative to the axis of the ultrasound beam as well as the difference in density between the blood cells and the surrounding plasma. Under laboratory conditions this effect cannot usually be observed at intensities less than about 0.5 W/cm^2 at 3 MHz (c.w.), and can be avoided at even higher intensities if the irradiating transducer is kept moving or if short pulses of ultrasound are used. Blood cell stasis prevents the normal circulation of erythrocytes and so tissue anoxia may result if stasis is maintained for prolonged periods.

Another major change in the acoustic exposure conditions brought about by the development of a standing wave field is the enhancement of the development of cavitational activity. Microbubbles smaller than resonant size are driven to the antinodes of pressure amplitude where they may grow to a resonant size. It is presumably these oscillating bubbles which were responsible for the mechanical disruption of the vascular endothelium reported by ter Haar et al. (1979) and the consolidation of the red cell band with fibrin to form an irreversible "plug" which does not break down when the acoustic field was turned off.

Lizzi et al. (1979) reported a novel reversible bio-effect in that the retinal blood supply of an albino rabbit was seen to blanch within the focal volume of a focused bowl transducer when it was subjected to an intensity/ time combination just below the level required to produce a (thermal) chorioretinal lesion. This blanched region disappeared when the ultrasound was turned off. At even lower intensities the blanching disappeared even though the 10 MHz ultrasonic field had not been switched off. It is not known if this transient blanching is due to mirovascular constriction (i.e. direct neural or neuromuscular stimulation by the ultrasound) or is a mechanical effect resulting from the compression of the nutrient capillaries by the radiation pressure forces emanating from the transducer.

A similar ultrasound-induced transient vasoconstriction within the microvasculature of the external ear of a guinea pig was observed by Zarod and Williams (unpublished observations). However, the effect was highly variable in its occurrence and was only observed under conditions where thermal damage to the pinna would be expected, and so the effect was not persued.

With the possible exception of prolonged blood cell stasis, it is unlikely that ultrasound-induced effects upon the vascular system will prove to be a hazard.

REFERENCES

Akopyan, V. B., Abuladze, N.K., 1982, Interspecific differences of erythrocytes ultrasonic resistivity of warm-blooded animals. Studia Biophys, 88: 119.

Chater, B.V., Williams, A. R., 1977, Platelet aggregation induced in vitro by therapeutic ultrasound. Thrombos Haemostas, 38: 640.

Chater, B. V., Williams, A.R., 1982, Absence of platelet damage in vivo following the exposure of non-turbulent blood to therapeutic ultrasound. Ultrasound Med Biol, 8: 85.

Crowell. J.A., Kusserow, B. K, Nyborg, W.L., 1977, Functional changes in white blood cells after microsonation. Ultrasound Med Biol, 3: 185.

Crum, L. A., 1979, Tensile strength of water. Nature, 278: 148.

Dyson, M., Pond, J. B., Woodward, B., Broadbent, J., 1974, The production of blood cell stasis and endothelial damage in the blood vessels of chick embryos treated with ultrasound in a stationary wave field. Ultrasound Med Biol, 1: 133.

Gross, D. R., Miller, D. L, Williams, A.R., 1985, A search for ultrasound cavitation within the canine cardiovascular system. Ultrasound Med Biol, 11: 85.

Hughes, D. E., Nyborg, W. L., 1962, Cell disruption by ultrasound. Science, 138: 108.

Lizzi, F. L., Coleman, D. J., Driller, J., Franzen, L. A., Jakobiec, F. A., 1978, Experimental ultrasonically induced lesions in the retina, choroid and sclera. Invest Ophthalmol Vis Sci, 17: 350.

Love, L. A., Kremkau, F.W., 1980, Intracellular temperature distribution produced by ultrasound. J Acoust Soc Amer, 67: 1045.

Ludlam, C. A., Moore, S., Bolton, A. E., Pepper, P. S., Cash, J. D., 1975, The release of human platelet-specific protein measured by a radioimmunoassay. Thrombos Res, 6: 543.

Lunan, K.D., Wen, A.C., Barfod, E.T., Edmonds P.D., Pratt, D. E., 1979, Decreased aggregation of mouse platelets after in vivo exposure to ultrasound. Thrombos Haemostasis, 40: 568.

Messino. D., Sette, D., Wanderlingh, F., 1963, Statistical approach to ultrasonic cavitation. J Acoust Soc Amer, 35: 1575.

Miller, D.L., Nyborg, W. L., Whitcomb, C. C., 1978, In vitro clumping of platelets exposed to low intensity ultrasound. In: Ultrasound in medicine, ed White DN, Lyons EA. New York, Plenum Press, 4: 545.

Miller, D. L., Nyborg, W.L., Whitcomb, C. C., 1979, Platelet aggregation induced by ultrasound under specialized conditions in vitro. Science, 205: 505.

Miller, D. L., Williams, A. R., Nyborg, W. L., 1979, Photochemical detection of platelet damage induced by low intensity ultrasound. Reflections, 5: 193.

Nyborg, W. L., 1965, Acoustic streaming. In: Physical acoustics, ed. Mason WP. New York, Academic Press.

Nyborg, W.L., 1978, Physical mechanisms for biological effects of ultrasound. USDHEW Publication (FDA) 78-8062: 1.

Roelandt, J., 1982 Contrast echocardiography. Ultrasound Med Biol, 8: 471.

Rooney, J.A., 1970, Hemolysis near an ultrasonically pulsating gas bubble. Science, 169: 869.

Sanada, M., Hattori, A., Watanabe, T., Shu, T., Kasahara, T., Ohn, M., Tamura. K. ,1977, The in vivo effect of ultrasound upon human blood platelets. Nikon Choompa Igakukai, Koen Rombunshu, Nov: 149.

Tarssanen, L., 1976, Hemolysis by ultrasound. Scand J Haematol, Suppl 29: 7.

ter Haar, G., Dyson, M., Smith, S.P., 1979, Ultrastructural changes in the mouse uterus brought about by ultrasonic irradiation at therapeutic intensities in standing wave fields. Ultrasound Med Biol, 5: 167.

Thomas, D., 1977, Haemostasis. Brit Med Bull, 33: 183.

Williams, A. R., 1974, Release of serotonin from human platelets by acoustic microstreaming. J Acoust Soc Amer, 56: 1640.

Williams, A. R., 1977, Intravascular mural thrombi produced by acoustic microstreaming. Ultrasound Med Biol, 3: 191.

Williams, A. R., 1981, In vivo thrombogenesis. In: The Rheology of Blood, Blood Vessels and Associated Tissues, ed. Gross DR, Hwang NHC. The Netherlands, Sijhoff and Noordhoff.

Williams, A.R., 1982, Absence of meaningful thresholds for bioeffect studies on cell suspensions in vitro. Brit J Cancer, 45: 192.

Williams, A. R., Chater, B. V., Allen, K. A, Sanderson, J. H., 1981, The use of β-Thromboglobulin to detect platelet damage by therapeutic ultrasound in vivo. J Clin Ultrasound, 9: 145.

Williams, A. R, Chater, B. V., Allen, K. A., Sherwood, M. R, Sanderson, J. H., 1978,Release of β-Thromboglobulin from human platelets by therapeutic intensities of ultrasound. Brit J Haematol, 40: 133.

Williams, A.R., Hughes, D.E., Nyborg, W. L., 1970,Hemolysis near a transversely oscillating wire. Science, 169: 871.

Williams, A. R., Miller, D.L., 1980, Photometric detection of ATP release from human erythrocytes exposed to ultrasonically activated gas-filled pores. Ultras Med Biol, 6: 251.

Williams, A. R., O'Brien, W.D., Coller, B. S., 1976a, Exposure to ultrasound decreases the recalcification time of platelet rich plasma. Ultrasound Med Biol, 2: 113.

Williams, A. R., Sykes, S.M, O'Brien, W. D., 1976b, Ultrasonic exposure modifies platelet morphology and function in vitro. Ultrasound Med Biol, 2: 311.

Wong, Y. S., Watmough, D.J., 1980, Haemolysis of red blood cells in vitro and in vivo caused by therapeutic ultrasound at 0.75 MH$_z$. Proc Ultrasound Interact Med Biol Symp. Reinhardsbrunn, E Germany, C 14.

Yaroniene G, 1978, Response of biological systems to low-intensity ultrasonic waves. Proc FASE 78, Warszawa: 13.

Zarod, A. P., Williams, A. R., 1977, Platelet aggregation in vivo by therapeutic ultrasound. Lancet, 2: 1266.

IMMUNOLOGICAL AND GENETIC EFFECTS

A.R. Williams

Department of Medical Biophysics
University of Manchester Medical School
Manchester, England

INTRODUCTION

The obvious importance of the immunological system in the protection from infection and the role of DNA as the store of genetic information for future generations means that both of these systems have been intensively investigated as potential "targets" for ultrasound interactions. In common with many other areas of biological investigation the majority of the published reports are concerned with the _in vitro_ exposure of isolated cells or even purified macromolecules. This is a reflection of the fact that it is often difficult to obtain a precise measurement of a given vital function _in vivo_ (partly because of the difficulty of access without perturbing the function you are trying to measure and partly because of the inherent homeostatic mechanisms which operate to prevent any change). Consequently, _in vitro_ exposure systems are favoured because they enable more sophisticated and/or quantifiable measurements to be performed.

(a)   Effects on the immunological system

Anderson and Barrett (1979) iradiated the spleens of anaesthetised mice _in vivo_ with ultrasound from a diagnostic apparatus (2MHz; SATA intensity 8.9 mW/cm^2; 691 pulses/sec) for 1.6, 3.3 or 5 min. The animals were subsequently challenged with sheep erythrocytes and the authors report a small decrease in the lgM compartment of the immunoglobulin response which was also reflected in a decreased number of direct antibody plaque-forming cells present in the spleen compared to sham treated controls. Stratmeyer and his collaborators (personal communication) and Child et al. (1981) have attempted to duplicate these observations at similar and higher acoustic intensities, but were unable to demonstrate a positive effect. It should be noted that the reactive capacity of the mammalian immunological system is so large that even if the small "desensitization" reported by Anderson and Barrett (1979) is subsequently shown to be a repeatable effect, this would not constitute a significant functional impairment of the system in its ability to combat an invading organism.

Anderson and Barrett (1981) have also investigated the effects of diagnostic intensities of ultrasound (SATA intensity 8.9 mW/cm^2 at 2 MHz, emitted by their same commercial apparatus - a Sperry echoencephalogram, type UM), on the ability of the reticuloendothelial system to phagocytose inert particles and bacteria. In one series of experiments they irradiated the livers of anaesthetized mice for either 1.6, 3.3 or 5 min. and investigated the rate at which particles of collidal carbon were being cleared from the animal's bloodstream. They reported that the half life of the exponential clearance curve was reduced when assayed immediately after the ultrasonic exposure, and that the magnitude of this reduction increased as the time interval between sonication and assay was increased. These observations are also perplexing in that there is an apparent negative "dose" correlation i.e. longer exposure times have less effect even though the animals have received more ultrasonic power. Their experimental protocol can be seriously criticized on the grounds that the carbon particles were injected as a suspension in 0.25 ml of water containing 0.5% gelatine. The entire blood volume of a mouse is only of the order of about 3 ml and so the injection of 0.25 ml of water will result in the immediate osmotic lysis of a number of erythrocytes and ultimately result in a significant reduction in the osmolarity of the animal's blood plasma. The measured clearance rates therefore reflect the rate at which carbon particles coated with gelatine are removed in a hypotonic environment in competition with free haemoglobin and cellular debris. These criticisms could be countered by repeating the experiments using carbon particles suspended in isotonic saline. These experiments have not been repeated in an independent laboratory, but Saad and Williams (1982) have found that continuous wave 0.75 MHz ultrasound began to affect the rate of clearance of blood-borne colloidal sulphur particles (injected in isotonic saline) in rats only at intensities greater than about 0.8 W/cm^2. The magnitude of this reversible change in the half life of removal increased with increasing intensity or exposure time and was proportional to the amount of ultrasonic energy deposited at the site of irradiation. A novel observation was that isolated lymphocytes irradiated with ultrasound in vitro and re-injected via the tail vein before the administration of the colloidal sulphur, also resulted in a similar decrease in the rate of removal of colloid whereas the re-injection of control lymphocytes did not (Saad and Williams, article in preparation).

In another series of experiments, Anderson and Barrett (1981) irradiated the shaved abdomen of anaesthetized mice for 10 min. using the same diagnostic apparatus described above and then isolated the free peritoneal macrophages by lavage. These macrophages were subsequently incubated with cultures of Staphylococcus aureus. It was found that a significantly larger fraction of the macrophages from the irradiated animals did not engulf bacteria which resulted in a lower net bacteriocidal rate. However, those sonicated macrophages which did engulf bacteria ingested approximately the same number of cells as their controls even though they were apparently less able to kill them once they were inside the body of the macrophage. These investigations merit being repeated in an independent laboratory.

Crowell et al. (1977) subjected white cell enriched canine plasma to the acoustic microstreaming field generated around a tungsten wire oscillating transversely at 20 kHz. They observed cell lysis at wire displacement amplitudes greater than 8 μm but also measured changes in phagocytic and bacteriocidal indices and metabolic activities at amplitudes significantly less than the value required to disrupt the cells. Visual observation of the number of bacteria engulfed by (and/or adhering to the surface of) the polymorphonuclear neutrophilic leucocytes showed that the average cell's phagocytic index increased with increasing displacement amplitude up to about 7 μm and thereafter decreased with increasing displacement amplitude. Other measurements showed that the number of bacteria killed by each leucocyte (i.e. its relative bacteriocidal capacity, did not exhibit this same trend but declined progressively with increasing displacement amplitude (as did the rate of oxygen utilisation by those same cells). Crowell et al. (1977) proposed that this discrepancy in their observations could have arisen if more bacterial were attached to the outside of the cells sheared at displacement amplitude less than about 7 μm, but that these bacteria were not engulfed by the "damaged" cells. This increased adhesion could be the result of changes in the distribution of the charges on the cell surface resulting from exposure to the microstreaming field.

Several other authors have observed similar changes after the leucocytes had been exposed to megahertz ultrasound _in vitro_. For example, in a preliminary communication, Saggio and Sommer (1980) report an increase in the phagocytic activity of macrophages, where Fung et al. (1978) report a decrease in the rate of uptake of labelled thymidine by human lymphocytes after they had been exposed to therapeutic intensities and frequencies of ultrasound. One criticism which can be levelled against most of the experiments performed using leucocytes is that the authors have usually not attempted to remove the majority of the platelets. These platelets are extremely fragile cells which are readily disrupted and/or activated by ultrasound _in vitro_ and release chemically active agents which can subsequently alter both their own functioning and that of other adjacent cells (Williams et al., 1976).

Ford et al. (1970) developed a sensitive technique for quantifying an animal's immunological competence by measuring the results of the competition between an animal's lymphocytes and foreign lymphocytes _in vivo_. A known number of foreign lymphocytes are injected into the hind foot pads of mice from which they migrate through the lymphatic system to the popliteal lymph nodes. Here, the host lymphocytes are attracted and proliferate and usually destroy the invaders. The gain in weight of this popliteal lymph node is measured (the node weight may increase by a factor of up to seventyfold). It was found that neither irradiation of the foreign lymphocytes _in vitro_ before injection nor irradiation of one of an animal's lymph nodes _in vivo_ after both hind limbs had been injected with the same number of foreign cells caused a measurable change in node weights indicating that the ultrasound (3 MHz, SATA intensity 0.8 W/cm^2, c.w.) did not appear to affect either the agressiveness of the invading lymphocytes or the ability of the host lymphocytes to recognise the invaders and to proliferate (Williams and Ford, article in preparation).

Thus, there is general agreement that ultrasound exposure (or the treatments and handling associated with the exposure) can alter the rate of functioning of various components of the immunological and reticuloendothelial system. However, since this system is designed to respond to a wide range of non-specific stimuli, it would be unusual if small changes similar to those described above could not be demonstrated. None of the observations reported to date give cause for concern that ultrasound exposure can impair the functioning of the immune system to the extent that it might pose an additional threat to the well-being of the animal.

(b)   Effects on DNA and the genetic apparatus

Several investigators have exposed isolated DNA or its constituent bases to ultrasound _in vitro_. High molecular weight DNA strands are cleaved into smaller fragments, presumably by the acoustic microstreaming fields associated with the various forms of cavitational activity. For example, Galperin-Lemaitre et al. (1975) reported the not unreasonable finding of the degradation of isolated DNA at intensities as low as 200 mW/cm^2 of MHz ultrasound, but unfortunately interpreted this as evidenced that ultrasound could possibly by "mutagenic". Wang (1977) showed that high therapeutic intsnsities of MHz ultrasound _in vitro_ could change the chemical composition of the purified bases present in DNA to yield products similar to those found after exposure to ultraviolet light or X-rays. This latter finding is the result of interaction of the bases with the highly reactive free radicals produced by cavitational activity within the solutions. However, neither of these studies should give cause for concern because the DNA inside a living cell is protected both from acoustic microstreaming fields (which would tend to disrupt the cell rendering it non-viable before the DNA itself is cleaved) and from the free radicals which would have to pass through the cell membranes and the cytoplasmic contents to reach the nucleus. In the case of ionizing radiation the free radicals may be produced within the nucleus, whereas in the case of ultrasound we have no evidence to suggest that cavitational activity could occur within the nucleus, or even that if it were to occur there that the cell could remain viable.

Nevertheless, some studies apparently indicate that ultrasound can alter the DNA within the intact cell. For example, Liebeskind et al. (1979a) exposed He La cells grown in tissue cultrue to diagnostic intensities of pulsed ultrasound and reported a variety of effects which included a small (but transient) increased immunoreactivity to antinucleoside antibodies for the cells in the G_1 phase. This result indicates the possible presence of single stranded or denatured DNA (even though the authors were unable to demonstrate DNA strand breakage by the moderately sensitive technique of alkaline-sucrose ultracentrifugation) which might reflect a low level of DNA repair synthesis. Complementary observations were reported by Pinamonti et al. (personal communication) who exposed human leucocytes in vitro to diagnostic intensities of pulsed ultrasound and then isolated their DNA and examined it using the electron microscope and by electrophoresis on Agarose gels. Pinamonti et al. reported that the DNA isolated from sonicated cells appeared to be more "tangled together" when the lysed nuclei were viewed under the electron microscope and that the sonicated DNA was cleaved into smaller fragments following digestion with nuclease S_1 which will digest any single-stranded portions of the DNA. Neither of these potentially significant biological effects has been confirmed in an independent laboratory.

If effects similar to those described above were commonly associated with ultrasound exposure, then it should be possible to detect them as a change in the mutation rate of an organism such as a bacterium or yeast. These organisms are used because they are readily available, have a short cell cycle so that many generations of the organism can be studied within a few days or weeks, and they are amenable to a number of well-established techniques to pinpoint the nature and exact locus of any ultrasound induced mutation. Combes (1975) could not detect an increase in the back-mutation of an auxotropic strain of Baccilus subtilis after it had been irradiated for 5 min. at 2 MHz at temporal peak intensities of up to 60 W/cm^2 (20 μs pulses, duty cycle 0.004). He was also unable to detect mutagenic lesions in vivo after transforming DNA had been irradiated in vitro. Thacker (1974) used the yeast Saccharomyces cerivisiae to test for ultrasound-induced mutation in nuclear genes and in mitochondrial DNA as well as for recombination of a nuclear gene. He used a variety of exposure conditions simulating diagnostic (20 μsec pulses with 5 μsec spaces and a peak pulse power of 10 W/cm^2, and therapeutic conditions (5 W/cm^2 continuous up to 30 min), and also even more powerful exposure regimes. These tests yielded no evidence for increased mutations or recombinations, even when only about 0.1% of the cells remained viable, provided that chemical agents such as hydrogen peroxide were not allowed to accumulate and that excessive heating was avoided.

In 1963 Dr Hubert J. Dyer induced an acoustic microstreaming field inside the apical protonema cells of the moss Physcomotrium hyriforme by the external application of a fine-pointed metal probe vibrating at 80 kHz (i.e. simulating the effects of an external stable cavitation bubble). These cells were all undergoing mitotic divisions of the nucleus at the time (ie. in their M phase) and 22 of these treated cells survived this and the subsequent handling and subculturing techniques and continued to grow. Two visibly detectable morphological mutants were found amongst the irradiated clones whereas none were found in the controls or in the many hundreds of subcultrues made of the original wild-type strain (Dyer, 1972). The subcultures derived from these abnormal mosses were also abnormal and some were still alive 18 years later (after 25-30 subcultures).   Preliminary biochemical investigations confirmed that there were many differences in chemical composition between the wild type and mutant strains indicating a widespread genetic "reorganisation" rather than a single point mutation (H.J. Dyer, personal communication).   One mutant contained more DNA than the original wild type whereas the other contained less DNA than the wild type.   It is tempting to speculate that these mutants could have arisen either by the inclusion of an additional chromosome or by the loss of one complete chromosome during cell division.   There was no evidence of mutant clones from cells irradiated during interphase.

Spencer (1952) reported a transmissible morphological change in plants grown from peas (<u>Pisum sativum</u>) which had been exposed to ultrasound before germination had become apparent.   Despite the high acoustic intensities (20 W/cm^2, c.w., O.5 MHz for 20 sec) most seeds were able to germinate and produced plants which were almost twice · as tall as their unsonicated controls.   Cross-breeding experiments showed that only the offspring of the female sonicated plants continued to grow as abnormally tall plants.   This indicates that the ultrasound has not produced a dominant genetic mutation, but instead has resulted in a change of some cytoplasmic factor which is transmitted through the cytoplasm of the seeds produced by the female plants.   The effects of these non-nuclear phenotype modifying factors (called dauermodifiers) may be transmitted through a number of successive genrations before gradually disappearing.

Suspensions of single cells have been widely used to demonstrate the genetic changes induced by ionizing radiation.   They offer many practical advantages in that they are readily available and are easy to culture, have a short cell cycle so that many generations of the organism can be studied within a few days or weeks.   These advantages are of course countered by some disadvantages in that the cells in suspension are more likely to be affected by cavitation-induced streaming than cells in a solid tissue whereas the role of heating will tend to be diminished.   Another potential experimental disadvantage is that if the damaging mechanism is a rotational torque arising from sudden discontinuities in intensity within the acoustic beam, then this would tend to rotate the entire cell if it is free in suspension whereas it would tend to rotate only the cellular contents if that cell was embedded within a tissue (this latter situation is closer to the conditions produced by Dyer, 1972).

The first startling reports of a potentially serious genetic effect induced by diagnostic intensities of ultrasound were the articles by Macintosh and Davey in 1970 and 1972 claiming that they had observed an increased incidence of chromosome aberrations in sonicated human lymphocytes.   The significance of these reports lay in the fact that this technique is used to assess the mutagenic potential of ionizing radiations.   Therefore, if diagnostic ultrasound is also able to induce chromosome aberrations then it may also be mutagenic, i.e. may be capable of inducing tumours.   These papers stimulated many other laboratories to attempt to duplicate these finding using a variety of frequencies, intensities, exposure systems and irradiation media.   A few articles also claimed positive results at diagnostic exposure levels (eg. Kunze-Muhl and Golob, 1972) while others reported inconclusive data which was not statistically significant but suggested that the effect might be real. However, the majority of the articles describing attempts to duplicate these studies found no increased incidence of chromosome abnormalities (see review by Williams, 1983), even though the ultrasonic exposure conditions ranged from the diagnostic through the therapeutic zones and in to the region where transient cavitation would be expected.

Thus, after many years of controversy the greatest weight of evidence seems to indicate that ultrasound does not cause chromosome abnormalities. But, how could the positive results have been obtained in the first place? The answer appears to lie in the experimental complexities inherent in the preparation of the chromosome spreads and in the difficulties the operator experiences in quantifying the aberrations. On a "real" slide prepared as part of any experiment the individual chromosomes are seldom completely spread out as shown in the "classical" photographs in textbooks. In practice, many of the chromosomes may overlap each other and the operator is frequently called upon to decide whether or not they are normal or abnormal. It is therefore imperative that the operator does not know if the slide that he or she is scoring is from a sonicated or a control series because it is a normal human tendency in the case of a marginal decision to say it is normal if you know that it is a control and to say abnormal if you know it has been sonicated and you believe that ultrasound can cause aberrations. The slides on which the Macintosh and Davey (1970) and (1972) articles were based were scored by Macintosh in the full knowledge of which samples had been sonicated and which were the controls. When he repeated this work using the same ultrasonic Doppler instrument and exposure system, but this time scoring the slides without knowing which was which (ie. the experiment was performed double-blind) he found no increase in chromosomal abnormalities (Macintosh et al., 1975).

In retrospect, the whole topic of chromosome aberrations probably received far more attention than it deserved, because as Thacker (1973) and Wells (1977) point out, if these chromatid and chromosome breaks were to occur in vivo (instead of during the preparation of cell smears in vitro) then they would most probably result in the death of that cell.

A similar flurry of research activity was initiated by the report of Leibeskind et al. (1979b) which described a small but statistically significant increase in the sister chromatid exchange (SCE) rate of human lymphocytes following exposure to diagnostic levels of ultrasound. An SCE is the exchange of homologous portions of each of the two chromatids in a chromosome and it can occur spontaneously. The biological significance of SCE's is unclear but it is presumed that an increased rate of SCE is indicative of chromosomal damage (Gebhart, 1981). The SCE rate can be measured with a high degree of precision but the interpretation of the results is complicated by the fact that some powerful mutagens, such as ionizing radiation and some chemicals, cause only small increases in SCE frequency whereas some weak mutagens cause a large increase in SCE rates.

Goss (1984) reviewed a total of 14 papers which attempted to confirm the SCE effects reported by Liebeskind et al. (1979b) as well as to extend the ultrasonic exposure conditions from the diagnostic into the therapeutic range and above. Haupt et al. (1981) and Ehlinger et al. (1981) both reported statistically significant increases in SCE rates whereas eleven other articles (which included a study by Liebeskind et al. on a different cell line) reported negative effects, ie. that ultrasound treatment did not cause an increase in SCE rates.

Thus, just as in the case of the chromosome aberrations described above, the majority of the published studies (including others not included in the Goss, 1984, article) indicate that diagnostic levels of ultrasound exposure do not cause an increase in SCE rates. However, two or more negative effect papers do not necessarily "cancel out" one positive effect report. Also, it is much more difficult in this case to pinpoint any single methodological error which could give rise to false positive, or alternatively false negative SCE results. In general, the different papers employed widely different experimental protocols, some being in vitro exposures while others were irradiated in vivo, they used different cell lines, different concentrations of bromo deoxyuridine which was added either before or after the ultrasound exposure, the cells were harvested at different times and were also expsoed to markedly different ultrasound "dosages" in a variety of different exposure vessels and media. These sources of variability preclude us from coming to any firm conclusion as to the possible effects of diagnostic intensities ofultrasound on the frequency of SCE's.

Despite the limited nature of the data base on SCE effects, the Bioeffects committee of the AIUM offered the following summary which was quoted as an appendix in Goss (1984):

> "If the SCE frequency is increased by ultrasound, it would appear on the basis of the studies discussed here (i.e. Goss, 1984) that the magnitudes of the effects are small, and that they occur only under unusual, and as yet largely undefined conditions in vitro. Even where an effect has been observed, the importance of the magnitude of that effect and its biological significance remain unknown. Although continuing studies of SCE and ultrasound in vivo are extremely important, there appears to be no basis at this time to alter presently held views of the safety of clinical ultrasound as described by the AIUM Statement on Clinical Safety of October 1983."

REFERENCES

Anderson, D. W. and Barrett, J. T., 1979, Ultrasound: a new immunosuppressant. Clin. Immunol. Immunopathol., 14: 18.

Anderson, D. W. and Barrett, J. T., 1981, Depression of phagocytosis by ultrasound, Ultrasound Med. Biol., 7: 267.

Child, S. Z., Hare, J. D., Carstensen, E. L., Vives, B., Davis, J., Adler, A. and Davis, H.T., 1981. Test for the effects of diagnostic levels of ultrasound on the immune response of mice, Clin. Immunol. Immunopathol., 18: 299.

Combes, R. D., 1975, Absence of mutation following ultrasonic treatment of Bacillus subtilis cells and transforming deoxyribonucleic acid, Brit. J. Radiol., 48: 306.

Crowell, J. A., Kusserow, B. K. and Nyborg, W. L., 1977, Functional changes in white cells after microsonation, Ultrasound Med. Biol., 3: 185.

Dyer, H. J., 1972, Structural effects of ultrasound on the cell, In "Interactions of Ultrasound and Biological Tissues", Eds. J. M. Reid and M. R. Sikov, DHEW Publication 73-8008, (FDA): 73.

Ehlinger, C. A., Katayama, P. K., Roester, M. R. and Mattingly, R. F., 1981, Diagnostic ultrasound increases sister chromatid exchange; preliminary report, Wisc. Med. J., 80: 21.

Ford, W. L., Burr, W. and Simonsen, M., 1970, A lymph node weight assay for the grafversus-host activity of rat lymphoid cells, Transplantation, 10: 258.

Fung, H., Cheung, K., Lyons, E.A. and Kay, N.E., 1978, The effect of low dose ultrasound on human peripheral lymphocyte function in vitro, In "Ultrasound in Medicine", Eds. D. N. White and E. A. Lyons, Plenum Press, N.Y., 4: 583.

Galperin-Lemaitre, H., Kirsch-Volders, M. and Levi, S., 1975, Ultrasound and mammalian DNA, Lancet, 2: 662.

Gebhart, E., 1981, Sister chromatid exchange (SCE) and structural chromosome aberration in mutagenicity testing (review article), Human Genetics, 58: 235.

Goss, S. A., 1984, Sister chromatid exchange and ultrasound, J. Ultrasound Med., 3: 463.

Haupt, M., Martin, N., Simpson, J. L., Iqbal, M., Elias, S., Dyere, A. and Sabbagha, R. E., 1981, Ultrasonic induction of sister chromatid exchanges in human lymphocytes, Human Genetics, 39: 221.

Kunze-Muhl, E. and Golob, E., 1972, Chromosomenanalysen nach Ultraschalleinwirkung, Humangenetik, 14; 237.

Liebeskind, D., Bases, R., Elequin, F., Neubort, S., Leifer, R., GOLDBERG, R. and Koenigsberg, M., 1979a Diagnostic ultrasound: effects on the DNA and growth patterns of animal cells, Radiology, 131: 177.

Liebeskind, D., Bases, R., Mendez, F., Elequin, F. and Koenigsberg, M., 1979b, Sister chromatid exchanges in lymphocytes after exposure to diagnostic ultrasound, Science, 205: 1273.

Macintosh, I. J. C., Brown, R. C. and Coakley, W. T., 1975, Ultrasound and in vitro chromosome aberrations, Brit. J. Radiol., 48: 230.

Macintosh, I. J. C. and Davey, D. A., 1970, Chromosome aberrations induced by an ultrasonic foetal pulse detector, Brit. Med. J., 4; 92.

Macintosh, I. J. C. and Davey, D. A., 1972, Relationship between intensity of ultrasound and induction of chromosome aberrations. Brit. J. Radiol., 45: 320.

Saad, A.H. and Williams, A.R., 1982, Effects on therapeutic ultrasound on clearance rate of blood borne colloidal particles in vivo, Brit. J. Cancer, 45: 202.

Spencer, J. L., 1952, Effects of intense ultrasonic vibrations on Pisum. II. Effects on growth and their inheritance, Growth, 16: 255.

Thacker, J., 1973, The possibility of genetic hazard from ultrasonic radiation, Curr. Topics. Rad. RES. Q., 8: 235.

Thacker, J., 1974, An assessment of ultrasonic radiation hazard using yeast genetic systems, Brit. J. Radiol., 47: 130.

Wang, S. Y., 1977, Ultrasonic radiation of nucleic acid components, Symp. Biol. Effects and Characterization of Ultrasound Sources, HEW Publication 78-8048: 196.

Wells, P. N. T., 1977, "Biomedical Ultrasonics", Academic Press, London, N.Y.

Williams, A. R., 1983, "Ultrasound: biological effects and potential hazards", Academic Press, London, N.Y.

Williams, A. R., Sykes, S. M., and O'Brien, W. D. J., 1976, Ultrasonic exposure modifies platelet morphology and function <u>in vitro</u>. <u>Ultrasound Med. Biol.</u>, 2: 311.

DEVELOPMENTAL AND TERATOGENIC EFFECTS OF ULTRASOUND

B.R. Fisher and M.E. Stratmeyer

Food and Drug Administration
Center for Devices and Radiological Health
5600 Fishers Lane (HFZ-112)
Rockville, Maryland 20857

INTRODUCTION

In obstetrics, the applications of ultrasound cover a broad spectrum. During pregnancy ultrasound is used alone to visualize and monitor fetal development, and it is also used as an adjunct with other procedures, such as amniocentesis, to determine the well-being of the developing fetus. Ultrasound is currently used to assist in chorionic villi sampling, a relatively recent technique designed to obtain genetic information on the fetus during earlier stages of gestation than is possible with amniocentesis. In general, the clinical applications of diagnostic ultrasonography are diverse and its potential use can be justified during virtually all stages of pregnancy.

There are two types of ultrasound used in fetal applications: continuous wave doppler ultrasound (CW) for fetal heart rate monitoring and pulse-echo for visualization. In addition, pulse doppler has found recent use for measuring fetal blood flow. There is an increased concern regarding potential biological consequences that may result from the levels at which these devices operate. Data from a recent survey indicates that some new devices operate at higher exposure levels than those known to have been used in the past (Stewart and Harris, in press). The level of concern is further heightened by the use of pulsed doppler devices to measure blood flow in the fetal heart, placenta, and umbilical vessels. The temporal average intensities of some of these devices approach therapeutic levels.

Possible risks associated with ultrasound exposure on the developing embryo or fetus is an important issue. Embryonic and fetal development is a dynamic process involving rapid growth, functional changes, and complex interaction of various cell populations and developing organ systems. It is essential that development follows its established spatial and temporal program to ensure normal intrauterine maturation. Soon after fertilization, cleavage segregates various portions of the zygote's cytoplasm into specific cell populations. Subsequent development is an intricate system of genetic expression combined with cellular interaction. At specific times during development, cells produce specific gene products. Through cell-to-cell interaction, chemical signals and messenger molecules are

195

transmitted and progressively the cells' fate is determined. This process of determining cellular characteristics through genetic expression is referred to as "cellular differentiation." At gastrulation there is a cellular rearrangement which begins giving shape and form to the embryo. Through the mechanisms of selective adhesion and cell migration, the embryonic cells move in very distinct patterns and contact and interact with other specific cell populations. The patterns of gastrulation vary between species, but the end result is the same; the axis of the embryo is determined, the primary germ layers are formed and the process of neurulation is initiated. Subsequent interactions between the germ layers "induce" the formation of embryonic organs and organs systems (organogenesis). The final embryonic pattern, the orderly arrangement of all the organ systems, is obtained by the complex interrelationship of morphogenetic and differentiative events which occur throughout the rest of gestation.

The susceptibility of an embryo or fetus to a physical or chemical agent is strongly determined by its stage of development. From the brief description above, it can be seen that the development from a zygote to a full-term fetus is the dynamic interaction of many systems working in unison. Any agent or insult that disrupts the normal developmental program could potentially jeopardize normal intrauterine development. Because the very young embryo consists of a limited number of cells, the introduction of a physical or chemical agent at this stage of gestation could have a major impact on development. During latter stages of development, if an agent is introduced which has a pronounced effect on cell migration or cellular interactions, it could potentially disrupt the induction of various organ systems and/or limb formation. Recently, German (1984) introduced the "Embryonic Stress Hypothesis of Teratogenesis." German postulates that if an agent alters the production of specific messenger molecules essential for normal development, this functional alteration could have an effect on subsequent cellular interactions. If the resultant developmental error was not lethal to the embryo, the effect could manifest itself as an anatomical malformation. This hypothesis provides a generalized concept by which a single agent can produce a spectrum of developmental alterations; the nature and severity of the defect being determined in part, by the period of gestation when the insult was received.

Rugh's work with x-rays (1968) supports this hypothesis. In the mouse, specific congenital malformations were produced depending on the period of gestation when the insult was given. Here again, a spectrum of developmental alterations was produced by a single agent. In general, x-ray exposures during very early stages of development tended to be embryolethal, whereas exposures latter in development resulted in structural malformations. In the case of maternal hyperthermia, some fetal effects are delayed and are expressed only after a latency period. Therefore, it is not only important to know which endpoint to observe, but also when to look for an alteration in a particular endpoint.

Since fetal ultrasonography is used throughout gestation, there is the risk associated with exposure during critical developmental periods. There is also the possibility that the fetus may receive multiple exposures from sonograms administered over the course of a pregnancy. The mammalian conceptus has little regulatory control over its environment. Factors, such as immature biological barriers, poor immunosurveillance, and relative lack of metabolic detoxification and thermoregulatory mechanisms, all contribute to the general increase in susceptibility of the fetus to physical and chemical agents (Brix, 1982).

A physical or chemical agent which has an adverse effect on development can act at one or more of three potential sites. The agent can directly affect the fetus or it can elicit its effect on the maternal or the placental system, either of which could indirectly disrupt normal fetal development (Beck, 1981). The possibility of an indirect effect on the fetus is accentuated because normal responses of the maternal system can be altered by other physiologic stresses associated with pregnancy. Potential direct fetal effects from ultrasound are of special concern because the fetus often receives whole body exposure during diagnostic imaging.

In reviewing the work of different investigators careful consideration must be given to various experimental parameters outlined in their studies. Particular attention should be given to actual exposure conditions and dosimetry. Early ultrasound studies provided few details about exposure conditions making it difficult to directly compare the results between different laboratories.

Most reviews on the developmental effects of ultrasound limit themselves to the developmental events between fertilization and birth, although, development does not end at birth. Many fetal systems, such as the neural, visual, endocrine, behavioral and reproductive systems, are immature at birth and development continues well into adolescence. This review considers "development" as a continuum and will be expanded to cover ultrasonic effects on the germ cells, as well as post-natal development. The reported studies are presented in sequence according to the stage of development during which exposure occurred. Because, in a single study, some investigators have exposed subjects at different stages of gestation, the same study may be discussed several times. Emphasis will be placed on experimental design and exposure conditions which may help to explain observed effects. Intensities discussed in the following studies will be stated as spatial average, temporal average (SATA) intensities unless otherwise indicated. Intensities will be stated as specifically as possible from the information supplied by the investigators. Thus, the spatial and temporal intensity characteristics will sometimes be stated, while only "average" or "peak" intensities are given in other instances.

NONMAMMALIAN SYSTEMS

A wide variety of nonmammalian systems including fish, amphibians, insects, and chickens have been used to investigate the developmental effects of ultrasound. Some of these systems pass through developmental stages that are different or absent in mammalian systems. Variation in yolk content among eggs of different species results in varying cleavage patterns. Polar cell formation and a syncytial developmental stage are unique to Drosophila eggs. Also, placentation and the interaction of maternal compensation are absent in nonmammalian systems. These systems do however, exhibit some basic developmental stages similar to mammals. In general, a great deal of information has been obtained on these systems and their early developmental programs are now well characterized. Therefore, not only do these systems provide useful information on the mechanisms by which ultrasound interacts with organized tissue, but they can also be utilized to obtain information on how ultrasound might potentially affect developmental processes.

In an early study, Selman and Jurand (1964) demonstrated that ultrasound caused intracellular damage in newts. Exposure of Triturus alpestris tadpoles to 1 MHz, CW ultrasound at intensities of 8 - 15 W/cm^2 for 5 minutes resulted in destruction of the epidermis and pycnosis of muscle and neural tube cells. Subsequent electron microscopy revealed disruption of nearly all the endoplasmic reticulum in the notochord cells. This effect appeared reversible and within 24 hours more than half the total endoplasmic reticulum had resumed normal configuration.

Andrew (1964) exposed perch spawn to 1.5 mW/cm^2 pulsed ultrasound, 48 hours postfertilization for 3 or 5 hours. There were no gross structural defects observed in the eyes or spinal cords of the perch after hatching. Frog eggs which were similarly exposed for 24 hours sometime during their first 11 days of development, showed differences in the rate of development when compared with controls. Unfortunately, information concerning intensity data and pulse parameters were not provided.

Sarvazyan et al. (1982) extensively investigated the effects of ultrasound on amphibian embryonic tissue. Embryos of Rana esculenta, Rana temporaria, and Xenopus laevis at various stages of development and ectomesodermal explants (EME) were exposed to CW and low-intensity pulsed ultrasound. An EME is a small piece of skin ectoderm with its underlying mesoderm, removed from the lateral part of an embryo just after neurulation. With the appropriate conditions, through a process resembling gastrulation, the explant rolls into a sphere resulting in a mesodermal cortex covered by epidermal ectoderm. Both the embryos and the EME's were exposed to 0.88 MHz ultrasound at SATA intensities ranging from 0.025 - 0.1 W/cm^2. Pulse repetition frequencies were varied between 10 - 1000 Hz with a constant duty factor of 0.5 and exposure times were between 2 and 30 minutes. The results showed that the sensitivity of the embryo, as well as localization of damage, were dependent on the embryos' stage of development. In general, sensitivity to ultrasound decreased with increased gestational age. In very early stages of development, ultrasonic exposure disrupted the distribution of yolk and pigment. Ultrasonic exposure at the late blastula-early gastrula stage resulted in complete cellular destruction with cells in the animal hemisphere exhibiting the greatest sensitivity. Regions of destruction at this stage were wide and often resulted in death of the embryo. Lesions following exposure at the neurula stage were generally less embryolethal and more localized, usually appearing as a small area of cell necrosis, mainly on the back of the embryo. While there was no observable effect on EME's exposed to CW ultrasound at intensities less than 100 mW/cm^2, exposure to pulsed ultrasound below this intensity produced extensive damage. The investigators concluded that pulse repetition frequency was the exposure characteristic that determined the extent of damage to the embryos and EME's. The influence of pulse repetition frequency on EME's also showed species variability with R. temporaria exhibiting maximal sensitivity at lower pulse repetition frequencies (maximum effect at 10 - 20 Hz) than X. laevis (maximum effect at 110 - 130 Hz). The authors concluded that even though results obtained from amphibian embryonic tissue cannot be directly translated to the clinical situation, serious consideration should be given to all exposure parameters (not just intensity) relevant to diagnostic applications of ultrasound.

The fruit fly, Drosophila melanogaster, has been used extensively to investigate the biological consequences of ultrasound. Early studies performed by Fritz-Niggli and Boni (1950) exposed Drosophila during various developmental stages to 0.8 MHz, CW ultrasound at intensities of 0.7 - 4.0 W/cm^2 for 5 seconds to 25 minutes. They found the eggs, larvae and early pupae were all sensitive stages and as metamorphosis progressed, resistance to ultrasound increased rapidly. They also observed that a large number of larvae and pre-pupae which survived irradiation and continued to develop, later died as late pupae just before emergence. This effect has been termed "delayed lethality" by other investigators.

Selman and Counce also used Drosophila to investigate the effects of ultrasonic treatment on embryonic development (Selman and Counce, 1953; Counce and Selman, 1955). Embryos at various stages of development were exposed for 30 seconds to 1 MHz, CW ultrasound at intensities of 0.3 - 0.5 W/cm^2. Direct effects on the embryos were confirmed by microscopic observations made during treatment and subsequent developmental effects were determined by preparations fixed at intervals up to 20 hours posttreatment. Exposure at 0.5 W/cm^2 resulted in a slow rotary movement of the central region of cleavage stage eggs. In some cases, death resulted from treatment at preblastoderm stages; in others, there was complete recovery and normal development. The authors proposed that these "vortex-like" disturbances produced by ultrasonic exposure could displace cellular contents resulting in abnormal development. Ultrasonic exposure of late cleavage eggs at intensities of 0.5 - 1.2 W/cm^2 produced structural malformations and induced polyploidy. Concurrent microscopic observation of embryos exposed at the syncytial blastoderm stage to intensities of 0.3 - 0.5 W/cm^2 showed most of the cytoplasmic disruption localized in the posterior region with the pole cells eliciting the greatest sensitivity. Delayed lethality similar to that observed by Fritz-Niggli and Boni (1950) was reported following ultrasonic treatment.

Child et al. (1980a) suggested that the effect seen by Fritz-Niggli and Boni could be explained by standing wave formation produced by their exposure system. They examined the killing of eggs exposed to 1 MHz traveling and standing wave ultrasound at intensities up to 5 W/cm^2 (SPTA). Although they were unable to confirm the delayed lethality effect others reported, they did report the killing of one third of the eggs exposed to traveling waves at 3 W/cm^2 and approximately 1 W/cm^2 standing wave ultrasound.

Pizzarello et al. (1978) exposed larval and pupal stages of Drosophila to 2.25 MHz, pulsed ultrasound for 2.5 minutes at a temporal average acoustic power of 1.5 mW using a commercial diagnostic unit. Lethality was high in late 3rd instar larvae and pupae under these conditions. Exposure of growing larvae and prepupae resulted in a growth inhibition which expressed itself in the formation of "miniature" adults.

This study suffers from a number of design and reporting flaws. The exposure conditions used in this study certainly guaranteed reflection, therefore, the larvae and pupae were probably exposed to intensities greater than originally planned. Also, meaningful intensity data is missing, "miniature" is not quantitatively defined and there is no statistical analysis of the data. Because of these deficiencies, the validity of the reported effects is questionable.

Due to the potential impact of reporting a biological effect at such a low temporal average intensity, Child et al. (1980b) attempted to repeat Pizzarello's study and an effort was made to replicate the exposure techniques as closely as possible. Child et al. found no effect on survival at 1.5 mW and were unable to confirm the production of miniature flies reported in the Pizzarello et al. study. Although,

when the temporal peak intensity (and the power) was increased ten-
fold, they observed delayed lethality in one fourth of the exposed
larvae.

Pay et al. (1978) demonstrated delayed lethality in pupae exposed
to 1 MHz, CW ultrasound. In another study, Pay et al. (1982) showed
that although longevity was unaffected, egg laying capacity and egg
survivability decreased in female flies exposed as pupae and tested
throughout their lifetime. In these studies pupae were exposed to
intensities ranging from 0.2 - 4.0 W/cm^2 for 10 minutes. Pay's findings are confirmed by the research of Carstensen and Child (1981) who
reported that death occurred in 70% of the Drosophila eggs exposed to
1 MHz, CW ultrasound at an intensity of 5 W/cm^2 for 30 seconds. To
determine if the observed lethality was due to a thermal mechanism,
egg sensitivity was tested against heat alone. The findings suggested
that the observed effects could not be attributed to heat production
and that some other biophysical mechanism of ultrasound must be
involved. Subsequent work by Child and Carstensen (1982) exposed
Drosophila eggs for 2.5 minutes to 2.25 MHz, pulsed ultrasound at
various stages of development. Intensities varied between 20 -
40 mW/cm^2 (SATA) or 40 - 100 W/cm^2 (SATP), with a pulse repetition
frequency of 500 Hz and a pulse duration of 1 μsec. The results from
this experiment demonstrated that eggs were very sensitive to the
effects of high peak pulsed ultrasound just prior to hatching. This
coincides with the stage of development involving tracheal formation
and its filling with air. It has been postulated that the interaction
of ultrasound with small stabilized gas bodies within the respiratory
system may be responsible for the killing observed in Drosophila.

This group has also investigated the killing of Drosophila larvae
by microsecond pulses of ultrasound, and the data indicated no obvious
relationship between carrier frequency and delayed lethality (Berg
et al., 1983). On the other hand, they demonstrated that larval
killing and delayed lethality are strongly dependent upon peak intensity (Child et al., 1981). Decreases in survival rates were observed
at SATP intensities of 13 W/cm^2 (6 mW/cm^2 SATA) or greater using
1 μsec bursts and pulse repetition frequencies ranging from 50 -
5000 Hz. Carstensen, Child and coworkers have concluded that temporal
average intensity is a poor indicator for these biological effects
(Child et al., 1981), and suggests that temporal peak intensities may
be the best predictor of nonthermal biological effects (Carstensen,
1983).

Although cavitation produced by the interaction of ultrasound with
small gas bodies within the tracheal system may be the postulated
mechanism used to explain the effects observed in Child's work, Pay
et al. (1985) have recently shown that eggs, 2 hours postfertilization, exposed to pulsed ultrasound (1 MHz, 90 W/cm^2 SPPA, 6.5 μsec
pulse duration) at SATA intensities greater than 35 mW/cm^2, fail to
develop. They reported decreased survival at SATA intensities as low
as 3 mW/cm^2 when eggs were exposed for 10 minutes. The mechanism of
ultrasonic action responsible for this high mortality is still
unknown. However, it cannot be attributed to ultrasound interacting
with air in the tracheal system because ultrasound exposure precedes
tracheal development by approximately 11 hours.

Yolk quantity varies greatly between the eggs of birds and mammals, yet their patterns of early embryonic development are quite similar. Both the mammalian and bird blastodisc consist of two layers;
the epiblast and the hypoblast. Gastrulation of mammals including
humans, resembles that of birds with the formation of a primitive

streak. Cells from the primitive streak subsequently migrate between the hypoblast and the epiblast, giving rise to a trilaminar embryo. Chick embryos have been used extensively in both developmental and teratological studies, because they are relatively inexpensive and easy to maintain. Not only are the developmental stages well documented, but the acoustical properties of both the egg white and yolk have been characterized (Javanaud et al., 1984).

It appears that the chick embryo would be an ideal system for investigating the developmental effects of ultrasound. However, because the embryo is surrounded by a hard shell, investigators have the problem of determining the most appropriate method for delivering ultrasound. Early use of ultrasound in the food industry revealed that ultrasound could be used to evaluate the quality of eggs and to clean the outer shells in preparation for market, but little information was available on what effect ultrasound might have on the eggs' contents. Nikolov (1970) demonstrated that these commercial sonicators could affect the physiochemical properties of eggs. The outer shells appeared quite normal after a 5 - 10 minute sonic exposure but the viscosity and optical density of the inner contents were altered.

Studies centered on development, using lower intensities, found no effect on the embryo if eggs were exposed intact (Vazquex, 1963). The outer shell and air space inside the egg cause significant attenuation and reflection of the ultrasound beam. The outer egg shell itself is impermeable to ultrasound at diagnostic frequencies and it has been estimated that only 1/10,000 of the total acoustic power applied to an intact egg ever reaches the embryo when 2 MHz ultrasound is used (Sofia and Lele, 1975).

There are different techniques used to deliver ultrasound energy directly to the embryo; each has benefits and drawbacks. First, a small window can be cut into the outer shell to expose the embryo. Although this technique minimizes the influence of external factors, it is difficult to define the exposure conditions. In an alternate method the shell is completely removed prior to ultrasound exposure. Eggs can be opened at various stages of incubation and the contents can then be carefully transferred and maintained in a vessel designed for ultrasonic exposure. Although this method may allow more control over the exposure conditions, it removes the embryo from its natural environment and subjects it to various physical factors, which alone may have an adverse effect on development.

Taylor and Dyson (1972) exposed excised chick embryos with 1 MHz, pulsed ultrasound. In this procedure, after the shell was removed, the embryo and its extraembryonic membranes were lifted from the yolk and transferred to an exposure receptacle. The internal contents were discarded and only the embryo and its associated membranes were placed in the ultrasound field. Exposure to "peak intensities" of 40 W/cm^2 (pulsed 20 usec on and 180 usec off) during the head process stage (18-20 hours incubation) resulted in an increased incidence of fetal abnormalities. This increase in abnormalities was not observed when the peak intensity was reduced to 10 W/cm^2 or when the embryos were exposed during a later stage of gestation (42+ hours incubation). These results support the concept of increased sensitivity of the embryo during early stages of gestation and suggests the importance of peak parameters in determining threshold intensities which might affect development. Barnett (1983) has pointed out that the effects observed by Taylor and Dyson could have been enhanced by their exposure conditions because they exposed chick embryos in glass beakers.

This could result in reflection of the ultrasound beam and possible formation of standing waves which subsequently could intensify the total dose delivered to the embryo.

Barnett (1983) exposed chick embryos through a small window cut into the outer shell. Embryos were exposed to 4.5 W/cm^2 (SPTA) pulsed and 100 W/cm^2 (SPTA) CW focused ultrasound at 18 - 26 hours incubation. This stage of chick development corresponds to the definitive streak blastoderm stage and is equivalent to approximately 3 weeks gestation in the human fetus. All exposures were for 5 minutes at a frequency of 3 MHz. The pulse exposures used an SPTP intensity of 100 W/cm^2 and a 1 usec pulse duration. Although occasional abnormalities were found in both the treated and sham exposed embryos, these were attributed to experimental manipulation of the eggs and not to ultrasound treatment. In general, no lethal or developmental effects were observed during the 72 hours following ultrasonic treatment.

Vazquex (1963) investigated cephalic changes in chick embryos exposed to 0.87 MHz, CW ultrasound. Chick embryos between 29 - 49 hours incubation were exposed through a shell window to intensities ranging from 0.5 - 3.0 W/cm^2 for up to 30 minutes. This stage of incubation corresponds to the closure of the neural tube and the initiation of morphogenetic events in auditory development. This ultrasonic exposure resulted in damage to the central nervous system, the auditory organ, oral cavity and facial features. Severity of the malformations was strongly dependent on the stage at which the embryo was exposed, with the earlier stages of gestation showing the greatest sensitivity.

Shpuntoff (1985) used the same exposure method and observed growth inhibition in chick embryos exposed to low frequency ultrasound (29 kHz) on day 5 of incubation. Although this frequency is not used in fetal diagnostic procedures it is used in the field of dentistry and the author cautions that the dental application of low frequency ultrasound may adversely affect rapidly developing oral tissues.

The chick embryo has been used to investigate the effects of ultrasound on a developing system. Positive results have been attributed to experimental manipulations affecting the embryo or exposure conditions which result in phenomena not expected to be major factors in diagnostic situations, e.g., standing wave formation or heat production. The chick embryo model has also been used to study endpoints that are not development oriented, e.g., blood stasis (Dyson et al., 1971, 1974; Dyson and Pond, 1973) and cardiac function (Ruckman et al., 1985). Discussion of these studies have been omitted in this review.

MAMMALIAN SYSTEMS

There are several distinct advantages to using mammalian systems in the evaluation of developmental effects of ultrasound. Mammals provide a system which more closely approximates the human situation than the nonmammalian systems discussed thus far. The influences of placental interaction and maternal compensation on fetal development can be evaluated. The pregnant mammal undergoes many physiologic changes to provide an environment optimal for fetal development. Ultrasound could affect normal maternal and/or placental functions resulting in a potential compromise on fetal development. The use of a mammalian system thereby increases the chances of detecting an indirect effect on the fetus. Although mammalian systems better approximate the human situation, extrapolating data beyond the scope of a study must be avoided. Because of variations in reproductive systems and cycles of mammalian species, developmental toxicity data obtained from one species may not be directly applicable to other species.

Developmental testing utilizing mammalian systems are not without its drawbacks. Experimental manipulation of the mother and/or the fetus can introduce stress or other physical factors which may alter the normal embryonic environment resulting in adverse effects on fetal development. In all mammals, including humans, the precise time of fertilization is difficult to determine. Even when timed mating of animals is performed, the method of calculating gestational age may vary among investigators. There is also the problem of accurately determining embryonic and fetal dose.

As mentioned above, there is a great deal of variation in the reproductive systems and cycles of various species. Table 1 compares the approximate gestation periods and developmental times of some important organ systems in humans and other animals compiled by Hoar and Monie (1981). Even within the same species, factors such as strain specificity, experimental manipulations, and varying exposure parameters make comparison of interlaboratory data difficult.

Because organogenesis is considered by many investigators to be a critical period of development, many studies investigating the embryotoxic or embryolethal potential of a drug or physical agent direct fetal exposure to this stage of gestation. Developmental ultrasound studies are no exception, with the bulk of available data coming from fetal exposures during this period. Traditionally, most basic texts on developmental biology begin with a discussion of the germ cells, followed by the processes involved in fertilization and then sequentially cover developmental events as they occur. The following review will summarize the reported effects of ultrasound on developing mammalian systems in a similar fashion; according to the stage of development during which exposure occurred.

I. The Germ Cells

The first section briefly discusses the effects on testicular and ovarian tissue that have been attributed to ultrasonic exposure. Possible genetic damage produced by ultrasound exposure will not be covered in this review. The endpoints of studies involving exposure of the testes and ovaries have concentrated on two areas, histological damage and functional integrity.

There is little doubt that ultrasound can cause histological damage, but the evidence for functional damage is less clear. Hyperthermia induced by a 5 minute exposure to 3 MHz, CW ultrasound (1 W/cm^2) resulted in a moderate disruption of spermatogenesis and destruction of over half the seminiferous tubules examined in exposed rat testes (Abadir et al., 1979). Ionizing radiation was shown to enhance the ultrasound effect resulting in complete disruption of spermatogenesis. Fry et al. (1978) demonstrated that if the exposure intensity was high enough, testicular exposure to 1.3 MHz ultrasound could produce mortality in adult mice. Mortality was observed in males exposed to 70 W/cm^2 (SPTA) for 20 seconds at each matrix location; 36 testicular exposure sites per animal. These investigators found testicular irradiation to CW ultrasound produced a higher mortality rate than pulsed ultrasonic exposure at the same average intensity. Exposed males that survived showed no significant difference in

TABLE 1. Comparative Development of Specific Organ Systems and Gestation Periods*

	Implantation	Primitive Streak	Neural Plate	Optic Vesicle Formation	S-shaped Heart	Lower Limb Bud	Embryonic Period	Gestation Period
Man	7.5	17.0	19.0	24.0	25.0	32.0	57.0	267.0
Macaque	9.0	17.0	20.0	23.0	25.0	28.0	46.0	167.0
Guinea Pig	6.5	13.0	13.5	15.5	16.0	18.5	26.0	67.0
Rabbit	7.5	7.5	8.0	9.0	9.5	11.0	19.5	32.0
Rat	6.0	9.0	9.5	10.5	10.0	12.0	17.0	22.0
Mouse	5.0	8.0	7.0	9.5	8.5	10.3	15.0	19.0
Hamster	5.0	7.0	7.5	8.0	8.5	9.75	12.0	16.0
Chicken	–	0.5	1.0	1.3	2.0	3.0	5.5	21.0

* Adapted from Hoar, R. M., and Monie, I. W., 1981, Comparative development of specific organ systems, in: Developmental Toxicology, C. A., Kimmel and J. Buelke-Sam, eds., Raven Press, New York.

fertility when compared to controls. Other investigators have demonstrated that gonadal function in mice is resistant to ultrasound exposure, even when the energies delivered were sufficient to produce burns (Kirsten et al., 1963). Lyon and Simpson (1974) reported similar findings. Male mice were exposed for 15 minutes to either CW or pulsed 1.5 MHz ultrasound. CW exposures were conducted at an intensity of 1.6 W/cm^2. Pulsed exposure were conducted at average intensities of 0.9 W/cm^2 or 1.6 W/cm^2 (45 W/cm^2 or 6.4 W/cm^2, peak) with pulse durations of 30 usec and 1 msec, respectively. After examination, treated males showed no indication of sterility and no decrease in testicular weight or sperm count when compared with controls.

Histological examination of the testes reveals that the degree of damage at the cellular level resulting from ultrasonic exposure varies with cell type. O'Brien et al. (1979) observed that ultrasound was capable of disrupting testicular tissue by affecting both spermatocytogenesis and spermogenesis. Contrary to the effects following exposure to ionizing radiation, 1 MHz ultrasound (25 W/cm^2 SPTA) for 30 seconds showed spermatocytes to be the more sensitive cell type in mice. Similar findings have been observed in rats. Spermatocytes and spermatids in testicular tissue exposed for 5 or 10 minutes to 1.1 MHz, CW ultrasound at an intensity of 1 W/cm^2, developed irregular membranes and their intracellular contents were released into the surrounding interstitium (Dumontier et al., 1977). Other cell types, spermatogonia, Sertoli and Leydig cells appear resistant to the effects of ultrasonic exposure (Dumontier et al., 1977; Bailey et al., 1981), and because these stem and support cells maintain their morphologic and functional integrity, only temporary sterility from ultrasonic exposure was observed (Dumontier et al., 1977).

It should be emphasized that the ultrasonic intensities and exposure durations utilized in these studies are well in excess of those used in diagnostic practice and the observed effects have been attributed to tissue heating. In a study which utilized lower intensities, Smyth (1966) exposed the testicular area of mice to 10 mW/cm^2, 2.25 MHz, pulsed ultrasound for 10 or 20 minutes on 5 consecutive days. Exposed mice exhibited no differences upon histological examination and no alteration in reproductive competence when compared to controls.

Similar results have been observed in the ovaries of female mice and rats. If ultrasonic intensities are high enough, bilateral sonication of mouse ovaries with 1.3 MHz, pulsed ultrasound can result in death (Fry et al., 1978). Mortality was observed in females exposed to 70 W/cm^2 (SPTA) for 20 seconds at each matrix site; each ovary was irradiated at five positions. When exposure intensities were lowered, there was no statistically significant difference in pup weights, number of late resorptions, and runts born to mothers exposed prior to mating. There was, although, a surprising increase in litter size of irradiated females when compared to controls. Lyon and Simpson (1974) found no induction of genetic dominant lethals and no significant alteration in pre-implantation viability in females subjected to ovarian irradiation of the same intensities that were used in the studies on testicular tissue discussed earlier.

Comparable to the observed testicular effects, the alterations observed in ovarian function and cellular architecture are generally attributed to exposure conditions and/or parameters which facilitate tissue heating. Bailey et al. (1983) accessed the ultrasonically induced morphologic damage to mouse ovaries. Mouse ovaries were exposed to 1 MHz, CW ultrasound at spatial peak intensities of 5 to

100 W/cm^2 for up to 5 minutes. These intensities are greater than
those typically used for clinical therapeutic applications. Observed
tissue alterations consisted of pycnosis and general disruption and
alteration of cytoplasm of cells and vacuolization of cells and
tissue, with the extent of damage varying with cell type. Luteinized
cells were found to be the most sensitive, whereas oocytes of all
types were the most resistant to ultrasonic insult. In subsequent
work, they evaluated the temperature elevation in exteriorized mouse
ovaries produced by ultrasonic exposure. Temperature elevations
resulting from exposure of 10 W/cm^2 (SPTA) or less were not sufficient
to produce ovarian tissue damage but 25 W/cm^2 (SPTA) or more resulted
in damaging thermal levels (Bailey et al., 1984).

Smyth (1966) used the same exposure regime previously described
with testicular tissue to investigate effects on the ovary resulting
from ultrasonic exposure at diagnostic power levels. Due to apparatus
limitations, only the right ovary of each mouse was exposed to ultrasound. Functional and histological results indicated there were no
deleterious effects associated with ultrasound.

From the data available, it appears unlikely that ultrasonic exposure to intensities in the diagnostic range produces any effect on the
structural or functional integrity of testicular or ovarian tissue.

II. From Fertilization to Organogenesis

There are a few studies which have focused on the effects of fetal
exposure during earlier stages of development. The major events in
the first seven days of fetal mouse development include cleavage, the
concurrent processes of gastrulation and implantation, followed by
formation of the primitive streak. With all these developmental
events occurring in what corresponds to the first trimester in rodents
and reports suggesting increased fetal sensitivity during earlier
stages of development, it is surprising more studies have not investigated the potential fetal effects resulting from ultrasonic exposure
during these early stages of gestation.

Investigating the effects of pulsed ultrasound on fetal development, Warwick et al. (1970) and Woodward et al. (1970) exposed pregnant mice on the first five days of gestation. The pregnant dams were
lightly anesthetized with ether, then semi-submerged over the transducer so that ultrasound could be delivered to their ventral side.
The animals were exposed for five consecutive days to either 1, 2 or
3 MHz, pulsed ultrasound, at time averaged intensities of 0.75 –
27.0 W/cm^2 (20 – 490 W/cm^2, SPTP) for up to 420 seconds. Repeated
exposures on each animal on five successive days were performed in an
attempt to maximize the chance of producing an effect. Although the
intensities used in these experiments are well above those used in
clinical practice, the authors found no significant effect on litter
size, incidence of resorptions, or abnormalities which could be
attributed to ultrasound exposure. This study does suffer from some
design flaws. The number of subjects in some exposure groups are
small, too small in some cases to detect a low probability event or to
generate meaningful statistical data.

Stolzenberg et al. (1980a) exposed mouse embryos in utero to various durations and power intensities of 2 MHz ultrasound. Either CW
or burst mode (20% duty factor, 1 or 10 msec bursts) ultrasound was
used. Various stages of gestation were chosen for exposure, each representing a critical period of embryonic or fetal development. Exposure of dams on either day 1 (approximately first cleavage), day 2

(2 cell to 4 cell stage), or day 4 (concurrent gastrulation and implantation), were performed to detect any alteration in development which might arise from ultrasonic exposure prior to organogenesis. The other stages of pregnancy on which exposures occurred were organogenesis and organ tissue differentiation, gestational days 8 and 13, respectively. They observed that the mammalian embryo is resistant to insult prior to implantation and that an insult severe enough to affect embryonic development would either kill the embryo outright or produce a growth inhibiting effect resulting in reduced fetal weight with no associated fetal malformation. They also emphasized the potential for an indirect effect on the embryo produced by damaging maternal tissue, such as the uterus, ovaries, or placenta, all of which influence implantation and the maintenance of pregnancy. No adverse effects were observed in the fetuses, placentae, or ovarian tissues of dams exposed to 1 W/cm^2 (either burst or CW) for exposures up to 100 seconds. If exposure durations were increased (200 - 400 seconds), deleterious fetal effects were only observed under exposure conditions which produced maternal effects. The authors concluded that the ultrasound produced an indirect effect on the fetus by altering maternal tissue and/or function. Under these exposure conditions, thermistor probes indicated uterine tissue temperature elevations in excess of 40°C; therefore, the effects were assumed to be thermally mediated.

Akamatsu (1981) used a flush method to remove preimplantation embryos from the oviducts of rats and mice. Embryos in the late morula or early blastula stage were subsequently exposed in vitro to ultrasonic or thermal insult. A significant increase in morphological abnormalities and developmental retardation was observed in embryos exposed to 3.0 W/cm^2 CW ultrasound at a frequency of 2 MHz for 60 minutes. Similar results were obtained at lower intensities (0.65, 1.0, 1.8 W/cm^2) when exposures were extended to 12 hours. Embryos irradiated with 2 MHz, pulsed ultrasound (0.03 - 0.6 W/cm^2, SATA; 11 - 200 W/cm^2, SPTP) appeared unaffected, whereas embryos exposed to CW ultrasound exhibited similar effects to embryos exposed to elevated temperatures. Again, the results suggest the thermal mechanism of action is responsible for producing the observed embryonic effects.

Stratmeyer et al. (1981) observed a significant weight reduction in mice exposed to ultrasound during early stages of gestation. Mice were exposed in utero to 1 MHz, CW ultrasound. Pregnant mice were exposed to either 0, 0.075, or 0.750 W/cm^2 for 120 seconds on days 4, 10, or 14 of gestation. The exposure conditions were designed to prevent an increase above normal maternal body temperature (Stratmeyer et al., 1984). Analysis of the data indicated a significant decrease in fetal weights of mice exposed on day 4, but not in the fetuses exposed on days 10 or 14 of gestation.

Pizzarello and coworkers (1978) have reported developmental effects in rat embryos exposed to 2.25 MHz, pulsed ultrasound at low temporal average intensities. Rat embryos were exposed in utero on days 3, 5, or 6 of gestation for 5 minutes with a commercial diagnostic unit delivering an average power output of 1.5 mW. After anesthetization, the uterus was exposed by a small medial incision made in the abdominal wall of the pregnant animal. This allowed the transducer to be placed in contact with the uterus and power delivered directly to the uterine wall. Exposure of the embryos produced a decrease in mean fetal dry weight and increased fetal abortion frequency. At an intensity this low, heating due to ultrasonic absorption can be ruled out. When ultrasonic exposure was performed at later stages of development (day 15), these effects were not observed.

The limitations in this study have previously been discussed in the Drosophila work of the nonmammalian section. Because of the clinical implications of Pizzarello's findings, an attempt has been made to replicate this study. Trying to duplicate the exposure conditions and using the same intensities, plus additional exposures at 10 times the peak and average intensity, Child et al. (1984) were unable to reproduce these effects.

Bang (1971) found no developmental effects when fetuses were exposed in utero to 2.25 MHz, CW ultrasound on days 4.5, 5.5 or 6.5. Pregnant dams were exposed to 0.1 - 1.7 W/cm^2 for a duration of 60 seconds or up to 4.3 W/cm^2 for 15 seconds. When the fetuses were removed and examined on day 18 of gestation, there was no significant difference in either the number of fetuses, the number of gross macroscopic or skeletal malformations between control and treated groups.

III. Organogenesis

Most data on ultrasonic developmental biological effects are from studies which concentrated on potential fetal effects produced from exposure during organogenesis. This is the period of gestation when organs and organ systems are developing. Exposures are performed during organogenesis to maximize the possibility of detecting an observable malformation induced by ultrasound.

Various effects associated with fetal development have been attributed to ultrasound exposure during organogenesis. Shoji et al. (1971, 1972, 1975) reported that maternal exposure to ultrasonic waves produced fetal malformations and an increased incidence of intrauterine death in mice. They experimented with two inbred mouse strains, DHS and A/HeMk. Pregnant mice were exposed on day 8 of gestation to 2.25 MHz, CW ultrasound, at an intensity of 40 mW/cm^2 for 5 hours. In these studies the day of plugging was considered gestational day 0, whereas in studies by other investigators the day of plugging was considered day 1 of gestation. In general, fetuses from the treated and sham treated groups had increases in malformations and deaths and decreases in fetal weights when compared with untreated controls. Because sham treatment conditions also induced fetal effects, it was concluded that adverse fetal development resulted from maternal stress produced by the exposure conditions. In subsequent research with rats, fetal effects produced by 100 mW/cm^2 elicited strain specificity. Brain hernia and hydrocephalus were among the abnormalities reported in fetuses of Wistar-King A rats exposed in utero. In contrast, Wistar rat fetuses similarly exposed, appeared resistant to the effects of ultrasound (Shoji and Murakami, 1974).

The experiments by Shoji and coworkers have also been criticized because of the exposure procedure used. In these studies the transducer, coupled with glycerine, was placed in direct contact with the ventral side of the pregnant mice as opposed to partially submersing the animal in a water bath. Because of the tissue-air interface on the dorsal side, essentially all the ultrasonic energy is trapped within the animal. Lele (1975) has reported that in mice exposure to 40 mW/cm^2 under these exposure conditions could produce a temperature rise in excess of 2.5°C; a temperature rise sufficient to account for any teratogenic effects observed in these experiments.

Garrison et al. (1973) investigated the influence of ovarian sonication on fetal development. These investigators pointed out that the ovaries are essential in maintaining pregnancy, and while most studies concentrate on fetal exposures, the ovaries were the primary target in

this investigation. Rats were exposed on day 8 of gestation to
1.9 MHz, pulsed ultrasound at intensities of 10 or 100 W/cm^2 (SATP).
Exposures of 10 minutes/ovary were delivered over the lateral abdominal regions transcutaneously or applied directly to surgically exposed
ovaries. The investigators found no statistically significant
increase in the percent of resorptions and concluded that ultrasound
exposure, under these conditions, produced no alteration in ovarian
function with regard to fetal development.

External, skeletal and visceral abnormalities have been reported
in mouse fetuses exposed on day 8 of gestation to CW ultrasound at a
frequency of 2 MHz (Hara, 1980). Fetuses exposed in utero to 2 W/cm^2
for 5 minutes exhibited a significant increase in the number of brain
hernia, anencephaly, cleft palate and skeletal variations when compared with controls.

Fry et al. (1976, 1978) exposed pregnant mice to either CW or
pulsed 1 MHz ultrasound. Maternal abdominal surfaces were exposed on
days 8 or 9 of gestation for 10 seconds – 10 minutes to CW intensities
ranging from 10 mW/cm^2 – 10 W/cm^2. The pulse exposure regime used the
same intensities plus higher intensities up to 150 W/cm^2. Relatively
long pulse durations, up to 30 μsec, were used. Exposure duration at
the highest intensity was limited to 20 seconds at each matrix site;
128 abdominal exposure sites per uterine horn using a beam width of
2 mm. These exposure parameters resulted in an increase in resorption
sites in the irradiated dams, but effects to viable fetuses were minimal. When teratogenicity did appear, a higher incidence was associated with CW than pulsed exposure.

In another study, mice were exposed on day 8 of gestation to
pulsed ultrasound with average intensities ranging from 0.058 –
0.586 W/cm^2 peak intensities; 3 – 10 μsec pulse duration) for 5
minutes (Takabayashi et al., 1981). Fetal anomalies were observed in
mouse embryos exposed to 59.4 W/cm^2 peak intensity with pulse durations greater than 5 microseconds. If either the peak intensity or
the pulse width was reduced, no deleterious effects were observed.
These results suggest that specific pulse characteristics, not temporal average intensity, may determine the teratogenic potential of
pulsed ultrasound. Unfortunately, this report is brief and important
details on methodology are missing. Ultrasonic frequency is not
specified and lack of dosimetry information makes replication of this
study difficult. Therefore, some caution should be used in the interpretation of these data and results.

O'Brien (1983) induced a significant fetal weight reduction in the
offspring of outbred, CF1 mice with 1 MHz, CW ultrasound. On day 8 of
gestation, pregnant females were exposed to spatial average intensities up to 5.5 W/cm^2 for varying durations. Fetal weight reduction of
exposed animals ranged from 5.3% – 17.5% compared to sham treated animals. When the dose parameter was defined as I^{2}t (where I represents
spatial average intensity and t represents exposure time) further
analysis of the data revealed that the average fetal weight exhibited
a linear dose effect relationship. No significant difference in fetal
weight was observed in pregnant hybrid LAF1/J mice irradiated at
2.5 W/cm^2 under similar exposure conditions (O'Brien, 1982). O'Brien
suggests that the hybrid dams and their progeny elicit greater resistance to the effects of ultrasound compared with outbred strains.

Stolzenberg et al. (1980b) found litter size to be unaffected in
mice exposed to 2 MHz, CW ultrasound. A decrease in mean uterine
weight was observed in the progeny of dams exposed to 0.5 W/cm^2 for

140 seconds or 1 W/cm^2 for 60 seconds. Exposure to a spatial average intensity of 1 W/cm^2 for 40 - 60 seconds produced a decrease in fetal weight when compared with controls but not when compared with sham-treated fetuses. On the other hand, exposure to 0.5 W/cm^2 for 180 seconds produced a significant reduction in neonatal body weight, but only on day 25 postcoitus. Subsequent necropsies revealed that selected organ weights were unaffected by ultrasonic exposure.

Kimmel et al. (1983) exposed mice to 1 MHz, CW ultrasound on day 8 of gestation. Dams were exposed in a 30°C water bath to 0.0, 0.05, 0.50, or 1.0 W/cm^2 for 120 seconds. Fetuses were removed by laparotomy on day 17 of gestation and were extensively examined for external, visceral and skeletal defects. Although the data indicated a slight increase in the incidence of fetal abnormalities, there were no statistically significant differences between groups which could be attributed to ultrasound.

Edmonds et al. (1979) investigated postpartum survival of mice exposed in utero to ultrasound on day 8 of gestation. Pregnant dams were exposed to 2 MHz, CW ultrasound at a spatial average intensity of 0.44 W/cm^2 in a water bath for 60 - 180 seconds. The investigators reported no effect on neonatal mortality and concluded that if the fetuses were affected by ultrasound exposure their viability returned to normal postnatal control values.

Brown et al. (1979, 1981) studied the postnatal behavior and development in mice exposed in utero on days 8 and 9 of gestation. In their earlier report (Brown et al., 1979), altered neurobehavioral development was observed in mouse pups exposed to 1 MHz, CW ultrasound at an intensity of 250 mW/cm^2. The abdominal area over the uterine horns were exposed in a 30°C water bath for 3 minutes on day 9 of gestation. The ultrasound irradiated pups had accelerated or retarded responses to a variety of reflex developmental tests. In their subsequent work (Brown et al., 1981), dams were exposed on day 8 of gestation, and intensities and exposure durations were slightly modified. The pups exposed in utero to 75 mW/cm^2 for 2 minutes exhibited no statistically significant difference in acquisition of conditioned reflexes. Also, pups exposed to 50 or 500 mW/cm^2 for 3 minutes exhibited no statistical difference in reflex development assessed by pivoting, walking, forelimb grip, accelerated righting, and a rotorod test.

Sikov and Hildebrand (1976a, 1977) tested the effects of both CW (0.71 and 3.2 MHz; 2.8-32.4 W/cm^2, SATA) and pulsed (2.5 MHz; 15 - 410 W/cm^2, SATP) ultrasound on development by exposing Wistar rat fetuses at day 9 of gestation. A midline incision was made in the anesthetized mother and the uterine horns were exteriorized. After the uterine horns were exteriorized, two implantation sites in each horn were selected for either ultrasonic or sham exposure. Utilizing this method individual fetuses could be exposed. Exposure times were 5 or 15 minutes and several intensities and pulse durations were used. After exposure the uterine horns were returned to the abdominal cavity and the incision closed. This procedure may produce more stress on the mother and uterine contents, but it allows ultrasonic energy to be delivered directly to the uterine wall. On day 20 of gestation, fetuses were removed, and the effects of sonication were evaluated by detailed teratologic examination. Exposure to sufficiently high levels of ultrasound adversely affected fetal development. The embryotoxic effect was found to be dependent on the mode of ultrasound administered (CW versus pulsed) and the relationship between intensity

and effect was dependent on ultrasonic frequency. From fetal mortality data, an LD_{50} intensity of 17.6 W/cm^2 and an "apparent threshold"
of 3.0 W/cm^2 was calculated. Surviving fetuses had no significant
differences in weight or body length although there was an increased
incidence in fetal malformations associated with exposure intensities
greater than 10.5 W/cm^2. The most prominent effect observed from
pulsed exposure was the production of fetal cardiac abnormalities.
The higher intensities produced increased incidence of septal defects
but this effect did not exhibit intensity dependence. In general,
fetal abnormalities associated with pulsed ultrasound exposure showed
a better correlation with peak intensity than average intensity. In a
subsequent investigation (Sikov et al., 1984) they demonstrated that
the embryotoxic effect observed in the study above was attributed to
heat produced by ultrasound attenuation.

Murai and coworkers (1975a) exposed pregnant rats to 2.3 MHz, CW
ultrasound at an intensity of 20 mW/cm^2. Exposures of 5 hours were
conducted on day 9 of gestation. No significant difference was
observed in physical development or orienting behavior of exposed
pups. Some delay in reflex development was observed between exposed
and untreated control pups; this effect was not observed when exposed
pups were compared with sham treated animals. Although no effect in
cognitive behavior was observed, the offspring of irradiated rats
showed significantly more distinct vocalization when handled and had
more distinct escape responses (Murai et al., 1975b). Because much of
the observed effects could be attributed to the exposure conditions,
it is difficult from this study alone to determine if prenatal ultrasound exposure affects postnatal development.

In an attempt to maximize the chances of producing effects, some
investigators perform multiple consecutive exposures on the same animal for several days. McClain et al. (1972) exposed rats to 2.5 MHz,
CW ultrasound at an intensity of 10 mW/cm^2. Animals were exposed on
days 8, 9 and 10 of gestation for 0.5 or 2.0 hours. The ultrasound
exposure had no effect on litter size or weight and fetuses exhibited
no significant soft tissue or skeletal abnormalities.

These findings are supported by the work of Warwick et al. (1970)
and Woodward et al. (1970), previously described. They found no
effect on litter size, mean resorption rate, or mean abnormality rate
in mice repeatedly exposed to pulsed ultrasound (1, 2 or 3 MHz, 0.75 –
27 W/cm^2, time averaged) on days 8 through 12 of gestation. In contrast, Muranaka et al. (1974) reported a significant increase in fetal
mortality in mothers exposed to 100 mW/cm^2 for 4 minutes daily on days
8 – 14 of gestation. Utilizing 2.3 MHz ultrasound, this exposure
regime and 80 mW/cm^2 for 10 minutes on the same days of gestation
resulted in a 50% reduction in fetal weight. When the intensity was
lowered to 20 mW/cm^2, there was no significant difference in fetal
mortality, growth rate, or external malformations even with daily
maternal exposures of 30 minutes.

Stratmeyer et al. (1977), utilizing a 1 MHz, CW source, performed
in utero fetal exposures in CF1 mice on day 10 of gestation. Anesthetized dams were exposed while in a 30°C water bath to 0.25 or 0.80
W/cm^2 for 120 seconds. Fetuses examined on day 18 postcoitus had no
significant difference in fetal weight. Examination of the live lit-
ters indicated a significant difference in several of the measures of
body and selected organ weights at 21, 36, and 51 days postcoitus,
although the trend in decreasing weight with increasing exposure was
not always consistent. In subsequent work (Stratmeyer et al., 1981,
1984), fetuses born to ICR mice exposed to 0.075 or 0.75 W/cm^2 on day

10 of gestation had a significant difference in some of the organ weights at 200 days postcoitus; again, organ weights were generally less in the exposed groups compared to nonexposed groups.

IV. Morphogenesis and the Late Stages of Development

McClain et al. (1972), Warwick et al. (1970), and Woodward et al. (1970) who all utilized experimental procedures previously described, exposed rats and mice repeatedly during later stages of gestations. Results from these studies were similar to their results obtained at earlier gestational exposures. Rats exposed in utero on days 11, 12, and 13 of gestation to CW ultrasound (2.5 MHz; 10 mW/cm^2; 0.5 or 2.0 hours) had no significant difference in the occurrence of soft tissue or skeletal abnormalities and there was no effect on litter size or weight (McClain et al., 1972). With pulsed ultrasound (1, 2, or 3 MHz; 0.75 - 27.0 W/cm^2, time average intensity; 300 - 420 seconds, exposure duration), no effect on litter size, mean resorption rate, or mean abnormality rate could be attributed to in utero exposure of mice exposed on days 12 - 16 of gestation (Warwick et al., 1970; Woodward et al., 1970).

Curto (1976) observed early postpartum mortality in mice exposed in utero on day 13 of gestation to 1 MHz, CW ultrasound. Mice were exposed in a 30°C water bath to 0.125 - 0.5 W/cm^2 for 3 minutes. Curto's results are different than those of Edmonds et al. (1979), who observed no effect on neonatal mortality; there were differences in methodology between the two studies (ultrasound frequency, time of gestational exposure) which make direct comparison of their results difficult.

Stratmeyer et al. (1984) observed no exposure related pattern of fetal weight or body and organ weights in mice exposed in utero on day 14 of gestation to 1 MHz, CW ultrasound (0.075 and 0.75 W/cm^2 for 120 seconds) and examined on day 200 postcoitus.

Sikov et al. (1976) observed an intensity related prenatal mortality in rats exposed on day 15 of gestation. CW ultrasound (0.95 MHz) up to 1.0 W/cm^2 was delivered to exteriorized uterine horns for 5 minutes. Consistent with the results of Edmonds et al. (1979), no postnatal mortality or reduced growth rate was observed; subsequent behavioral testing of the offspring indicated a general delay in neuromuscular development of the exposed animals, although no persistent neuromuscular deficits were observed.

As part of a larger study, Smith (1966) exposed mice to 2.25 MHz at 10 mW/cm^2 for 10 minutes per day. In the teratogenic portion of this study, Smith exposed both males and females for 5 consecutive days before mating; during 10 days of mating, and then pregnant females alone throughout gestation until 2 days before delivery. These conditions, multiple CW ultrasound exposures at diagnostic levels, produced no congenital malformations in the offspring born to the exposed group or in the offspring born to the second generation of the exposure group.

CONCLUSIONS

In recent years, as technology has advanced, new medical devices and procedures have evolved with increased capability of monitoring fetal development, even at very early stages of development. Ultrasound is essential in many of these procedures, however some of the newer diagnostic ultrasound instruments operate at higher intensity levels than earlier instruments. For these reasons, it is more imperative than ever that we understand how, and under what conditions, ultrasound affects biological development.

A review of studies of the effects of ultrasound on developing organisms indicates that the biological data is highly variable and often inconclusive. Most studies reporting deleterious effects have used either intensity levels or exposure conditions which resulted in in situ exposures far in excess of those expected under clinical ultrasound diagnosis and are associated with elevated tissue temperatures. Often studies did not include sham-controls making it impossible to determine if experimental procedures other than ultrasound (maternal manipulation, anesthesia, restraint, etc.) may have produced maternal stress responsible for the observed effects. Few of the endpoints which have been examined involved functional deficits, which are sometimes more sensitive indicators of damage than are anatomic lesions. In general, the biology in the ultrasound bioeffects literature is not contemporary.

Because the current data are inadequate to exclude the existence of immediate effects with low probability of occurrence or delayed developmental effects, future research should concentrate on determining if such effects exist under conditions relevant to diagnostic ultrasound. Ideally, such research efforts would be conducted under a coordinated program designed to utilize the knowledge and methodology of contemporary developmental biology and the established expertise of ultrasound physics and dosimetry. Until more adequate information is available, a prudent approach to using obstetrical ultrasound would be to obtain the necessary diagnostic information using the least possible exposure (a combination of intensity or power and time). Because this approach demands a great deal of judgement on behalf of the clinician, it goes without saying that it also demands a great degree of understanding of the biology and physics of ultrasound exposure.

REFERENCES

Abadir, R., Harman, J., and Fahim, M., 1979, Enhancement of ionizing radiation effect on the testes of rats by microwave or ultrasound-induced hyperthermia, J Med., 10(1+2):1-12.
Akamatsu, N., 1981, Ultrasound irradiation effects on pre-implantation embryos, Acta Obstet Gynaecol Jpn., 33(7):969-78.
Andrew, D. S., 1964, Ultrasonography in pregnancy - an inquiry into its safety, Br J Radiol., 37(435):185-6.
Bailey, K. I., O'Brien, W. D., Jr., and Dunn, F., 1981, Ultrasonically induced, in vivo morphological damage in mouse testicular tissue, Arch Androl., 6:301-6.
Bailey, K. I., O'Brien, W. D., Jr., and Dunn, F., 1983, Ultrasonically induced morphological damage to mouse ovaries, Ultrasound Med Biol., 9(1):25-31.
Bailey, K. I., O'Brien, W. D., Jr., and Dunn F., 1984, Ultrasonically induced temperature elevation in mouse ovary, Ultrasound Med Biol., 10(4):L492-99.
Bang, J., 1971, The effects of continuous ultrasound on pregnant mice and measurement of intra-uterine energy levels, Ultrasonographia Medica., 1:495-501.
Barnett, S. B., 1983, The influence of ultrasound on embryonic development, Ultrasound Med Biol., 9(1):19-24.
Beck, F., 1981, Comparative placental morphology and function, in: "Developmental Toxicology," C. A. Kimmel and J. Buelke-Sam, eds., Raven Press, New York.

Berg, R. B., Child, S. Z., and Carstensen, E. L., 1983, The influence of carrier frequency on the killing of Drosophila larvae by microsecond pulses of ultrasound, Ultrasound Med Biol., 9(4):L448-51.

Brix, K. A., 1982, Environmental and occupational hazards to the fetus, J Reprod Med., 27(9):577-583.

Brown, N. T., Galloway, W. D., Monahan, J. C., and Fisher, B. R., 1979, Postnatal behavior and development following in utero exposure of mice to ultrasound and microwave radiation, in: "Proceeding of the Fifth FDA Science Symposium," Arlington, VA, 161-3.

Brown, N. T., Galloway, W. D., and Henton, W. W., 1981, Reflex development following in utero exposure to ultrasound, in: "Proceedings of the 26th Annual Meeting of the American Institute of Ultrasound in Medicine," San Francisco, CA, 119.

Carstensen, E. L., and Child, S. Z., 1980, Effects of ultrasound on Drosophila - II. The heating mechanism, Ultrasound Med Biol., 6:257-61.

Carstensen, E. L., Berg, R. B., and Child, S. Z., 1983, Pulse average versus maximum intensity, Ultrasound Med Biol., 9(4):L451-5.

Child, S. Z., Carstensen, E. L., and Smachlo, K., 1980(a), Effects of ultrasound on Drosophila - I. Killing of eggs exposed to traveling and standing wave fields, Ultrasound Med Biol., 6:127-30.

Child, S. Z., Carstensen, E. L., and Davis, H. T., 1980(b), A test for "miniature flies" following exposure of Drosophila melanogaster larvae to diagnostic levels of ultrasound, Exp Cell Biol., 48:461-6.

Child, S. Z., Carstensen, E. L., and Lam, S. K., 1981, Effects of ultrasound on Drosophila: III. Exposure of larvae to low-temporal-average-intensity, pulsed irradiation, Ultrasound Med Biol., 7:167-73.

Child, S. Z., and Carstensen, E. L., 1982, Effects of ultrasound on Drosophila - IV. Pulsed exposures of eggs, Ultrasound Med Biol., 8(3):311-2.

Child, S. Z., Carstensen, E. L., and Davis, H., 1984, A test for the effects of low-temporal-average-intensity pulsed ultrasound on the rat fetus, Exp Cell Biol., 52:207-10.

Counce, S. J., and Selman, G. G., 1955, The effects of ultrasonic treatment on embryonic development of Drosophila melanogaster, J Embryol Exp Morph., 3(2):121-41.

Curto, K. A., 1976, Early postpartum mortality following ultrasound radiation, in: "Proceedings of the 20th Annual Meeting of the American Institute of Ultrasound in Medicine," D. White and R. Barnes, eds., Ultrasound in Medicine, New York, 2:535-6.

Dumontier, A., Burdick, A., Ewigman, B., and Fahim, M. S., 1977, Effects of sonication on mature rat testes, Fertility and Sterility, 28(2):195-204.

Dyson, M., Woodward, B., and Pond, J B., 1971, Flow of red blood cells stopped by ultrasound, Nature, 232:572-3.

Dyson, M., and Pond, J. B., 1973, The effects of ultrasound on circulation, Physiotherapy, 59(9):284-7.

Dyson, M., Pond, J. B., Woodward, B., and Broadbent, J., 1974, The production of blood cell stasis and endothelial damage in the blood vessels of chick embryos treated with ultrasound in a stationary wave field, Ultrasound Med Biol., 1:133-48.

Edmonds, P. D., Stolzenberg, S. J., Torbit, C. A., Madan, S. M., and Pratt, D. E., 1979, Postpartum survival of mice exposed in utero to ultrasound, J Acoust Soc Am., 66(2):590-3.

Fritz-Niggli, H., and Boni, A., 1950, Biological experiments on Drosophila melanogaster and supersonic vibrations, Science, 112:120-2.

Fry, F. J., Dunn, F., Brady, J., Erdmann, W. D., and Strang, P., 1976, Ultrasonic toxicity study of the mouse reproductive system and the pregnant uterus, in: "Proceedings of the 20th Annual Meeting of the American Institute of Ultrasound in Medicine," D. White and R. Barnes, eds., Ultrasound in Medicine, New York, 2:533-4.

Fry, F. J., Erdmann, W. A., Johnson, L. K., and Baird, A. I., 1978, Ultrasonic toxicity study, Ultrasound Med Biol., 3:351-66.

Garrison, B. M., Bo, W. J., Krueger, W. A., Kremkau, F. W., and McKinney, W. M., 1973, The influence of ovarian sonication on fetal development in the rat, J Clin Ultrasound, 1(4):316-9.

German, J., 1984, Embryonic stress hypothesis of teratogenesis, Am J Med., 76:293-301.

Hara, K., 1980, Effects of ultrasonic irradiation on chromosomes, cell division and developing embryos, Acta Obstet Gynaecol Jpn., 32(1):61-8.

Hoar, R., and Monie, I. W., 1981, Comparative development of specific organ systems, in: "Developmental Toxicology," C. A. Kimmel and J. Buelke-Sam, eds., Raven Press, New York.

Javanaud, C., Ragalkar, R. R., and Richmond, P., 1984, Measurement of speed and attenuation of ultrasound in egg white and egg yolk, J Acoust Soc Am., 76(3):670-5.

Kimmel, C. A., Stratmeyer, M. E., Galloway, W. D., LaBorde, J. B., Brown, N. T., and Pinkavitch, F., 1983, The embryotoxic effects of ultrasound exposure in pregnant ICR mice, Teratology, 27:245-51.

Kirsten, E. I., Zinserr, H. H., and Aeid, J. M., 1963, Effect of 1 Mc ultrasound on the genetics of mice, IEEE Transact Ultrasonics Eng., 22:112-116.

Lele, P. P., 1975, Ultrasonic teratology in mouse and man, in: "Proceedings of the 2nd European Congress of Ultrasonics in Medicine," Excerpta Medica., Amsterdam, Holland.

McClain, R. M., Hoar, R. M., and Saltzman, M. B., 1972, Teratologic study of rats exposed to ultrasound, Am J Obstet Gynecol., 114(1):39-42.

Murai, N., Hoshi, K., and Nakamura, T., 1975(a), Effects of diagnostic ultrasound irradiated during fetal stage on development of orienting behavior and reflex ontogeny in rats, Tohoku J Exp Med., 116:17-24.

Murai, N., Hoshi, K., Kang, C. H., and Suzuki, M., 1975(b), Effects of diagnostic ultrasound irradiated during foetal stage on emotional and cognitive behavior in rats, Tohoku J Exp Med., 117:225-35.

Muranaka, A., Tachibana, M., and Suzuki, M., 1974, Effects of ultrasound on embryonic development and fetal growth in mice, Teratology, 10(1):91.

Nikolov, S. K. H., 1970, Hygienic evaluation of hens' eggs processed with low-frequency ultrasound, Gig Sanit., 35(8):38-41.

O'Brien, W. D., Jr., Brady, J. K., and Dunn, F., 1979, Morphological changes to mouse testicular tissue from in vivo ultrasonic irradiation, Ultrasound Med Biol., 5:(1C)35-43.

O'Brien, W. D., Jr., Januzik, S. J., and Dunn, F., 1982, Ultrasound biologic effects: A suggestion of strain specificity, J Ultrasound Med., 1:367-70.

O'Brien, W. D., Jr., 1983, Dose-dependent effect of ultrasound on fetal weight in mice, J Ultrasound Med., 2:1-8.

Pay, T. L., Andersen, F. A., and Jessup, G. L., Jr., 1978, Survival of Drosophila melanogaster pupa exposed to ultrasound, Rad Research, 75:236-41.

Pay, T. L., Hellman, K. B., and Sternthal, P. M., 1982, Effects of
    ultrasound on the longevity and reproductivity capacity of the
    female fruit fly Drosophila melanogaster, Ultrasound Med Biol.,
    8:549–52.
Pay, T. L., Stratmeyer, M. E., and Barrick, M. K., 1985, The effects
    of high peak short pulsed ultrasound on the eggs of Drosophila
    melanogaster, J Ultrasound Med., 4(10):23.
Pizzarello, D. J., Vivino, A., Madden, B., Wolsky, A., Keegan, A. F.,
    and Becker, M., 1978, Effect of pulsed low-power ultrasound on
    growing tissues I. Developing mammalian and insect tissue, Exp
    Cell Biol., 46:179–91.
Ruckman, R. N., Stratmeyer, M. E., O'Donnell, R. M., Morse, D. E., and
    Getson, P. R., in press, The effects of ultrasound on embryonic
    heart function, UFFC Trans.
Rugh, R., 1968, in: "The Mouse: Its Reproduction and Development,"
    Burgess Publishing Company, Minneapolis, MN.
Sarvazyan, A. P., Beloussov, L. V., Petropavlovskaya, M. N., and
    Ostroumova, T. V., 1982, The action of low-intensity pulsed
    ultrasound on amphibian embryonic tissues, Ultrasound Med
    Biol., 8(6):639–54.
Selman, G. G., and Counce, S. J., 1953, Abnormal embryonic development
    in Drosophila induced by ultrasonic treatment, Nature,
    172:503–4.
Selman, G. G., and Jurand, A., 1964, An electron microscope study of
    the endoplasmic reticulum in newt notochord cells after dis-
    turbance with ultrasonic treatment and subsequent regeneration,
    J Cell Biol., 20:175–83.
Shoji, R., Momma, E., Shimizu, T., and Matsuda, S., 1971, An experi-
    mental study on the effect of low-intensity ultrasound on
    developing mouse embryos, J Fac Sci Hokkaido Univ Scr Vl,
    Zool., 18(1):51–6.
Shoji, R., Momma, E., Shimizu, T., and Matsuda, S., 1972, Experimental
    studies on the effect of ultrasound on mouse embryos,
    Teratology, 6:119.
Shoji, R., and Murakami, U., 1974, Further studies on the effect of
    ultrasound on mouse and rat embryos, Teratology, 10:97.
Shoji, R., Murakami, U., and Shimizu, T., 1975, Influence of low-
    intensity ultrasonic irradiation on prenatal development of two
    inbred mouse strains, Teratology, 12(3):227–31.
Shpuntoff, H., and Wuchinich, D., 1984, Embryotoxic and teratogenic
    effect of high intensity, low frequency ultrasonic vibration on
    chicken embryos, Ultrasound Med Biol., 10(6):697–700.
Sikov, M. R., and Hildebrand, B. P., 1976(a), Effects of ultrasound on
    the prenatal development of the rat. Part 1. 3.2 MHZ continuous
    wave at nine days of gestation, J Clin Ultrasound, 4(5):357–63.
Sikov, M. R., Hildebrand, B. P, and Stearns, J. D., 1976(b), Postnatal
    sequelae of ultrasound exposure at fifteen days of gestation in
    the rat, in: "Proceedings of the 1st Triennial Meeting of the
    World Federation for Ultrasound in Medicine and Biology,"
    D. White and R. E. Brown, eds., Ultrasound In Medicine, New
    York, 3B Eng Aspects:2017–23.
Sikov, M. R., and Hildebrand, B. P., 1977, Embryotoxicity of ultra-
    sound exposure at nine days of gestation in the rat, in: "Pro-
    ceedings of the 1st Triennial Meeting of the World Federation
    for Ultrasound in Medicine and Biology," D. White and R. E.
    Brown, eds., Ultrasound in Medicine, New York, 3B:2009–16.
Sikov, M. R., Collins, D. H., and Carr, D. B., 1984, Measurement of
    temperature rise in prenatal rats during exposure of the exter-
    iorized uterus to ultrasound, IEEE Trans Sonics and
    Ultrasonics, SU-31(5):497–503.

216

Smyth, M. G., 1966, Animal toxicity studies with ultrasound at diagnostic power levels, in: "Diagnostic Ultrasound," C. C. Grossman, J. H. Holmes, C. Joyner and E. W. Purnell, eds., Plenum Press, New York, 296-9.

Sofia, J. W., and Lele, P. P., 1975, Avian egg as a test system for ultrasonic teratology studies, in: "Proceedings of the III New England Bioengineering Conference," Tufts University.

Stark, C. R., Orleans, M., Haverkamp, A. D., and Murphy, J., 1984, Short- and long-term risks after exposure to diagnostic ultrasound in utero, Obstet Gynecol., 63(2):194-200.

Stewart, H. F., and Harris, G. R., in press, Characterization of acoustic output from diagnostic ultrasound equipment, in: "Proceedings of Ultrasonics International '85," Ultrasonics, July 1-3, 1985, London, England.

Stolzenberg, S. J., Torbit, C. A., Edmonds, P. D., and Taenzer, J. C., 1980(a), Effects of ultrasound on the mouse exposed at different stages of gestation: acute studies, Radiat Environ Biophys., 17:245-70.

Stolzenberg, S. J., Torbit, C. A., Pryor, G. T., and Edmonds, P. D., 1980(b), Toxicity of ultrasound in mice: neonatal studies, Radiat Environ Biophys., 18:37-44.

Stratmeyer, M. E., Pinkavitch, F. Z., Simmons, L. R., and Sternthal, P., 1981, In utero effects of ultrasound exposure in mice, in: "Proceedings of the 26th Annual Meeting of the American Institute of Ultrasound in Medicine," San Francisco, CA, 121.

Stratmeyer, M. E., Simmons, L. R., Jessup, G. L., O'Brien, W. D., Jr., and Pinkavitch, F. Z., 1977, Growth and development in mice exposed in utero to ultrasound, in: "Symposium on Biological Effects and Characterization of Ultrasound Sources," Bureau of Radiological Health, DHEW Publication No. HEW (FDA) 78-8048, Rockville, MD, 140-5.

Stratmeyer, M. E., Pinkavitch, F. Z., Simmons, L. R., and Sternthal, P., 1981, Effects of in utero ultrasound exposure on the growth and development of mice, 1981, in: "Fifth Annual Meeting of Ultrasound in Medicine and Biology," Puschino, Russia.

Stratmeyer, M. E., Galloway, W. D., Brown, N. T., and Tully, M. J., 1984, In utero effects of ultrasound exposure in ICR mice, J Ultrasound Med., 3(9):31.

Takabayashi, T., Abe, Y., Sato, S., Sato, A., and Suzuki, M., 1981, Effects of pulse-wave ultrasonic irradiation on mouse embryos, Tokoho J Exp Med., 8(4):281.

Taylor, K. J. W., and Dyson, M., 1972, Possible hazards of diagnostic ultrasound, Br J Hosp Med., 573-7.

Vazquex, S., 1963, Cephalic changes in chick embryos under the action of ultrasound, Ann Otol Rhinol Laryngol., 72:103-12.

Warwick, R., Pond, J. B., Woodward, B., and Connolly, C. C., 1970, Hazards of diagnostic ultrasonography - a study with mice, IEEE Trans Sonics Ultrasonics, SU-17(3):158-64.

Woodward, B., Pond, J. B., and Warwick, R., 1970, How safe is diagnostic sonar?, Br J Radiol., 43(514):719-25.

EXPOSURE TO MEDICAL ULTRASOUND: STUDIES OF HUMAN EFFECTS

M.E. Stratmeyer and B.R. Fisher

Food and Drug Administration
Center for Devices and Radiological Health
5600 Fishers Lane (HFZ-112)
Rockville, MD 20857

INTRODUCTION

During the last three decades, medical ultrasound has grown from a new imaging tool used by only a few clinical pioneers to a diagnostic science now used worldwide in several clinical specialities. In one medical speciality alone, obstetrics, estimates of the percentage of pregnant women in the United States examined by diagnostic ultrasound range from 15-40% (NIH, 1984); in some countries, diagnostic ultrasound is a recommended routine prenatal procedure (NIH, 1984). The rapid development and expansion in the use of diagnostic ultrasound has been largely due to the perceived safety and medical benefits of this technology.

The perceived safety of ultrasound is heavily based on the lack of any clinically observed adverse effects attributed to ultrasound exposure. This perception has been reinforced by several widely held concepts regarding diagnostic ultrasound. It was once thought that diagnostic ultrasound devices produced temporal average intensities ranging from a few mW/cm^2 to tens of mW/cm^2 and temporal peak intensities ranging from a few W/cm^2 to about 100 W/cm^2. Such temporal average intensities were considered to be too low to cause heating under the usual conditions of clinical use, and the temporal peak intensities of microseconds duration were not considered to be capable of causing cavitation in mammalian tissue. Furthermore, it was believed by some that a threshold level would have to be exceeded before tissue damage would be likely to occur and that "all of the tissue in the suprathreshold region would be affected in contrast with the scattered atoms affected by x-irradiation" (White, 1973); thus, any ultrasound damage should be more easily detected than damage induced by x-irradiation.

We are now aware that some diagnostic ultrasound devices produce temporal average and temporal peak intensities orders of magnitude greater than those reported in the past (Stewart and Harris, in press). The high spatial average intensities of some of today's diagnostic ultrasound devices are theoretically capable of producing temperature rises in tissue of over $1^\circ C$ (NCRP, 1983). Although the significance of such a temperature increase may be debated, the temporal average intensity of diagnostic ultrasound devices is no longer an acoustic parameter that can be ignored. The apparent increase in temporal peak intensities has elicited considerable interest in recent years in the phenomenon of cavitation as a possible mechanism for producing biological effects. Flynn (1982) has shown the theoretical plausibility of producing transient cavitation with microsecond duration pulses of ultrasound with temporal peak intensities in the range produced by diagnostic ultrasound devices. Recent studies (Edmonds and Sancier, 1983; Reisz et al., 1985) have reported free radical formation from exposure to temporal peak intensities of ultrasound in the range produced by diagnostic devices. There is also indirect evidence that ultrasound-produced free radicals are present inside the cell (Armour and Corry, 1982). Free radical production provides a hypothetical model for inducing isolated ultrasound damage (e.g., point mutations) analagous to that of ionizing radiation. Thus, the higher than anticipated intensities used by current diagnostic devices, coupled with our now expanded (but still inadequate) understanding of the mechanisms of action of ultrasound are sufficient cause to reexamine the available information on which the perceptions of the safety of ultrasound are based.

The studies surveyed in this review, the endpoints examined, the major findings, and the type of ultrasound used (pulsed or continuous wave ultrasound) are listed in Table 1. Only studies involving in vivo human exposure were reviewed. The study design, results, investigators' conclusions, and limitations of each study will be briefly discussed in the text. The type of ultrasound (pulsed or continuous wave) and its intended use (diagnostic or therapeutic) will be mentioned, but specific intensity information is not included because instrument intensity values often were not measured and in situ intensities and exposure times are unknown and undoubtedly vary widely among subjects in any given study. The reader may wish to refer to other reviews (Scheidt and Lundin, 1978; NIH, 1984). Because of the complexities and the difficulties in evaluating clinical data, it is strongly recommended that the original literature be examined.

GERM CELL EXPOSURE

Although diagnostic ultrasound is increasingly being used to estimate follicular development and to examine ovarian blood flow, only one study was found that investigated the effect of ultrasound exposure on human germ cells. Testart et al. (1982) examined the effect of ultrasonography on the interval between ovulatory stimulus and follicle rupture in 68 cycles of 60 women. Ovarian ultrasonography performed during the three days before expected ovulation was associated with premature follicle rupture (p <0.01). The investigators suggested that ultrasound exposure should be avoided during this period if conception is desired. They also pointed out that this observed effect may not be a direct effect of ultrasound, but rather an indirect effect due to physical or psychological stress associated with the ultrasound procedure. Prior ultrasound exposure histories of the patients were not presented; however, there did not appear to be any dose-dependent exposure effect in this limited study.

EMBRYONIC AND FETAL EXPOSURES

Most studies of human effects were designed to examine the impact of ultrasound exposure on the embryo and fetus. However, most of the data involved exposures during the fetal period, with very little data on exposure during the embryonic period. This lack of data on embryonic exposure is unfortunate. Although until recently, ultrasonography has been performed primarily in the second and third trimesters, there now appears to be a trend toward using ultrasonography at earlier stages of pregnancy.

220

One of the first attempts to investigate the effect of ultrasound exposure on the human conceptus was that of Bernstine (1969). This study involved 720 obstetric patients who had Doppler ultrasound examinations. The study population was comprised of two groups: women with no complications of pregnancy and women who were hospitalized with complications. The number of patients in each group was not given. No adverse effect on fetal survival was observed. There was no increased incidence of prematurity (3.8% in the study versus 7.9%, U.S. Navy statistics). Nor was there an increased incidence of fetal anomalies (0.55% in the study versus 1.3%, U.S. Navy statistics). One problem with interpreting these data is the lack of evidence that the study groups and U.S. Navy obstetric population are comparable. Furthermore, since only 80 patients were exposed in the first 2-14 weeks of gestation, gross structural abnormalities would not be expected because most exposures were after the period of major organogenesis.

Hellman et al. (1970) assessed the incidence of fetal abnormalities in 1,114 obstetric patients in New York City (U.S.), Glasgow (Scotland), and Lund (Sweden). Most of the patients were examined with pulsed ultrasound (93%); a few were examined with continuous wave ultrasound (4%), or both (3%) (NIH, 1984). Neither frequency of the ultrasound examination nor gestational age at time of first examination appeared to increase the incidence of fetal abnormalities, nor was the incidence of abnormalities greater than in the general U.S. population (2.7% versus 4.8%). However, the number of exposures during the first ten weeks of gestation, the period of major organogenesis, is small (146) and only about one-half of these (77/146) had multiple exposures. Thus, this study is considered to be of extremely low statistical power (NIH, 1984). The investigators pointed out that the study population is not representative of a general population since only patients who were considered to have normal pregnancies at the time of examination were included in the study.

In one of the first studies with postnatal follow-up examinations, Koranyi et al. (1972) examined 171 children in Budapest (Hungary) ranging in age from 6 months to 3 years who had been exposed in utero to pulsed ultrasound. The investigators reported that body weights and lengths, with few exceptions, were between the 10th and 90th percentiles using the anthropometric chart of Boston University. They also indicated that the children had better than average mental and emotional development, although it was not mentioned to what population the study group was compared. The incidence of congenital defects reported did not differ significantly from that of the general population of Budapest. However, only 10 of the 259 ultrasound examinations of the study group occurred during the 8th-12th weeks period of pregnancy. This study is weakened by a low follow-up rate; only 43% (171/400) of the eligible population participated in the follow-up examinations. It should also be noted that the study population apparently was of high socioeconomic status, which may not be representative of the comparison groups.

Scheidt et al. (1978) analyzed 123 variables in newborn and 1 year examinations of infants from 1,952 women. The study population consisted of three groups: 303 women who received amniocentesis and ultrasound examination for placental localization, 679 who received amniocentesis only, and 970 controls who had neither amniocentesis nor ultrasound examination. Results of the newborn and 1 year examinations were similar in the three groups. The amniocentesis with ultrasound group had a significantly higher proportion of infants with abnormal grasp and tonic neck reflexes compared to the control group. However, the investigators pointed out that when examining 123 variables, some statistically significant values can be expected due to chance alone. They also noted other limitations of the study. Most exposures were performed during 13th-20th weeks of gestation; thus, these results do not apply to possible risks during organogenesis or other periods of gestation. Also, only relatively large increases in the frequency of abnormal conditions would be observed due to the relatively small number of subjects. Table 2 illustrates this limitation, given the number of subjects in the study and an event that normally occurs at a 1% frequency. It also has been noted that because ultrasound was not randomly assigned, a possible association between ultrasound exposure and poor outcome could have been obscured by a possible bias of higher socioeconomic class in the ultrasound groups (NIH, 1984).

A study of children exposed to pulsed diagnostic ultrasound at three Denver (U.S.) hospitals in a four year period between 1968-72 represents the longest follow-up period to date. Stark et al. (1984) reported on 425 exposed children and 381 matched control children examined at birth and again at 7-12 years of age. Body weights and lengths, head circumferences, gestational ages, Apgar scores, congenital anomalies, and congenital infections were recorded at birth. Hearing, vision, cognitive function and behavior were tested at the 7-12 year examination. The numbers of hospitalizations between birth and the 7-12 year examination were also recorded. No significant exposed versus nonexposed differences were found in the outcome measures used. There were nonsignificant increases in the incidence of dyslexia and the number of hospitalizations among exposed children; however, the authors concluded that both findings may be explained by the greater number of pregnancy complications in the exposed group. It was noted that the percentage of dyslexic children was higher in the ultrasound-exposed children at all three hospitals; although the differences were not statistically significant at the individual hospitals, the difference was statistically significant ($p < 0.01$) when the data for the three hospitals was combined (NIH, 1984). The investigators pointed out that only 23 subjects were exposed during organogenesis, so little can be inferred about ultrasound exposure during this period. Because the response rate was quite low (27%), the high rate of attrition in the study groups could possibly impact on the outcome measures. It should also be noted that controls were selected using two sets of criteria.

Moore et al. (1982) analyzed different subsets of the eligible study population from the Stark et al. Denver study described above for the possible association between diagnostic ultrasound exposure and birthweight. They examined the prenatal and birth records on 2,135 single births (1,061 exposed and 1,074 nonexposed) in two of the hospitals. The third hospital was not included because the criteria for matching exposed and unexposed infants differed from that used at the other two. A crude association between ultrasound and low birthweight (≤ 2500 grams) was found ($p < 0.005$). A more detailed analysis was done for a subpopulation of 527 births (285 exposed and 242 nonexposed) to test this association while controlling for potential confounding factors. The analyses yielded significant differences between the exposed and nonexposed groups. When the analyses were further refined by restricting the subpopulation of those births of 37 weeks or more, the logistic regression model still yielded significant differences, but results of the multiple linear regression model were no longer significant, although the mean birthweight of the exposed group was still lower than the unexposed group. The NIH Consensus Development Panel on Diagnostic Ultrasound Imaging in Pregnancy concluded that a significant association of ultrasound exposure with low birthweight was demonstrated in the Denver study. They also indicated that the matching procedures were probably not sufficient to make them comparable in terms of complications that affect birthweight; thus, the association cannot be assumed to be causal (DHEW, 1984).

A summary of the birthweights of infants delivered by two physicians who held differing views on the value of routine diagnostic ultrasound during pregnancy was presented by Smith (1984). There was no apparent difference between the average weights of infants exposed to routine diagnostic ultrasound (315 subjects) and those who were not (1,080 subjects). However, "routine" and "not routine" exposures were not defined; there is probably no true unexposed group for comparison. There are several other limitations to this study. There is no indication of the time of exposure, except that they were antenatal exposures, nor is there any indication of the number of exposures. In addition, birthweight figures were unadjusted for factors known to affect birthweight. Because of these limitations, no definitive statement can be made regarding the effect of ultrasound on birthweight based on this study.

Using data from the 1980 National Natality Survey (Placek, 1984), Madden et al. (1985) explored the multivariate relationship between birthweight and demographic, health, and pregnancy variables, including ultrasound exposure. They analyzed 7,316 cases of single live births to married women whose gestation ranged from 28–45 weeks. About one-third of these women had at least one ultrasound examination. A detailed analysis of the relationship between ultrasound exposure and adjusted birthweight was also performed on a subset of this population comprising 3,469 single births to married women with no medical or pregnancy complications and whose gestation was 38–42 weeks. Of the variables examined, smoking had the greatest effect on birthweight; ultrasound exposure appeared to have little effect on birthweight. Some of the limitations of this study include: missing data was inputed (except for ultrasound exposure), which could possibly be a source of bias if the imputation procedures were inadequate; the study only examines the effect of ultrasound on one endpoint, birthweight; and the number of cases exposed during early gestation is limited (<2% during the first 10 weeks of pregnancy). However, the results supported the investigators' conclusion that diagnostic ultrasound exposure had little or no measurable effect on fetal birthweight.

Using data from the Oxford Survey of Childhood Cancers on 1,731 children who died of cancer in the United Kingdom between 1972–81 and 1,731 matched controls, Wilson and Waterhouse (1984) identified 103 cases and 103 controls with verified claims of exposure or no exposure to ultrasound during the pregnancy. Both exposure to pulsed diagnostic ultrasound and continuous wave Doppler were included in the study. The investigators concluded that diagnostic ultrasound did not increase the risk of solid tumors and leukemia between birth and 6 years of age. However, because of a slight preponderance of ultrasound exposure in the cases exposed in the early 1970's, the question regarding the onset of cancers and deaths after 6 years remained unresolved. As the authors pointed out, a possible selection bias of abnormal pregnancies cannot be ruled out in the ultrasound exposed cases, thus the relationship may not be causal. One obvious limitation of this study is the relatively small number of ultrasound exposed case/control pairs. A more minor consideration is that although gestational age at exposure and "dosage" were stated to be similar between case and control mothers, no data was presented. If the study could be expanded, it would also be useful to analyze the data based on the numbers of children exposed to pulse-echo only, Doppler only, and both pulse-echo and Doppler ultrasound. Depending upon the relevance of high temporal peak intensity compared to low temporal average intensity, this might be a significant confounder.

A similar study of data from the Inter-Regional Epidemiological Study of Childhood Cancers analyzed information on 555 children with malignancy diagnosed between 1980–83 and 1,110 control children (Cartwright et al.,

1984). They concluded that ultrasound exposure did not significantly
raise the estimated relative risks for malignancies in either the 0-4
years of age or in the 5 years and older groups. Nor was there any apparent trend in estimated relative risks with increased number of ultrasound exposures. Wilson and Waterhouse (1984) suggested that the difference in their findings and this study might be due to the fact that this
study is limited to three regions in the United Kingdom and that the former study included the entire United Kingdom. Both studies have several
of the same limitations: the number of ultrasound exposed cases and controls is relatively small; there is no indication of gestational age at
exposure; and the type of ultrasound exposure (pulse-echo or Doppler or
both) is not stated. Again, depending on relative importance of possible
mechanisms of action of ultrasound, this could be a significant limitation.

In 1975, David et al. reported that Doppler ultrasound used for fetal
monitoring increased fetal activity. The study design included three
groups of patients. Fifteen patients were studied for 30 minutes with
the ultrasound monitor activated (unknown to the patient) during the last
15 minutes. Six patients were studied for 30 minutes without activating
the ultrasound monitor (sham-exposed). Fifteen patients were studied for
three successive 15 minute periods: first with an attenuating air cell
between the activated ultrasound transducer and the abdomen, then with
the air cell and the unactivated transducer, and finally with the activated transducer and no air cell. There was a significant increase
(p <0.001) in fetal activity when the fetus was exposed to the ultrasound. The study did have several limitations: the study groups were
relatively small; the study was not performed double blind (with neither
the patient nor the investigator being aware if the ultrasound was on or
off) to eliminate unintentional maternal or investigator bias; and the
sequence of ultrasound and control periods were not randomized. The last
design limitation may be particularly important based on Murrills et al.
(1983) study that demonstrated an increase in fetal movements with increased movement recording time.

The David et al. (1975) study stimulated several investigations of
the possibility that ultrasound could stimulate fetal activity (Hertz
et al., 1979; Powell-Phillips and Towell, 1979; Murrills et al., 1983).
These studies attempted to refine the experimental design of David et al.
(1975). In an effort to measure fetal movement more objectively, some
investigators used tocodynamometers and some used a double blind design.
With the exception of the study by Murrills et al. (1983), the numbers of
subjects in the other studies were quite small, particularly considering
the variability of the measurements. None of these studies detected an
effect of ultrasound exposure on fetal movement.

Murrills et al. (1983) performed a randomized, double blind study
using 100 subjects and 50 controls. The 150 mothers recorded fetal movement over a 30 minute period. The ultrasound transducer was activated at
random for either the first or second 15 minutes of the test period.
Exposure to fetal Doppler ultrasound caused no significant maternally detected fetal activity. The authors suggested that the progressive increase in fetal activity observed in their pilot study may indicate that
the positive results in the David et al. (1975) study conceivably could
have been due to increased awareness to fetal movement by the mother and
observer rather than an actual increase in fetal movement. Although investigators found a close correlation between maternal and observer measurements, this apparently well designed study could have perhaps been
improved by using a more objective measure than maternal awareness of
fetal movement.

NEONATAL EXPOSURE

Although ultrasonic diagnosis is commonly used on the newborn, including imaging of the brain, research on the possible effects of exposure has received little attention to date. The only known study was
reported in 1967 (Kohorn et al.). Twenty normal babies were studied during their first 3 days of life to determine whether pulsed diagnostic
ultrasound exposure might alter their cerebral electrical activity. A
bilateral electroencephalographic (EEG) recording was made on 8 infants
for 3 minutes before ultrasound exposure, for 10 minutes during ultrasound application from one side of the head, and for 5 minutes following
ultrasound exposure. A unilateral EEG recording was made on 10 other
infants for 3 minutes before exposure, for 3 minutes during ultrasound
application from one side of the head, for 2 minutes during application
from the other side, and for 5 minutes following exposure. Using a different ultrasound probe, a unilateral EEG recording was made on the remaining 2 infants for 3 minutes before exposure, fok 5 minutes during
ultrasound application from one side of the head, for 5 minutes during
application from the other side, and for 5 minutes following exposure.
The investigators observed no change in the EEG patterns during exposure
to diagnostic ultrasound. However, the EEG recordings were not interpreted blind with respect to exposure. Any definitive conclusions of
safety or lack of an effect are quite tenuous because two different
probes were used; the exposure duration, probe positioning, and EEG electrode positioning were variable; and the study group sizes were quite
small.

ADULT EXPOSURE

Most of the studies of ultrasound effects in humans have involved
exposure during the fetal period because of obvious scientific, social
and emotional reasons. There are, however, a few studies involving exposure of adults, most of which have investigated the effects of ultrasound
exposure on blood components.

Anderson and Barrett (1979) reported an immunosuppressive effect in
mice following splenic exposure to pulsed diagnostic ultrasound which
prompted Berthold et al. (1982) to investigate this possiblility in human
volunteers. Forty-one healthy women (tested anti-Rubella antibody-nega-
tive) received Rubella vaccine. The spleens of 20 women were exposed to
pulsed ultrasound for 5 minutes under routine diagnostic conditions. The
following parameters were measured in both the exposed and the control
patients: blood cell count, IgA, IgM, IgG, isoagglutinins, anti-Rubella
hemagglutinin and hemolysin titers, complement C3, granulocyte oxidative
metabolism, skin tests to mumps and tuberculin antigens, T lymphocytes
(and esterase positive and negative subsets), B lymphocytes and O lymphocytes. There was a significant (p <0.01) increase 7 days after immuniza-
tion in peripheral O lymphocytes in the control group that was not seen
in the experimental group, but the investigators cautioned that this
finding should not be overinterpreted. The authors concluded that the
results of this study "were essentially negative" and provided "no evidence of an immunosuppressive effect of ultrasound in man." Although
this study is relevant to the clinical conditions as described, its
results are not directly comparable to those of Anderson and Barrett
(1979). The in situ intensity in the human spleen would be considerably
less than that in the mouse and the energy per unit mass of spleen tissue
(intensity x time/tissue weight) would be even further reduced.

Sanada et al. (1977) exposed 10 patients with indications of cardiac abnormalities to pulsed diagnostic ultrasound and examined the morphology, adherence, and clotting properties of their platelets. They reported an increased number of platelets with altered morphology (development of pseudopodia) after 5 minutes of exposure, which reached a maximum after 15 minutes, and then tended to decrease toward preexposure levels. They also reported that blood platelet counts were significantly reduced after 10-15 minutes of exposure and proposed that the platelets were becoming lodged in the blood capillaries. These results are difficult to evaluate because of the small size of the study group and the lack of statistical analysis of the data. The greatest shortcoming of the study, however, was the absence of a sham-exposed group to determine if the effect was due to the blood collection apparatus, which remained in place during exposure.

Using β-thromboglobulin (β-TG) as an index of damage, Williams et al. (1981) investigated the effect of continuous wave therapeutic ultrasound on platelets. Sequential blood samples were taken (prior to, during, and following exposure) from 10 volunteers via a catheter placed in an arm vein just downstream of the ultrasound transducer. Blood samples were taken in the same manner from 7 sham-exposed volunteers. No elevation of β-TG was detected. The investigators pointed out that the detection of an effect was minimized by the short residence time of any given platelet in the most intense portion of the ultrasound beam (approximately 1 second) and the short time between exposure and platelet inactivation (approximately 3 seconds). For these reasons, as well as the relatively small group sizes and the large variability in the data, it is unlikely that anything but a large effect could be detected.

The effect of Doppler ultrasound monitoring on maternal erythrocyte fragility was studied by Bause et al. (1983). Predelivery (prior to Doppler monitoring in the exposed group) and postpartum blood samples were taken from 16 women exposed to Doppler monitoring during labor and 8 unmonitored control women. Erythrocyte fragility was measured using the incubated osmotic fragility test because it was believed to be a sensitive indicator of damage related to erythrocyte membrane permeability. Although there was no significant change in erythrocyte fragility, the investigators observed a trend toward increased fragility in patients with more than 7 hours of exposure. The mean time of labor for those patients exposed for more than 7 hours was approximately 10 hours compared to approximately only 1 hour for the unexposed patients. Because of this rather large selection bias and the additional uncontrolled variables of drug types and quantities administered to the study subjects, any conclusions regarding an effect of ultrasound are tenuous, at best.

Becher et al. (1983) studied the sister chromatid exchange (SCE) frequency and cell proliferation patterns of stimulated lymphocytes in vitro before and after in vivo exposure to pulsed diagnostic ultrasound. The abdominal and pelvic organs of 15 males with histories of testicular cancer were exposed for 50-60 minutes. The peripheral lymphocytes were obtained immediately before and after exposure. There were no statistically significant differences in SCE incidences before or after ultrasound exposure. Nor were there any statistically significant differences in cell cycle specific metaphase patterns before or after ultrasound exposure; thus, there was no evidence of cell growth inhibition. The interpretation of these results is limited by several factors. The study size (stated as 15 patients but data was presented for only 14 patients) is quite small, particularly considering the large variability of the data (e.g., the frequency of M_1 metaphases ranged from 6.4-69.0% in different individuals). The prior ultrasound exposure history of the

patients was not included. No positive controls were included to demonstrate that the cells were functioning as expected. Finally, it was not
stated if the slides were scored blind. For these reasons, little can be
concluded from the results regarding any possible genetic effects of
diagnostic ultrasound exposure.

Another study of the possible effect of ultrasound exposure on SCE
induction in lymphocytes was conducted by Stella et al. (1984). The
study involved 10 patients, each of whom received 8-20 applications of
continuous wave therapeutic ultrasound. Various portions of the body,
depending on the patients' symptoms, were exposed for 5-6 minutes per
application. Blood samples were obtained before ultrasound therapy
started, about halfway through the treatment cycle, and at the end of
therapy. Blood samples of 7 patients were also obtained 3 months after
the last treatment. The number of SCE's at mid-treatment was significantly increased in all patients (p <0.02). Although there was no
additional increase in SCE frequency at the end of therapy, the SCE frequency remained elevated in all patients (p <0.05). For the 7 patients
tested three months posttherapy, the frequencies of SCE's had returned to
the pretherapy baseline levels. There were no significant increases in
chromosomal aberrations in lymphocyte cultures from 5 of the patients.
Nor was there a consistent trend in the distribution of first, second,
and third division metaphases in the lymphocyte cultures from another
group of 5 patients. The authors suggested there may have been a retardation of the cell proliferation cycle, which was indicated by increased
first division metaphases and decreased second and third division metaphases in some of the 5 patients. It cannot be determined from this
study if the reported effect is induced by a direct effect of ultrasound
or an indirect effect, i.e., heating. Because of the variability in the
data, the relatively small increases in the SCE frequency, and the unresolved questions regarding the possible significance of SCE's to human
health, these results should not be overinterpreted. However, this study
should stimulate further research.

CONCLUSIONS

Most of the attention regarding possible adverse effects of exposing
humans to medical ultrasound has centered on its applications during
pregnancy. This is not surprising when one considers the biological consequences and emotional impact of permanently damaging a fetus. Compared
even to the recent past, diagnostic ultrasound is being used more extensively and earlier in pregnancy and even prior to conception. Unfortunately, there still are almost no data on the effects of exposure during
these periods. Most of the existing information is from exposures during
the second and third trimesters of pregnancy, after the critical period
of organogenesis. A major difficulty with interpreting even this data is
establishing a causal association between ultrasound exposure and an observed effect. Is an effect caused by ultrasound, or is an effect caused
by some risk factor that coincidently led to the use of a diagnostic
ultrasound procedure?

One major limitation of many of the investigations is the relatively
few subjects who were studied in a given protocol. Because of the limited group sizes in many if these investigations, only relatively large
increases in the frequency of abnormal events could have been detected.
For example, in the study by Bernstine (1969) of 720 exposed pregnancies,
the observed incidence of prematurity would have had to be more than 20%
greater than the U.S. Navy-wide incidence of prematurity for the difference to achieve statistical significance (NCRP, 1983).

TABLE 1. Human Exposure to Medical Ultrasound

Reference	Effect studied	Presence or absence of an observed effect	Type of Ultrasound*
GERM CELL EXPOSURE			
Testart et al., 1982	Ovulation	Pos	P
EMBRYONIC AND FETAL EXPOSURE			
Bernstine, 1969	Fetal abnormalities	Neg	CW
Hellman et al., 1970	Fetal abnormalities	Neg	P, CW
Koranyi et al., 1972	Physical/psychological development	Neg	P
Scheidt et al., 1978	123 variables in newborn covering and 1 year examinations	Neg*	P
Stark et al., 1984	Fetal abnormalities, neurological/physical development	Neg	P
Moore et al., 1982	Birthweight	Pos	P
Smith, 1984	Birthweight	Neg**	P
Madden et al., 1985	Birthweight	Neg**	P, CW
Wilson and Waterhouse, 1984	Childhood cancer	Neg	P, CW
Cartwright et al., 1984	Childhood cancer	Neg	P, CW
David et al., 1975	Fetal movement	Pos	CW

Reference	Effect studied	Presence or absence of an observed effect	Type of Ultrasound*
Hertz et al.,	Fetal movement	Neg	CW
Powell-Phillips and Towell, 1979	Fetal movement	Neg	CW
Murrills et al., 1983	Fetal movement	Neg	CW
NEONATAL EXPOSURE			
Kohorn et al., 1967	Cerebral electrical activity	Neg	P
ADULT EXPOSURE			
Berthold et al., 1982	Immune reactions	Neg**	P
Sanada et al., 1977	Platelet morphology	Pos	P
Williams et al., 1981	Platelet damage	Neg	CW
Bause et al., 1983	Erythrocyte fragility	Neg**	P
Becher et al., 1983	SCEs and cell cycle patterns	Neg	P
Stella et al., 1984	SCEs	Pos	CW

* Type of ultrasound: CW = continuous wave, P = pulsed
** Negative, with qualifications

TABLE 2. Possibility of Detecting Small Increases in the Frequency
          of Abnormal Conditions

Normal Frequency	Increased Frequency	Probability of Detection at p = 0.05
1%	3%	75%
1%	2%	37%

Source: Scheidt et al., 1978.

Based on the evaluation of the data from available studies on the
possible effects of ultrasound in humans, the following conclusion can be
drawn with reasonable certainty: diagnostic exposures have not resulted
in any highly evident effects, i.e., no acute, highly visible adverse
effects have occurred with any great frequency. This is not a meaning-
less conclusion, and it is somewhat reassuring; however, it does not
obviate the need for meaningful information on possible long-term, low
frequency or less obvious adverse effects of ultrasound exposure.

REFERENCES

Anderson, D. W., and Barrett, J. T., 1979, Ultrasound: a new immuno-suppressant, Clin Immunol Immunopathol., 14:18-29.

Armour, E. P., and Corry, P. M., 1982, Cytotoxic effects of ultrasound in vitro dependence on gas content, frequency, radical scavengers, and attachment, Radiat Res., 89:369-80.

Bause, G. S., Niebyl, J. R., and Sanders, R. C., 1983, Doppler ultrasound and maternal erythrocyte fragility, Obstet Gynecol., 62:7-10.

Becher, R., Zimmer, G., Schmidt, C. G., and Sandberg, A. A., 1983, Sister chromatid exchange and proliferation pattern after ultrasound exposure in vivo, Am J Human Genet., 35:932-7.

Bernstine, R. L., 1969, Safety studies with ultrasonic doppler studies, a clinical follow-up of patients and tissue culture study, Obstet Gynecol., 34:707-9.

Berthold, F., Berthold, R., Matter, I., Reither, M., Rother, U., Skvaril, F., and Willems, W. R., 1982, Effect of spleen exposure to ultra-sound on cellular and antibody-mediated immune reactions in man, Immunobiol., 162:46-55.

Cartwright, R. A., McKinney, P. A., Hopton, P. A., Birch, J. M., Hartley, A. L., Mann, J. R., Waterhouse, J. A. H., Johnston, H. E., Draper, G. J., and Stiller, C., 1984, Ultrasound examinations in pregnancy and childhood cancer, Lancet, ii:999-1000.

David, H., Weaver, J. B., and Pearson, F., 1975, Doppler ultrasound and fetal activity, Br Med J., 2:62-4.

Edmonds, P. D., and Sancier, K. M., 1983, Evidence for free radical pro-duction by ultrasonic cavitation in biological media, Ultrasound Med Biol., 9:635-9.

Flynn, H. G., 1982, Generation of transient cavities in liquids by micro-second pulses of ultrasound, J Acoust Soc Am., 72:1926-1932.

Hellman, L. M., Duffus, G. M., Donald, I., and Sunden, B., 1970, Safety of diagnostic ultrasound in obstetrics, Lancet, 1:1133-5.

Hertz, R. H., Timor-Tritsch, I., Dierker, J., Jr., Chik, L., and Rosen, M. G., 1979, Continuous ultrasound and fetal movement, Am J Obstet Gynecol., 133:152-4.

Kohorn, E. I., Pritchard, J. W., and Hobbins, J. C., 1967, The safety of clinical ultrasound examination, Obstet Gynecol., 29:272-4.

Koranyi, G., Falus, M., Sobel, M., Pesti, E., and van Bao, T., 1972, Follow-up examination of children exposed to ultrasound in utero, Acta Paediatriea Academiae Scientarium Hungaricae, 13:231-8.

Madden, D. A., Chiacchierini, R. P., Stratmeyer, M. E., Dworkin, F. H., and Roney, P. L., 1985, Relationship between birthweight, in utero ultrasound exposure and other variables, presented at the American Statistical Association Annual Meeting, Las Vegas, NV.

Moore, R. M., Barrick, M. K., and Hamilton, P. M., 1982, Effects of sonic radiation on growth and development (Abstr), Am Epidemiology., 116:571.

Murrills, A. J., Barrington, P., Harris, P. D., and Wheeler, T., 1983, Influence of doppler ultrasound on fetal activity, Br Med J., 286:1009-12.

NCRP, 1983, "Biological effects of ultrasound: mechanisms and clinical implications," Report No. 74 of the National Council on Radiation Protection and Measurements, NCRP Publications, Bethesda, MD.

NIH, 1984, The task force report. IV. epidemiological studies, in: "Diagnostic Ultrasound Imaging in Pregnancy, Report of a Consensus Development Conference," U.S. Department of Health and Human Services, Public Health Service, National Institutes of Health, NIH Publication No. 84-667, Bethesda, MD.

Phillips, W. D. P., and Towell, M. E., 1979, Doppler ultrasound and subjective assessment of fetal activity, Br Med J., 2:101-2.

Placek, P. J., 1984, The 1980 national natality survey, a national fetal mortality survey -- methods used and PHS agency participation, Public Health Reports, 99:11-116.

Riesz, P., Berdahl, D., and Christman, C. L., 1985, Free radical generation by ultrasound in aqueous and nonaqueous solutions, Environ Health Perspect, 64:233-52.

Sanada, M., Hattori, A., Watanabe, T., Shu, T., Kasahara, T., Ohn, M., and Tamura, K., 1977, The in vitro effect of ultrasound upon human blood platelets, Nihon Choompa Igakukai, Koen Rombunshu, Nov:149-50.

Scheidt, P. C., and Lundin, F. E., 1977, Investigations for effects of intrauterine ultrasound in humans, in: "Symposium on Biological Effects and Characterizations of Ultrasound Sources," Bureau of Radiological Health, DHEW Publication (FDA) No. 78-8048, Rockville, MD.

Scheidt, P. C., Stanley, F., Bryla, D. A., 1978, One-year follow-up of infants exposed to ultrasound in utero, Am J Obstet Gynecol., 131:743-8.

Smith, C. B., 1984, Birthweights of fetuses exposed to diagnostic ultrasound, J Ultrasound Med., 3:395-6.

Stark, C. R., Orleans, M., Haverkamp, A. D., and Murphy, J., 1984, Short- and long-term risks after exposure to diagnostic ultrasound in utero, Obstet Gynecol., 63:194-200.

Stella, M., Trevisan, L., Montaldi, A., Zaccaria, G., Rossi, G., Bianchi, V., and Levis, A. G., 1984, Induction of sister chromatid exchanges in human lymphocytes exposed in vitro and in vivo to therapeutic ultrasound, Mutat Res., 138:75-85.

Stewart, H. F., and Harris, G. R., in press, Characterization of acoustic output from diagnostic ultrasound equipment, in: "Proceedings of Ultrasonics International '85," Ultrasonics, July 1-3, 1985, London.

Testart, J., Thebault, A., Souderes, E., and Frydman, R., 1982, Premature ovulation after ovarian ultrasonography, Br J Obstet Gynaecol., 89:694-700.

White, D. N., 1973, The toxicity of ultrasonic and x-ray energy (from computerized axial tomography and its implications for ultrasonic encephalography), in: "Ultrasonics in Medicine, Proceedings of the Second World Congress on Ultrasonics in Medicine," Excerpta Medica, Amsterdam.

Williams, A. R., Chater, B. V., Allen, K. A., and Sanderson, J. H., 1981, The use of β-thromboglobulin to detect platelet damage by therapeutic ultrasound in vivo, J Clin Ultrasound, 9:145-51.

Wilson, L. M. K., and Waterhouse, J. A. H., 1984, Obstetric ultrasound and childhood malignancies, Lancet, ii:997-9.

STANDARDS AND RECOMMENDATIONS ON

ULTRASOUND EXPOSURE

Michael H. Repacholi

Chief Scientist, Royal Adelaide Hospital
Adelaide, South Australia 5000

1. INTRODUCTION

This paper presents a review of published standards and recommendations or policy statements that exist for equipment design and performance, and for limiting human exposure to ultrasound. Recommendations on research priorities identified by various institutions form the basis of a separate publication in this text by Dr. Nyborg. General guidelines or policy statements have been issued by various professional, national and international organisations and these will be described and discussed. Earlier reviews of standards and recommendations can be found in Repacholi and Benwell (1982), IRPA/WHO (1982), NCRP (1983) and Nyborg and Ziskin (1985).

2. STANDARDS

A standard is a general term, incorporating both regulations and guidelines, and is defined as a set of specifications for equipment or rules laid down to promote the safety of an individual or group of people. A regulation is normally promulgated under a legal statute and is referred to as a mandatory standard. A guideline does not generally have any legal force and is issued for guidance only - a voluntary standard. Statements of policy on the safe use of ultrasound are considered to be guidelines.

Standards can specify limits of exposure and other safety rules for personal protection, and/or specify details on the performance, construction, design, or functioning of a device, or methods of testing its performance. Alternatively they may take the general form of a policy statement indicating that certain people should not be exposed to ultrasound (e.g. models for demonstration), or that ultrasound exposures should only take place under a given set of conditions.

It was stated that "with expanding services in ultrasound diagnosis, the frequency of human exposure is increasing with the potential that the major part of the entire population (of some countries) may be exposed" (IRPA, 1977). The US Center for Devices and Radiological Health, using available data on the growth rate of sales of diagnostic ultrasound equipment, forecasted that the majority of the children born in the USA after the early 1980s could be exposed to ultrasound in utero (Stewart & Stratmeyer, 1982). This has proven to be the case - most industrialised countries now routinely scan pregnant patients at least once during pregnancy. Thus it is most important that the safety of ultrasound is assured.

Standards development should preferably be preceded by the preparation of, or reference to a document that identifies the hazard of human exposure to ultrasound. Such a document would summarize the experimental data on exposure of various biological systems, the known mechanisms of interactions of ultrasound with biological systems, a health-hazard analysis, and an assessment of the various national and international standards. Such an assessment forms an important basis for recommendations.

3. DIAGNOSTIC EQUIPMENT

Since our knowledge of ultrasound biological effects is sufficiently incomplete that a definitive risk assessment of exposure to ultrasound cannot be made, and it will take some time before enough information is available, many organisations have developed standards aimed at accurately characterising the equipment output. These standards, in the form of hydrophone, transducer or ultrasound equipment specifications, have the benefit of formulating acceptable measurement procedures and lead to a better understanding of the actual exposures received by patients. Thus, when a health-risk assessment can be made, the extent of the problem will be clearer.

Other standards pertain to quality assurance - ensuring that if people are exposed, diagnostically useful images are obtained. Good quality assurance has the obvious benefit of tending to maximise the quality with lower exposures.

The International Radiation Protection Association developed a health criteria document in conjunction with the World Health Organisation (IRPA/WHO, 1982). The purpose of this document was to give an in-depth review of the biological effects literature and give a health risk assessment of human exposure to ultrasound. Part of this review was a summary of standards that existed in various countries. One of the key recommendations based on this review was: "The establishment of guidelines on the performance of diagnostic ultrasound equipment is recommended - including requirements concerning image quality and stability, and quality assurance measures.

At present there does not appear to be a need to limit the output exposure levels of diagnostic ultrasound

234

equipment, other than to recommend strongly that the lowest output levels be used commensurate with image quality, adequate to obtain the necessary diagnostic information".

The European Regional Office for WHO has reinforced this view (Hill and ter Haar, 1982), but went one step further when it was stated that: "Protection measures should not be so restrictive as to unduly hamper the development, or to place any unjustified limitation on the use of the procedure. However, it appears at present that, with suitable existing equipment and techniques, many diagnostic procedures can be carried out entirely satisfactorily under conditions such that the patient is exposed to a relatively low beam intensity, such as $100W/m^2$ temporal-spatial average of less".

The International Electrotechnical Commission is in the process of developing guidelines on methods of measuring the performance of ultrasonic pulse-echo diagnostic equipment (IEC, 1985a) and drafting standards for ultrasound medical equipment in general (IEC, 1980, 1982).

At the national level, the American Institute of Ultrasound in Medicine (AIUM), through its standards committee, has been very active in the diagnostic ultrasound field. The following are examples of diagnostic ultrasound standards that exist or are being developed:

(i)   100 Millimeter Test Object, including standard procedure for its use (AIUM, 1974);

(ii)   American Institute of Ultrasound in Medicine standard on presentation and labelling of ultrasound image (AIUM, 1978);

(iii) Standard specification of echoscope sensitivity and noise level including recommended practice for such measurements (AIUM, 1979);

(iv)   American Association of Physicists in Medicine (AAPM) ultrasound instrument quality control procedures (AAPM, 1979);

(v)   Recommended nomenclature: physics and engineering (AIUM, 1980);

(vi)   Pulse echo ultrasound imaging systems; performance tests and criteria (AAPM, 1980);

(vii) American Institute of Ultrasound in Medicine standard for transducer characterization (AIUM, 1981);

(viii) AIUM interim standard on methods for testing single-element pulse-echo ultrasonic transducers (AIUM, 1982);

(ix)   AIUM-NEMA safety standard for diagnostic ultrasound equipment (AIUM, 1983).

Probably the most definitive standard for diagnostic ultrasound equipment is the AIUM/NEMA standard. It has been described in detail in AIUM (1983). The purpose of the standard was to set precise definitions of parameters primarily related to acoustic output levels, specify labelling requirements for acoustic output parameters (with test methods were appropriate), set electrical and mechanical safety guidelines. Qualitative ultrasound safety guidelines relating to equipment characteristics and information are provided to the users and information on known or suspected biological effects is also given. The standard covers all ultrasonic echo ranging, through transmission devices, Doppler echo equipment and combinations of these. Details related to performance characteristics of equipment as they pertain to patient exposure and safety are included, but use, medical efficacy and performance parameters unrelated to exposure and safety are not considered.

The National Council on Radiation Protection and Measurement (NCRP, 1983) has produced a very detailed account of the biological effects of ultrasound, interaction mechanisms, characteristics of ultrasound, measurement methods and reviews of clinical safety. Details of their recommendations are given by Dr. Nyborg elsewhere in this text. Regarding diagnostic equipment, the NCRP recommends that: (1) Manufacturers of equipment for diagnostic ultrasound should make public their data on exposure parameters, including those specified by the AIUM-NEMA standard (AIUM, 1983).

(2) (a) Ultrasound equipment should be designed so that the maximum levels of the various intensities which the equipment can produce are as low as practicable for the anticipated uses of the equipment.

   (b) Where such flexibility is consistent with reasonable cost and performance of the system, operators should be able to adjust controls to use the minimum acoustical intensities required to image the desired organs on each patient.

   (c) As a matter of prudence, users of the equipment should be encouraged by the manufacturer to minimise the acoustical intensities to the patient and to minimise the dwell times, within the limits of obtaining necessary diagnostic information.

The Non-Ionizing Radiation Section of Health and Welfare Canada was one of the first to look at the overall problem of human ultrasound exposure with a view to identifying if exposure standards were necessary. In its publication "Guidelines for the safe use of ultrasound Part 1 - Medical and Paramedical applications" (H & WC, 1980), details of biological effects, applications of ultrasound, recommended exposure levels and safe-use guidelines are given. The code recommends that manufacturers endeavour to design and construct equipment to function at SATA intensities of less than $100mW/cm^2$. In any case intensities should be kept as low as readily achievable. A labelling system is specified for SPTA intensities less than or equal to 100mW/cm^2 (for non focused transducers) and up to 250mW/cm^2 (for focused transducers). For intensities above these values a total power indicator and elapse exposure timer is also recommended. It is understood that the Canadians are presently reviewing these recommendations.

The only country to have mandatory requirements limiting the output of diagnostic ultrasound equipment is Japan. The Japanese Standards Association (JSA) has several industrial standards for diagnostic ultrasound devices. These include standards for A-mode (JSA, 1984a), manual scanning B-mode (JSA, 1984b), fetal Doppler (JSA, 1984c) and M-mode (JSA, 1984d). Besides safety requirements on electrical parameters, construction, design, and testing procedures, there are specifications on performance (sensitivity, resolution, dynamic range etc), including limits the SATA intensity for the various types of diagnostic equipment. The limitations on the output (SATA intensity) of each probe when measured under free field conditions are given below:

A mode	100mW/cm^2
Manual Scan B mode	10mW/cm^2
M mode	40mW/cm^2
Fetal Doppler	10mW/cm^2

The rationale for setting these output limits is not entirely clear, although it is believed that experimental data collected in Japan form the basis for the limits. These have been discussed by Maeda (1985) - see section 5.

In France, a standard for diagnostic ultrasound devices, which includes specifications on construction, labelling, use, and conditions for approval was published in 1982 (Association francaise de Normalisation, 1982).

4. THERAPEUTIC EQUIPMENT

Ultrasound has been used since the 1930s in physiotherapy. Though the biological mechanisms of ultrasound therapy have not received systematic investigations, many standards have been developed for therapeutic ultrasound devices. For example, there are both French (Association Francaise de Normalisation, 1963) and Australian Standards (SAA, 1969) on ultrasonic therapy equipment, which indicate ultrasonic output tests and techniques or measurement.

Both Canada and the USA have published mandatory regulations on ultrasound therapy devices under their respective radiation control acts (Health and Welfare Canada, 1981; US Food and Drug Administration, 1978). Standards incorporating accuracy specifications for the acoustic output power and intensity and for the timer were identified as necessary in the US and Canada, since these directly affect the amount of exposure received by the patient. The labelling of individual applicators is necessary to prevent transducers from being connected to the wrong generator, and thereby probably causing significant discrepancies between the acoustic output and the dial indication.

The Canadian ultrasound therapy device regulations is essentially same as that in the United States except the maximum SATA intensity from the transducer is limited to $3W/cm^2$ in Canada. The rationale for this limitation in the Canadian regulation is as follows:

(i)   Survey data indicate that $3W/cm^2$ is commonly found as the maximum nominal intensity available for most devices.

(ii)   This intensity has been accepted by European manufacturers for many years as the maximum necessary for therapy.

(iii)   Research data indicate that even this value is already within the adverse bioeffects range so it seems prudent to restrict new devices from producing even greater intensities.

Support for the $3W/cm^2$ intensity in the Canadian standard is to be found in the chapter on ultrasound drafted by Hill and ter Haar (1982) for the WHO Regional Office for Europe. In this document it states: "Since ultrasound is often used therapeutically under relatively uncontrolled conditions, the current practice apparently demonstrates that levels higher than $30kW/m^2$ ($3W/cm^2$) are not needed for treatment, there does not seem to be any justification for using such higher exposure levels".

IRPA/WHO (1982) has tended to be a little more conservative about recommending an upper limit for therapy when it states: "There are arguments for and against setting upper limits to the intensity of the beam of an ultrasound therapy device. It should be remembered that physiotherapists want to produce an effect on the region of injury, and they require an appropriate amount of ultrasound energy to achieve this aim. An upper limit might be constructed as a "safe level" for exposure, thus encouraging its use. Above $3W/cm^2$, the heat generated is generally unbearable for most patients; moreover such an intensity has been reported to retard bone growth (Kolar et al., 1965). In addition, cavitation, which may cause significant tissue damage, is increasingly possible at intensities above this level".

5.   STATEMENTS AND RECOMMENDATIONS

One of the first organisations to publish a statement to give guidance on the scientific literature was the American Institute of Ultrasound in Medicine (AIUM). This AIUM Bioeffects Statement, was first published in 1976,

modified in 1978 and reaffirmed in 1982 and is presently as
follows:

"In the low megahertz frequency range there have been
(as of this date) no independently confirmed significant
biological   effects   in mammalian tissues exposed to
intensities (a*) below 100mW/cm^2.   Furthermore, for
ultrasonic exposure times (b**) less than 500 seconds and
greater than one second, such effects have not been
demonstrated even at higher intensities, when the product
of intensity (a) and exposure (b)   is less than 50
joules/cm^2.

*   (a)   Spatial peak, temporal average as measured in a
            free field in water.   The spatial peak intensity
            should be determined with a device, such as a
            calibrated miniature hydrophone, for which the
            dimensions of the sensitive area are smaller than
            the distance over   the   local value of the
            ultrasound field intensity shows a significant
            variation.

**   (b)   Total time; this include off-time as well as
            on-time for a repeated pulse regime.

This statement applies to all existing   data   on
biological   changes   produced in mammalian tissues by
ultrasound in the frequency range from about 0.5 to 10MHz.
All seemingly reliable data were included   from   the
literature as well as results of satisfactory quality that
have been published more recently.   However, in any
application of the Statement to decisions concerning the
safety of human beings, attention should be given to the
following considerations.

Most of the data apply to mammals other than man, and
it   is not clear how to relate them to them human
situation.   However, the Statement is helpful in arriving
at recommendations for the use of ultrasound in medicine.
The Statement does not, in itself, imply specific advice on
"safe   levels"   which   might be universally valid.
Determination of recommended maximum levels will require
consideration of such difficult topics as: adequacy of
present knowledge of bioeffects; expected reliability of
equipment specifications; assessment of patient benefits;
and others.   So far these matters have not been treated
systematically.

The AIUM Bioeffects Statement was widely misconstrued
as a statement of safety in clinical diagnosis and in many
cases   misinterpreted regarding the biological effects
evaluation.   To remedy this situation, the AIUM issued a
statement on Clinical Safety /AIUM (1983), which is as
follows:

"Diagnostic   ultrasound has been in use for over
twenty-five years.   Given its known benefits and recognised
efficacy for medical diagnosis, including use during human
pregnancy, the American Institute of Ultrasound in Medicine
herein addresses the clinical safety of such use.

No confirmed biological effects on patients or instrument operators caused by exposure at intensities typical of present diagnostic ultrasound instruments have ever been reported. Although the possibility exists that such biological effects may be identified in the future, current data indicate that the benefits to patients of the prudent use of diagnosis ultrasound outweigh the risks, if any that may be present".

The Committee for Standards on Ultrasonic Medical Equipment, Japanese Society of Ultrasonics in Medicine, stated its "Views on Safety of Diagnostic Ultrasound" in 1983 (Maeda, 1985). This Committee concluded that the minimum intensity of ultrasound showing reproducible biological effects, when the irradiation time ranged from 10 sec to 1.5 hr in the frequency range of a few MHz, was approx. $1W/cm^2$ when using CW ultrasound and approx. $240mW/cm^2$ (SPTA) using pulsed ultrasound. The Committee on Medical Engineering of the Japanese Society of Obstetrics and Gynaecology stated in 1985 that the ultrasonic diagnosis of the pregnant women, fetus and newborn using real-time B-mode device should not be limited when clinically indicated (including the necessary screening of the fetus), however, use for other than medical purposes should not be permitted (Maeda, 1985).

The rationale for the Japanese statements was given by Maeda (1985). He reported on bioeffects studies in Japan that investigated changes of chromosome, cell growth, fertilized animal ovum, the fetal animal etc. After exposure to CW ultrasound, anomalous changes of the fetus of animals was observed at an intensity of about $1W/cm^2$ or more, and cultured cell growth was suppressed at about the same intensity. For pulsed ultrasound, cultured cell growth was the most sensitive, but no effect was observed when the SPTA intensity was $240mW/cm^2$ or less. Statistics showed no increase of neonatal anomaly rate after introduction of antepartum ultrasound diagnosis. The fertilized rat ovum was exposed to pulsed diagnostic ultrasound for 12 hrs, and the ovum was transferred into the animal uterus, resulting in normal fetal growth without anomaly.

In 1983, the Australian Society for Ultrasound in Medicine (ASUM, 1983) issued a policy on ultrasound services which stated:

1. At present there have been no independently verified studies that have demonstrated any biological effect of diagnostic ultrasound in vivo in humans. As a matter of principle patients should be examined only by competent personnel and only as much as is necessary to provide the required diagnostic information.

2. Ultrasound services should be provided only by those Medical Practitioners who have competence in the specific examinations they undertake. Such examinations must be in the best interest of the

patients and carried out using appropriate equipment.

3. Patient identification. The date of service and name of the Medical Practitioner or Medical Practice responsible for the conduct of the ultrasound examination should be imprinted in, or otherwise recorded with, each film or other record.

4. A written report should be issued on all ultrasound examinations by the responsible Medical Practitioner and the report should be made available with copies of the films or other records in response to a legitimate request.

5. A register of ultrasound examinations performed should be kept by each medical practice.

6. Specialists in ultrasound should collaborate in undergraduate and postgraduate education and in the education of other Medical Practitioners and Sonographers.

7. While all Medical Practitioners should be free to request ultrasound investigations dependent on their clinical experience and judgement, a specialist in diagnostic ultrasound has a duty to decide whether a requested investigation is appropriate, having regard to the level of diagnosis required, risks involved and cost effectiveness.

8. Sonographers should not practice independently of Medical Practitioners.

The Royal College of Obstetrics and Gynaecology (RCOG, 1984) in England formed a working party on routine ultrasound examination in pregnancy. A summary of their more pertinant recommendations is given below:

1. The present evidence for the safety of ultrasound based on over 20 years of experience and research is sufficiently convincing for us not to recommend a change in the common practice of routine ultrasound examination between 16-18 weeks or pregnancy. However, pregnant women should not be persuaded to have an ultrasound examination against their wishes. While we do not consider that written informed consent to routine ultrasound examination is necessary, such an examination must be accompanied by a written explanation as to why the procedure is recommended. Scanning personnel should ensure that mothers have read and understood the content of the written explanation.

2. There should be a diploma of obstetric ultrasound which all personnel performing unsupervised antenatal scanning should hold. The organisation of the examination and the award of the diploma should be the responsibility of the RCOG and the Royal College of Radiologists.

3. a) At present, there are no beam intensity standards
        for ultrasound equipment sold in the U.K.

    b) Manufacturers should publish maximum SPTA and SPTP
        intensity values for their equipment.

    c) A government agency should carry out random checks
        on the power output.

    d) Beam intensity standards should be established for
        all ultrasound scanning equipment to ensure that
        the minimum power is used to achieve a
        satisfactory image.

The present status of human exposure to ultrasound was
reveiwed at a special seminar on Safety and Standardisation
of Diagnostic Ultrasound in Obstetrics (Sydney, July, 1985)
sponsored by WFUMB. The purpose of the meeting was to
provide a forum at which an international group of experts
could determine areas in which international consensus
exists, and to identify matters on which agreement has not
been reached and set directions for future studies and
research. The theme of the meeting was restricted to
discussion on the safety of clinical ultrasound and
development of quantitative exposure criteria.

It was agreed that there was no verified evidence of
significant effects in mammalian tissue following exposure
to pulsed ultrasound as used in diagnostic imaging.
However, a number of areas of biological research needed to
be addressed, particularly where high intensity pulsed
ultrasound is used in some modern Doppler devices (Barnett
and Kossoff, 1985).

CONCLUSIONS

It is generally agreed that diagnostic ultrasound at
present levels is safe. However, modern Doppler devices
are using increasingly higher peak pulse intensities.
These devices are being studied particularly to determine
if adverse biological effects are being produced.
Therapeutic ultrasound requires intensities high enough to
produce an effect - hopefully beneficial.

Standards - both regulations and guidelines, have
tended to be more cautionary than restrictive in that more
complete and accurate information is required rather than
specifying that the devices not do certain things (such as
go above given output levels). Japan is the only exception
to this for diagnostic devices, requiring that the
transducers remain below set SATA intensities. Canada is
presently the only country to have mandatory restrictions
on the output of therapy devices, although the upper limit
set is not a problem for therapists.

REFERENCES

AAPM (1979). Ultrasound instrument quality control procedures. American Association of Physicists in Medicine, Chemical Rubber Publishing Co., p. 45 (CRP Report Series - Report 3) Cleveland, Ohio.

AAPM (1980). Pulse echo ultrasound imaging systems: Performance tests and criteria. American Institute of Physics (American Association of Physicists in Medicine Report No. 8) New York.

AIUM (1974). 100 millimeter test object including standard procedure for its use. American Institute of Ultrasound in Medicine, Washington, DC.

AIUM (1978). American Institute of Ultrasound in Medicine standard on presentation and labelling of ultrasound images. Reflections, 4: 70-75.

AIUM (1979). Standard specification of echoscope sensitivity and noise level including recommended practice for such measurements, American Institute of Ultrasound in Medicine, Washington, DC.

AIUM (1980). Recommended nomenclature: Physics and engineering, American Institute of Ultrasound in Medicine, Washington, DC.

AIUM (1981). American Institute of Ultrasound in Medicine standard for transducer characterization, American Institute of Ultrasound in Medicine, Washington, DC.

AIUM (1982). Interim standard on methods for testing single-element pulse-echo ultrasonic transducers. Suppl. to J. Ultrasound Med. 1(7), September issue.

AIUM (1983). Safety standard for diagnostic ultrasound equipment, AIUM/NEMA Standards Publication/No. UL1-1981. J. Ultrasound Med. 2(4): S1-S50 (special supplement).

AIUM (1984). Safety considerations for diagnostic ultrasound. Bioeffects Committee of AIUM, AIUM, 4405 East-West Highway, Bethesda, Maryland, USA.

Association Francaise de Normalisation (1963). Appareils a ultrasons, (Norme francaise NF C 74-306). Paris, France.

Association Francaise de Normalisation (1982). Appareils a ultrasons utilises en diagnostic, (Norme francaise NF C 74-335), Paris, France.

ASUM (1983). Standards of practice : Policy on Ultrasound Services Society August newsletter, Australian Society for Ultrasound in Medicine, P.O. Box R374, Royal Exchange, Sydney, Australia 2000.

Barnett, S.B. and Kossoff, G. (1985). Current
    international policy on the use of diagnostic
    ultrasound imaging in pregnancy. Rad. Protect. in
    Australia, 3(4): 145-147.

H & WC (1980). Guidelines for the safe-use of ultrasound,
    Part I - Medical and paramedical applications. Safety
    Code-23 (Health and Welfare, Canada, Publication,
    80-EHD-59).

Health and Welfare Canada (1981). Ultrasound therapy
    devices regulation. Canada Gaz., Part II, 115 (8):
    1121-1126.

Hill, C.R. & ter Haar, G. (1982). Ultrasound. In: Suess,
    M.J., ed. Nonionizing radiation protection.
    Copenhagen, World Health Organisation Regional Office
    for Europe (WHO Regional Publications, European Series
    No. 10).

IEC (1980). Draft: IEC Standard Publication 601-2-XX
    Ultrasonic Medical Diagnostic Equipment, Part 2.
    Particular requirements for safety (IEC/TC 62D (Sec)
    31, Dec. 1980).

IEC (1982). Draft: Methods of measuring the performance of
    ultrasonic pulse-echo diagnostic equipment (IEC/TC
    29/SC 29D (Central Office) 16, February 1982).

IEC (1985a). Methods of measuring the performance of
    ultrasonic pulse-echo diagnostic equipment
    (29D(CO)16). Draft: International Electrochemical
    Commission, Geneva.

IEC (1985b). Characteristics and calibration of
    hydrophones for operation in the frequency range 0.5MHz
    to 15MHz (29D(CO)19). Draft: International
    Electrochemical Commission, Geneva.

IRPA (1977). Overviews on non-ionizing radiation.
    International Radiation Protection Association, US
    Dept. of Health, Education and Welfare, Washington,
    DC. pp. 42-59.

IRPA/WHO (1982). Ultrasound, Environmental Health Criteria
    No 22, United Nations Environment Programme, World
    Health Organisation, International Radiation Protection
    Association, WHO, Geneva.

JSA (1984a). Japanese Industrial Standard, A-mode
    ultrasonic diagnostic equipment. Japanese Standards
    Association. Tokyo, Japan.

JSA (1984b). Japanese Industrial Standards, Manual
    scanning B-mode ultrasonic diagnostic equipment.
    Japanese Standards Association, Tokyo, Japan.

JSA (1984c). Japanese Industrial Standard. Ultrasonic
    Doppler fetal diagnostic equipment. Japanese Standards
    Association. Tokyo, Japan.

JSA (1984d). Japanese Industrial Standard. M-mode
    ultrasonic diagnostic equipment.   Japanese Standards
    Association, Tokyo, Japan.

Kolar, J., Babickj, A., Kaslova, J., & Kasi, J. (1965).
    The effect of ultrasound on the mineral metabolism of
    bones.   Travmatol. protezinov., 26 (8): 43-51 (in
    Russian).

Maeda, K. (1985). Japanese policy and statement.
    Abstract. World Federation of Ultrasound in Medicine
    and biology Seminar on Safety and Standardisation of
    Diagnostic Ultrasound in Obstetrics. Sydney, July.

NCRP (1983). Biological effects of ultrasound :
    Mechanisms and clinical implications. National Council
    on Radiation Protection and Measurements, 7810 Woodmont
    Ave, Bethesda, Maryland USA 20814.

RCOG (1984). Royal College of Obstetrics and Gynaecology,
    Report of the RCOG working party on routine ultrasound
    examination in pregnancy. Chameleon Press Ltd. London.

Repacholi, M.H. and Benwell, D.A. (1982).   Ultrasound
    standards : Regulations and guidelines.   In: Essentials
    of medical ultrasound. edited M.H. Repacholi and D.A.
    Benwell, Human Press, Clifton, New Jersey, p 281-304.

SAA (1969). Ultrasonic therapy equipment, Standards
    Assoc.   of   Australia   (Pub. AST40-1969). Sydney,
    Australia.

Stewart, H.F. & Stratmeyer, M.E. (1982). An overview of
    ultrasound: Theory, measurement, medical applications
    and biological effects, DC, US Dept. of Health and
    Human Services DHEW Pub. (FDA) 82-8190, Washington, DC.

US Food and Drug Administration (1978).   Performance
    standard for ultrasonic therapy products. Fed. REg.,
    43(34): 7166-7172.

Ziskin, M.C. and Nyborg, W.L. (1985). Standards and
    guidelines for medical ultrasound.   In: Biological
    effects of ultrasound.   edited W.L. Nyborg and M.C.
    Ziskin, Churchill Livingstone, New York, p169-174.

PROTECTIVE MEASURES FOR ULTRASOUND EXPOSURE

Deirdre A. Benwell

Radiation Protection Bureau, Health and Welfare Canada
Room 233, Environmental Health Centre
Tunney's Pasture, Ottawa, Ontario, K1A OL2, Canada

INTRODUCTION

In this work specific guidelines are given for the safe use of ultrasound equipment. The physical principles forming the basis for these protective measures are briefly described. In addition, the types of regulatory measures that may be used to enforce these procedures are also described.

In conjunction with protective measures, great care should be taken in the selection of safety limits of ultrasound radiation that are protective but that do not unduly restrict technological progress. In medical uses of ultrasound, ultrasound exposure is part of the diagnosis or treatment and thus protection is used in the sense of balancing risk and benefit. It is also important that adequate standards for measurement and calibration techniques be accepted at an international level to ensure a basic level of uniformity of labelling and performance of instrumentation and terminology world-wide (Repacholi 1982).

PHYSICAL BASIS FOR PROTECTIVE MEASURES

All protective measures for reducing ultrasound exposure rely on one or both of the following physical factors: (1) At high frequencies, air is an effective attenuator of ultrasound, and (2) interfaces with major discontinuities in acoustic impedance act as effective barriers to the transmission of ultrasound (WHO 1982b).

Physical protective measures for ultrasound exposure are divided into two distinct categories: those for airborne ultrasound (generally in the kilohertz frequency range), and those for solid - or liquid borne ultrasound (usually in the Megahertz frequency range) (NHW 1980a and b).

For airborne ultrasound, the critical organ to be protected is generally agreed to be the ear and the auditory system (Grigoreva 1966, Acton 68 and 73, Parrack 69, NHW 1980b). Protective measures are, therefore, modelled on procedures established for the audible frequency range (WHO 1982a and b, NHW 1980b). If ambient levels cannot be kept below certain limits by redesign, relocation, or construction of physical sound absorbers or sound barriers, then adequate ear protection is provided. Most ear protection suitable for audible sound will also be suitable for airborne ultrasound (WHO 1982b, NHW 1980b).

The most potentially dangerous situation for solid or liquid-borne ultrasound is when high power levels of ultrasound are present in any liquid media as this provides good acoustic coupling to the human body (eg. ultrasonic cleaning tanks). The transmission of ultrasound from the liquid or solid depends on the materials involved and the degree of contact with the skin. Common protective measures are limiting occupancy of such dangerous areas, personnel training, posting warning signs and labels (NHW 1980b).

REGULATORY AND ENFORCEMENT PROCEDURES

The various ways in which standards are enforced by a country depend upon many factors including the magnitude and probability of the hazard to health and the legislative practices of the country. There are two general types of standards used to protect the general population, patients and persons occupationally exposed to ultrasound. These are: (1) exposure standards and (2) emissions standards, described as follows (Repacholi and Benwell 1982):

(1) Emissions standards that refer to equipment or devices and specify maximum emission or leakage radiation from a device, usually at a specified distance. Detailed specifications on the design, construction, functioning, and performance of the device are usually given to ensure that the maximum exposure or leakage levels are not exceeded.

(2) Exposure standards apply to personnel protection and generally refer to maximum levels to which whole or partial body exposure is permitted. This type of standard has greater applicability in industry where, for example, exposure standards may limit the intensity of airborne ultrasound around one or more cleaning tanks.

The following list of common enforcement procedures is given in WHO (1982(b)):
>   Licensing of installations or devices
>   Statutory regulations
>   Registration
>   Notification
>   Voluntary Procedures
>   Guidelines and recommendations
>   Quality assurance programs
>   Certification

To date, apart from ultrasound therapy regulations in North America (Canada 1984, USA 1978), countries have inclined towards voluntary procedures, guidelines, quality assurance and certification to ensure adequate protection for medical ultrasound. No protective regulations for industrial and commercial ultrasound applications are known at present to the author.

PROCEDURES FOR SAFE USE

Ultrasound has a very good record for safety, to date, (AIUM 1984) inferring that the general procedures followed for its safe use, together with the exposure levels used, appear to be satisfactory. To continue such a good record of safety, however, it is important to continually monitor safe use procedures.

Safe use procedures are divided into three general categories: (1) care of equipment, (2) use of equipment, and (3) operator training and education. The procedures used obviously differ depending on the type of ultrasound device and its application.

Care of equipment

All ultrasound devices, as with almost any electrical device, should be regularly calibrated and maintained. Canadian safe use guidelines (NHW 1980a) recommend that this be done by trained technicians, and/or manufacturers, at least once a year. Ultrasound physical therapy devices should generally have the ultrasound power output and timer accuracy included in the calibration.

Use of equipment

In the case of medical ultrasound, the patient exposure should be minimized as much as possible without the loss of medical benefit. A further protective measure along these lines is to keep ultrasound exposure records for each patient. This provides a data base on which future epidemiological studies for risk assessment can be based while at the same time recording cumulative data per patient. In addition, exposure records provide a data base for the estimation of the minimum exposure required to achieve the desired medical benefit. This should tend to encourage the use of lower ultrasound exposure levels.

Other protective measures involving use of equipment are divided into various categories of ultrasound applications as follows:

Physical Therapy. Measures for the protection of the operator include: (a) not touching the ultrasound applicator face when the device is switched on, (b) the operator should not immerse any part of him/her in a water bath containing an operating ultrasound therapy device applicator; (c) ultrasound therapy device applicators should only be turned on when the face of the applicator is in contact with the patient, and the operator is holding the applicator by the handle.

Measures to protect the patient exposed to therapeutic ultrasound include testing the patient skin for normal reactions to heat and cold. It is advisable to use an alternative type of treatment for patients deficient in this sensation. In addition coupling media should always be used between the applicator surface and the patient for good ultrasound transmission. An important protective measure is the continual movement of the applicator during the course of treatment over the area to be treated to minimize the risks of causing hot spots (undue temperature rise in a single volume of tissue receiving excessive exposure) (Stewart and Stratmeyer 1982, NHW 1980a).

The final protective measure with respect to ultrasound therapeutic equipment use is to heed accepted contraindications (NHW 1980a). For example, ultrasound therapy must not be applied such that the beam could irradiate the uterus of a pregnant woman.

Diagnosis. Limitations on the use of diagnostic ultrasound are a controversial issue. "There is no firm evidence that any physiological change, beneficial or not, is produced in patients by exposure to ultrasound during a diagnostic examination" (NCRP 1983a). However since ultrasound at diagnostic levels can cause biological effects in cells and in animals, and although the extrapolation to effects on human beings is not possible at present, some caution in the use of diagnostic ultrasound would seem advisable. The statement made at the National Institute of

Health Conference in February 1984 (NIH 1984) supports this view:
"...taking into account the available bioeffects
literature, data on clinical efficacy, and with concern
for psychosocial, economic, and legal/ethical issues, it
is the consensus of the panel that ultrasound
examination in pregnancy should be performed for a
specific medical indication. The data on clinical
efficacy and safety do not allow a recommendation for
routine screening at this time.

Ultrasound examinations performed solely to satisfy
the family's desire to know the fetal sex, to view the
fetus, or to obtain a picture of the fetus should be
discouraged. In addition, visualization of the fetus
solely for educational or commercial demonstrations
without medical benefit to the patient should not be
performed."

There are advocates of increased use of diagnostic ultrasound
such as the routine use of ultrasound in pregnancy although at
present there is no conclusive proof of benefit. The evidence can
be quite persuasive, when considering remote populated areas with
no readily available physician, hospital, or medical help in the
vicinity. However there is no clear indication of necessity in
areas where the pregnant woman has easy access to a physician.

The National Institute of Health statement (NIH 1984) also
advocates informing patients of the clinical indication for
ultrasound and the specific benefit to be gained, as well as
potential risk and alternatives, if any. This seems to be a
reasonable approach. In addition, if the patient requests further
information on the ultrasound exposure, such as frequency
intensity, time, it should be available.

Dentistry. Protective measures in dental ultrasound depend
greatly on the use of the equipment. The main application in
dentistry is the cleaning of teeth and their interproximal
crevices. It is important that cooling measures (eg. water
cooling) are used at all times when the device is being used.
Care should be taken that the water flow is sufficient to prevent
a buildup of heat. In addition the tool tip should be kept moving
to prevent local spot heating of the tooth surface, and caution
should be taken that only that part of the dental work being
treated is in contact with the tool tip. The angle of the tool
tip and the force of application are two other parameters that
should be carefully controlled.

Surgery. Few general protective measures in terms of safe
use procedures can be given for this application due to the
critical dependence of the interaction of ultrasound with tissues
in each surgical procedure. Quality assurance procedures and
quality control in manufacturing are required to meet and maintain
the manufacturer's performance specifications. Ultrasound surgery
should be used only when clinically indicated, by well trained and
skilled surgeons.

Industry - High Power Ultrasound. The main protective
measure for high power industrial ultrasound is to avoid contact
exposure at all times. Situations which are particularly
dangerous are those for which high power levels of ultrasound are
present in liquid media as described in the section on Physical

Factors. Canadian safe use guidelines also recommend limited occupancy, responsibility of personnel using high power ultrasound devices, warning signs at the entrances to areas containing high power ultrasound devices, and labelling of the devices themselves (NHW 1980b).

Industry - Low Power Ultrasound. Cautionary procedures are advised. For example, the user should not touch any part of the ultrasound equipment while operating. Cautionary signs should be on the equipment (NHW 1980b).

Airborne Ultrasound. This may be present in applications of high and low power ultrasound as well as specific ultrasound applications where it is the only source. Safety procedures are the same as for protective measures in the audible sound frequency range. The objective is to ensure that ambient airborne ultrasound levels are not excessive. Since the mechanism for harm due to airborne ultrasound seems to be exclusively through the ear and auditory mechanism, if safety procedures for audible sound or noise are followed, personnel should also be protected for airborne ultrasound. This is due to the facts that (i) acoustic waves travel poorly through air at ultrasound frequencies, and higher levels can be tolerated, and (ii) ears appear very much less sensitive to ultrasound frequencies (20 kHz). However extreme care should be taken in the instrumentation used and the location of measurement of airborne ultrasound since there are very few instruments accurate above 20 kHz and the ultrasound emissions are very directional. Exposure limits for the safe use of airborne ultrasound are given in the Canadian safe use guidelines (NHW 1980b). This specifies one-third octave band limits of 80 dB at or below the 20 kHz one-third octave band, and a limit of 110 dB at one-third octave bands of 25 kHz and above. Similar limits are given in Switzerland (Cahiers suisse 1982).

Operator training and education

This is an important protective measure for all applications of ultrasound. In the field of medicine, ultrasound therapy training is included in physiotherapy programs at Canadian universities but diagnostic ultrasound training is less formalized. Canadian safe use guidelines recommend 6 months for formal training of diagnostic ultrasound operators (technicians or doctors) (NHW 1980a, NHW 1984). This is often completed at "on the job" or in the ultrasound facility of a large hospital. Common sources of training are one week manufacturers' courses introducing the fundamentals of ultrasonic imaging. In North America, the American Registry of Diagnostic Medical Sonographers has administered examinations in diagnostic ultrasound since 1975. These follow guidelines outlined by the American Society of Ultrasound Technical Specialists and include the requirement of at least 1 year's experience in ultrasound.

Dental ultrasound also requires training on the part of the operator and it would be advisable to include ultrasonic dental cleaning techniques in dentistry course work particularly for dental technicians.

Training and education for operators are similarly advisable for industrial and commercial uses of ultrasound so that operators are aware of potential hazards, safe use practices and the need for calibration and maintenance.

SUMMARY AND CONCLUSIONS

An overall description has been given of the various protective measures for ultrasound exposure. The one notable area omitted is that of setting specific maximum allowable limits for the use of ultrasound. These would vary depending upon the mode of ultrasound and its application. It is debatable, at this stage, whether there is sufficient knowledge to define such exposure standards. The importance of uniformity of instrumentation and terminology is generally accepted. However specific international measurement and calibration techniques are still under discussion.

REFERENCES

Acton, W.I. (1968), A criterion for the prediction of auditory and subjective effects of airborne noise from industrial sources, Brit. J. Indust. Rad., Vol.24, pp.297-304.

Acton, W.I. (1974), The effects of industrial airborne ultrasound on humans, Ultrasonics, May, pp.124-128.

AIUM (1984), "Safety Considerations for Diagnostic Ultrasound", American Institute of Ultrasound in Medicine, 4405 East-West Suite 504, Bethesda, MD, U.S.A. 20814.

Cahiers suisse (1982), "Bruit des installations a ultrasons", Caise national suisse d'assurance en cas d'accidents, 6002 Lucerne.

Canada (1984), Canada Gazette Part II. Radiation Emitting Devices Regulations Part XIII. Ultrasound Therapy Devices PC.1981-908 April 2, 1981. Amended November 22, 1984 by PC.1984-3737.

Grigroreva, V.M. (1966), Ultrasound and the question of occupational hazards, Maschinstreochiya, No.8, p.32, Abstract in Ultrasonics, Vol.4, p.214.

NCRP (1983a), "NCRP Report No.74. Biological Effects of Ultrasound: Mechanisms and Clinical Applications", National Council on Radiation Protection and Measurements. 7910 Woodmont Avenue, Bethesda, MD, U.S.A. 20814.

NCRP (1983b), "NCRP Report No.73. Protection in Nuclear Medicine and Ultrasound Diagnostic Procedures in Children", National Council on Radiation Protection and Measurements. 7910 Woodmont Avenue, Bethesda, MD, U.S.A. 20814.

NHW (1980a), "Safety Code 23. Guidelines for the Safe Use of Ultrasound. Part I. Medical and Paramedical Applications". 80-EHD-59, Information Directorate, National Health and Welfare Canada, Brooke Claxton Building, Ottawa, Ontario, K1A OK9.

NHW (1980b), "Safety Code 24. Guidelines for the Safe Use of Ultrasound. Part II. Commercial and Industrial Applications". 80-EHD-60. National Health and Welfare Canada, Brooke Claxton Building, Ottawa, Ontario, K1A OK9.

NHW (1984), "Diagnostic Facilities in Hospitals". Report of the Subcommittee on special services in hospitals. Guidelines for establishing standards for special services in hospitals. Health Services Directorate, Health Services and Promotion Branch, National Health and Welfare Canada, Tunney's Pasture, Ottawa, Ont.

NIH (1984), "Diagnostic Ultrasound Imaging in Pregnancy", NIH Publn. No.84-667, National Institute of Health, Bethesda, MD, U.S.A.

Parrack, H.O. (1969), Letter to Aram Glorig, dated Nov.15, 1967, Subject "Standards Working Group 53-4" (Distributed as attachment to letter to members of S3-W40, dated 31 December 1969 from Aram Glorig, M.D.).

Repacholi, M.H., Benwell, D.A. (1982), "Essentials of Medical
    Ultrasound. A Practical Introduction to the Principles,
    Techniques and Biomedical Applications". Humana Press,
    Clifton, NJ, U.S.A. 07015.
Stewart, H.F., Stratmeyer, M.E. (Eds.) (1982), "An Overview of
    Ultrasound: Theory, Measurement, Medical Applications and
    Biological Effects". HHS Publn. FDA 82-82190, Centre for
    Devices and Radiological Health, Rockville, MD, U.S.A. 20857.
USA (1978), Dept. of Health and Human Services. Ultrasound Therapy
    Performance Standard. U.S. Federal Register 43(34).
WHO (1982a), "Environmental Health Criteria 22 Ultrasound", World
    Health Organization, Geneva.
WHO (1982b), "WHO Regional Publications European Series No.10.
    Nonionizing Radiation Protection". Ed. M.J. Suess, World Health
    Organization Regional Office for Europe, Copenhagen, Denmark.

RESEARCH PRIORITIES IN ULTRASOUND

Wesley L. Nyborg

Physics Department
University of Vermont
Burlington, VT   05405   USA

In the last few years several reports have been published
which include recommendations for research. One of these
(BRH, 1982) is a publication of the U.S. Department of Health
and Human Services, Bureau of Radiological Health (BRH), prepared by government scientists. The BRH report contains a
comprehensive tabulation and discussion of literature on biological effects of ultrasound, especially where these bear on
safety of medical ultrasound. On the basis of the literature
survey, areas were identified in which further research is
needed. The BRH report, including the research recommendations, was reviewed before publication by many individuals,
within the government and outside. Their section entitled
"Recommendations for further research" is here reproduced
(essentially) verbatim.

RECOMMENDATIONS FROM THE BRH REPORT

In the introductory paragraph it is explained that these
recommendations are not listed in order of priority.

(1)   Measurement of Internal Ultrasonics Fields

The spatial and temporal characteristics of ultrasound
fields radiated by clinical devices into water is relatively well established. Fundamental characteristics of
ultrasound tissue interactions, such as attenuation,
velocity, and impedance, have been measured but because
of differences in these values from one tissue to the
next and because of differences in the geometry of experimental animals, and the anisotropic nature of the
acoustic properties of many biological materials, this
information is difficult to use in obtaining reliable
estimates of internal exposure fields. Therefore additional work is needed to develop instrumentation and
techniques capable of measuring internal exposure parameters. In the development of these detectors, interaction mechansims are likely to be an important design
consideration. For example, a detector that measures
absorbed energy would be useful for quantifying effects

that are due to thermal mechanisms, but a detector that responds to peak pressure amplitude may be more useful for quantifying cavitation phenomena. Much work is required in this area including the development of adequate phantoms.

(2)   Instrument Development and Measurements

With regard to clinical instrumentation there is a dual need. First, instrumentation should be developed to provide methods of measuring the exposure levels from diagnostic ultrasound equipment. Instruments and methods for field measurement of the temporal and spatial intensities need to be developed. Second, there must be more complete knowledge of the intensities to which patients are exposed by currently available devices and the many new devices being introduced each year.

(3)   Studies of Mechanisms of Action

The degree of importance of various physical mechanisms in producing biological effects needs systematic investigation. At higher intensities, the absorption of ultrasonic energy by conversion to heat is well recognized as a mechanism causing biological effects. Not so thoroughly examined have been nonthermal interactions such as cavitation and viscous stresses. The latter includes microstreaming and shear stresses, radiation forces, radiation torques, and stresses associated with particle acceleration.

(4)   In Vitro Studies

Investigations at the level of macromolecules and cells offer promise as a screening technique to evaluate the relative importance of various physical mechanisms of interaction and clarify the need for further study at higher levels of biological organization. Alterations to cell membrane structure have been reported by a number of investigators. Some alterations include increased density of microvilli and ruffles in cell membrane following exposure that may alter growth characteristics. Studies are needed to establish the mechanisms causing these effects and their potential significance. The persistence of a hereditable disturbances in cell motility after ultrasound exposure is especially important and investiga tions need to be conducted to determine if these effects occur in vivo.

(5)   Developmental Studies

Animal studies have shown potential effects on fetuses, such as fetal weight reduction and cardiac defects and other fetal anomalies in rodents, following in utero exposure. Some of the reported effects, such as fetal abnormalities have been questioned and further work is needed to establish cause and effect. Studies are needed to determine the relative biological importance of the high temporal peak intensities and other parameters associated with pulse-echo diagnostic equipment.

(6) Hematological Studies

Investigators have reported effects both in vivo and
in vitro at diagnostic and therapeutic intensities
suggestive of perturbations of the hematologic system in
laboratory animals and in human patients. Systematic
research should be conducted to thoroughly investigate
reported effects such as formation of thrombi which could
have adverse consequences in vivo, effects on platelets
and increased fragility of blood cells after long exposure, such as that involved in fetal monitoring.

(7) Genetic Studies

Although hereditable genetic effects from ultrasound have
not been demonstrated in vivo, additional investigations
are needed, not only to substantiate or refute some
reported effects on genetic material, such as increased
sister-chromatid exchange frequency, unscheduled DNA
synthesis, and alterations to nucleic acid percursor
uptake, but also to determine their significance. For
example, for other types of insults, sister-chromatid
assay has been suggested to be a sensitive measure of
genetic damage, because the frequency of exchange increases after exposure of the cell to known mutagens and
carcinogens. Of particular importance are investigations
of effects from high peak intensities and other parameters associated with diagnostic ultrasound equipment as
compared to potential effects that might be caused by the
lower time-averaged intensities from continuous wave
exposures.

(8) Immunological Studies

These studies suggest that ultrasound may affect immunological responses in laboratory animals and in humans.
Considering the fundamental importance of the immune
system, it is important that these effects be confirmed
or refuted. Investigation of possible effects of ultrasound on the immune system could have applicability in
both the diagnostic and therapeutic areas.

(9) Behavioral Studies

Some experiments with rodents suggest that behavioral
effects may be shown by neonates exposed in utero. This
has proven to be a difficult area of research because of
problems in obtaining reproducible experimental results.
If some of these difficulties can be overcome this may
prove to be a very fruitful area of research for identi
fying potential consequences to the human fetus exposed
in utero.

(10) Human Studies

Retrospective and prospective investigations are
needed to observe effects on both mother and newborn
exposed in utero and appropriate long-term follow-up
should be conducted. An added difficulty to these
types of studies is that control populations of unexposed neonates are rapidly disappearing as the use of

ultrasound diagnosis increases. This fact provides further incentive toward prompt initiation of these studies. The importance of studies on the fetus is even more urgent since the introduction of ultrasound exposure to developing Graffian follicle for ovulation timing for in vivo fertilization. Short-term studies with specific end points, such as hematological and immunological investigations, should also be conducted.

RECOMMENDATIONS FROM THE NCRP

Another source of research recommendations is a publication (NCRP, 1983) of the National Council of Radiation Protection and Measurements (NCRP), a private organization chartered by the U.S. Congress. In accordance with NCRP procedures, the publication was prepared by a committee appointed specifically for the purpose (SC-66). It received critical review, within and outside the NCRP, before final approval. This report (like the BRH report) includes an extensive discussion of evidence for change produced by ultrasound in living systems, and the implications of this evidence for clinical use of ultrasound. In addressing the implications, emphasis is given to statistical analysis of existing human surveys and to detailed comparison of conditions for laboratory experiments with those for clinical situations. In making these comparisons, considerable importance is attached to understanding basic mechanisms for biological effects. Among the 50 recommendations contained in the NCRP publication, those listed below deal with research needs. In the report the lists of recommendations are preceded by discussions of background which serve as rationale for them.

(1) A sustained research effort should be maintained to widen the data base and to increase the understanding of biological effects of ultrasound. The activities should include a balance between (a) those whose aim is to gain general insight and (b) those directed to more immediate clinical needs. Among the former (a) are investigations of basic principles of the interaction between ultrasound and living matter. Clearly indicated here are thermal and cavitational mechanisms but investigators should be alert to others, such as the effects of radiation forces. Among the latter activities (b) are investigations into biological effects which occur under conditions of frequency, intensity and pulsing parameters typical of clinical practice.

(2) Research should be carried out to investigate the possibility that biologically significant cavitation or bubble activity occurs in human tissue under conditions of diagnostic and therapeutic medical ultrasound. Such studies should include (a) physical studies of the response of bubbles (cavitation "nuclei") to short high-intensity repeated pulses characteristic of pulse-echo techniques; (2) investigations of the potential of mammalian tissue for containing bubbles or nuclei; and (c) the biological significance of any bubble activity produced by medical ultrasound in tissue.

(3) Studies should be made of temperature distributions produced in the body by ultrasound, and of the biological

significance of temperature elevation.

(4) Studies should be undertaken to clarify certain effects already reported in the literature (e.g., fetal weight reduction in mice) but which lack sufficient information on dose-response relationships and mechanisms of action.

(5) Studies should be carried out to determine the extent to which effects accumulate in successive exposures. If any cumulative effects are found, it will be most important to determine their mechanism of action.

(6) Studies should be made of physiological factors which might predispose to ultrasonically induced bio-effects. These factors include hypoxia, reduced blood-flow, mechanical trauma, nutritional deficiencies, drugs, and hyperthermia produced by fever or by other means.

(7) Epidemiological surveys can yield important information that sometimes cannot be obtained in any other way. Unfortunately, they tend to be very expensive and time-consuming. Nevertheless, such surveys should be encouraged when the following conditions are satisfied:
i) Suitable endpoints have been identified;
ii) The studies will employ ultrasound equipment with well-specified exposure parameters;
iii) The survey will be large enough to detect significant changes;
iv) It has been determined that the results will be important whether positive or negative;
v) The survey can be executed in a cost-effective manner; and
vi) Sufficient care is taken to avoid errors caused by exposure-unrelated differences in health status of patients who receive ultrasound examinations.
When condition (ii) is satisfied, information on the in fluence of exposure parameters can be sought by dividing the population into subgroups according to the applicable ranges of these parameters.

(8) Experiments in which biological effects of diagnostic ultrasound on laboratory animals are sought must be well planned in order to yield meaningful results. Since the probability of an effect appears small, a priori, the number of animals must be large enough to provide a significant demonstration of either a positive or negative result. Suitable steps must be taken to avoid observer bias. In particular, adequate sham exposures and controls are essential for meaningful interpretation of results.

(9) Encouragement should be given to participation of investigators and investigative teams with different scientific backgrounds and approaches. Investigators must be knowledgeable and facilities adequate for both the biological and the physical aspects of the research.

(10) Published reports of bio-effects should include detailed specification of ultrasonic, and other pertinent parameters, to facilitate replication of experiments and to permit comparison of effects as a function of such para-

meters. The ultrasonic parameters may include in situ values of intensities or other field quantities which are relevant to the particular investigation. They may also, or alternatively, include exposure parameters which give free-field characteristics of the ultrasonic equipment used.

(11) Research and development should continue on techniques and instrumentation for characterizing focused and pulsed ultrasonic fields.

(12) Forceful encouragement should be provided for in vivo measurements of ultrasonic attenuation, absorption, scattering, velocity and characteristic acoustic impedance. In so far as possible, measurements on humans should be conducted; where not possible, and this may be in the majority of cases, demonstrated mammalian analogues should be studied. A much greater variety of tissues and organs is to be treated, over that now appearing in the literature, to reflect the clinical involvement currently receiving attention. Further, the full range of pathological states of these tissues and organs, appearing clinically, must also be examined, at the least to determine how their propagation properties differ from those of the normal state.

(13) Investigators should be encouraged to devote attention to those measurements and measurement techniques that provide data which can be related directly to bio-effects studies which are clinically relevant, and to clinical practice generally.

(14) Investigations should be made in which the diagnostic capabilities of ultrasonic equipment and procedures are assessed and related to the intensities and dwell times used. Such information is needed to guide manufacturers and users in choosing exposure parameters which yield maximum information with minimum risk.

(15) The development of various phantoms and test objects for evaluating instruments should be encouraged. Critical physical parameters, such as spatial resolution, sensitivity, and beam patterns are normally best evaluated with these objects.

(16) The establishment of a complete system of optimum exposure parameters for balancing benefit against risk should be accepted as a long range goal, at least for those situations where it is found that there is a reasonable expectation of significant risk. Such a system would have to distinguish between different kinds of equipment and different applications and would allow for new technological and medical developments and for clinical judgment in individual cases.

RECOMMENDATIONS FROM THE NIH

A third report (NIH, 1984) is a publication of the U.S. Department of Health and Human Services, National Institutes of Health (NIH). It is based, in large part, on a draft document prepared by a Panel (14 members) commissioned by several U.S. governement agencies. The draft document, dealing with issues concerning the use of diagnostic ultrasound in pregnancy, was distributed widely for comment and, finally, was presented to the general public at a Consensus Development Conference on February 6-8, 1984. One of the five specific questions which the report addresses is "What further studies are needed of efficacy and safety of use of ultrasound in pregnancy?" The response to this question, as published in the report, is as follows:

"It is critical, in view of the existing data and the special considerations affecting fetal and embryonic development, to encourage and support a sustained research effort aimed specifically at test systems that can help provide a better data base for developing reasonable estimates of bioeffects and of risk. In particular, we recommend:

(1) The study of fundamental mechanisms leading to bioeffects.

(2) Laboratory experiments that focus especially on those cellular processes that are most likely to be affected during embryonic and fetal development.

(3) Postnatal studies in animals after in utero exposure to ultrasound.

(4) Exploration of interactions between administered ultrasound and such developmentally significant agents as drugs, nutrition, ionizing radiation, hyperthermia, and hypoxia.

(5) Development of improved dosimetry.

A long-term follow-up of infants involved in a randomized clinical trial would help clarify questions about the effect of ultrasound on development in humans, and other epidemiological studies using a wide variety of methods should be considered. Studies of the psychosocial, ethical, and legal aspects of ultrasound use are also needed.

Further nonexperimental studies that seek to establish the clinical efficacy of ultrasound should address the question of its contribution to reducing morbidity and mortality. Randomized, controlled clinical trials of routine ultrasound screening in pregnancy should be conducted in the United States."

NICHD REQUEST FOR APPLICATIONS

Most convincing of all recommendations for research are probably those which are accompanied by indications that financial support might be available. The announcement reproduced below appeared recently in a publication of the U.S. Department of Health and Human Services, via the NIH Guide for Grants and Contracts, Vol. 14, No. 3, March 1, 1985. While the deadline (15 July 1985) for this request for application (RFA) is past, the text of the announcement still has considerable interest as an expression of research needs.

"The Genetics and Teratology Branch (GT) of the Center for Research for Mothers and Children (CRMC) of the National

Institute of Child Health and Human Development (NICHD) invites research project grant applications for studies of the bioeffects of ultrasound on developing organisms.

I.   Background Information

The use of ultrasound in the management of pregnancies has since its introduction into obstetric practice in the 1950's become a highly sophisticated technology that is capable of detecting many structural and functional abnormalities of the developing fetus. It may be employed to determine fetal size and gestational age, assess fetal structural anomalies, detect multiple and ectopic pregnancy, and as a guide in fetal therapy. The technology has overcome the many limitations of roentgenology and has virtually eliminated the need for fetal exposure to ionizing radiation.

Because of these advantages, the use of diagnostic ultrasound has grown rapidly until today about one-third to one-half of all pregnant women, and therefore at least one million developing fetuses, are exposed to ultrasound radiation in the United States each year. Yet it is not clear if diagnostic ultrasound usage during pregnancy is free of risk to the developing fetus. There have been no reports of clinically observed adverse effects associated with the prenatal use of ultrasound, but clinical impressions, although valuable, do not establish conclusively that the use of ultrasound involves no risks. Past epidemiological studies have not yielded conclusive evidence regarding safety or adverse effects of ultrasound because of inadequate study design. Animal and cellular studies have also been unable to rule out or suggest harmful ultrasound effects and some studies could not be repeated. Furthermore, information on exposure conditions of previous ultrasound bioeffects studies is frequently incomplete.

The extraordinary acceptance of ultrasonography as an indispensible prenatal diagnostic tool that might soon result in prenatal exposure of a majority of infants to ultrasound in utero, as well as the lack of the necessary bioeffects information, lead NICHD to encourage ultrasound research. A better data base for reasonable estimates of bioeffects and risks of ultrasound on developing organisms should result in the near future.

II. Research Goals and Scope

This RFA solicits applications from qualified investigators for interdisciplinary studies to advance our understanding of potential bioeffects of ultrasound that might be initiated in developing organisms before birth. Investigations should search for ultrasound effects covering the organisms' earliest developmental periods and on through embryogenesis, fetal and postnatal stages to maturity. Studies may include potential defects, whether they are immediate or delayed, at all levels of biological organization to determine possible molecular, cellular, as well as tissue and organ-level, key developmental processes that might be affected. This should include examination of differential gene action, of all cellular morphogenetic processes, and of determination and differentiation that specify the organism's maturation. Investigations may utilize appropriate animal models for ultrasound effect determinations and/or cell, tissue, organ or embryo culture methods to carry out such studies. Epidemiological studies are also encouraged to exclude major ultrasound effects, to examine for subtle ultrasound effects, and to determine frequencies of potential lasting effects, should some be discovered. Clinical investigations are sought that contribute to improved prenatal use of the ultrasound technology, but efficacy of such studies is not an objective of this RFA. Investigations of fundamental ultrasound interaction mechanisms with developing biological systems and separation of different causes of potential adverse developmental outcomes as well as of appropriate ultrasound dosimetry are also encouraged."

REFERENCES

BRH, 1982, "An Overview of Ultrasound: Theory, Measurement, Medical Applications, and Biological Effects," H. F. Stewart and M. E. Stratmeyer, eds., HHS Publication FDA 82-8190, Bureau of Radiological Health, Rockville, MD 20857.

NCRP, 1983, "Biological Effects of Ultrasound: Mechanisms and Clinical Implications," National Council of Radiation Protection and Measurements Report No. 74, NCRP Publications, 7910 Woodmont Ave., Suite 1016, Bethesda, MD 20814.

NIH, 1984, "Diagnostic Ultrasound Imaging in Pregnancy," NIH Publication No. 84-667, Superintendent of Documents, U.S. Government Printing Office, Washington, DC 20402.

TISSUE REGENERATION

Gail ter Haar

Physics Department
Institute of Cancer Research
Sutton, Surrey, U.K.

INTRODUCTION

Ultrasound finds widespread use by physical therapists for the treatment of soft tissue lesions.   Many users believe it to have considerable beneficial effects (for example, Middlemast and Chatterjee (1978), Oakley (1982)), while others find it less effective (Pizzarello et al (1975), Shamberger et al (1981)).

The repair of soft tissue injuries can best be described in terms of three overlapping phases: an inflammatory phase, a proliferative phase and a remodelling phase.   These different phases will be outlined here, and any known effect of ultrasound on each stage described.

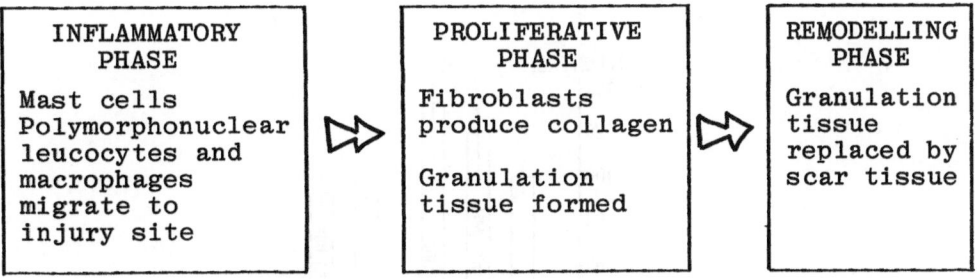

Fig. 1.   Block diagram showing the phases in tissue regeneration.

1. Inflammatory Phase

During the inflammatory phase, there is a rapid migration of mast cells, polymorphonuclear leucocytes and macrophages clear the site of pathogens and debris, wound factors are released, and the processes of tissue regeneration are set into motion.   Ultrasound has been shown to stimulate histamine release from mast cells (Fyfe and Chahl, 1984).   If it also stimulates release of other wound factors, then this important

first, inflammatory phase may be accelerated.   Phagocytic
activity by macrophages may also be altered by ultrasonically
induced shear stresses (Crowell et al, 1977).

2.   Proliferative Phase

During the proliferative phase, cells migrate to the
injured site, and start to divide.   Granulation tissue is
formed, and fibroblasts start to produce collagen.   The wound
strength begins to increase, and specially adapted fibroblasts,
myofibroblasts, cause the wound to contract.

Ultrasound has been shown to interact in a number of ways
with components of this phase of healing.   The synthesis of
collagen may be stimulated when fibroblasts are irradiated by
ultrasound either _in vivo_ or _in vitro_.   Harvey et al (1975)
showed that when primary diploid human fibroblasts were
irradiated with ultrasound, the amount of protein synthesized
was increased.   A significantly increased rate of synthesis
was found when spatial peak intensities greater than $0.5Wcm^{-2}$
were used at 3MHz for 5 minute exposure times.   Pulsed beams
(2ms on:8ms off), also enhanced the amount of protein synthesized, as shown in Fig.2.

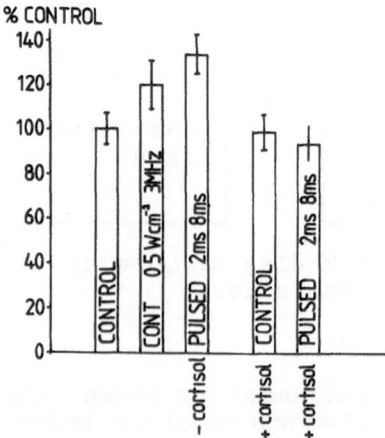

Fig.2.   Graph showing effect of ultrasound on total protein
synthesis (expressed as a percentage of control values).
The effect of cortisol is also shown.   Exposure parameters: 3MHz; $0.5Wcm^{-2}$ (spatial peak); 5 mins
(Adapted from Harvey et al, 1975).

In subsequent papers this group has shown that this effect may be mediated by cavitation (Webster et al, 1978, Webster et al, 1980). The stimulatory effect was suppressed by the addition of cortisol to the culture medium (Fig.2). Cortisol is known to stabilize lysosomal membranes. The permeability of lysosomal membranes is thought to be altered by ultrasonic irradiation (Harvey et al, 1975). Electron microscopic studies of fibroblasts irradiated in vitro revealed that, in comparison to control cells, there were more free ribosomes, more dilatation of rough endoplasmic reticulum, more cytoplasmic vacuolation, more autophagic vacuoles, and more damage to lysosomal membranes and mitochondria. Increased collagen synthesis has also been demonstrated following ultrasonic irradiation in vivo (Webster et al, 1979). Seven days after treatment of cryosurgical lesions on rat flanks with 3MHz $0.5Wcm^{-2}$ ultrasound, pulsed 2ms on:8ms off for 5 minutes, the collagen content was found to have increased by 20% over that of the untreated scar. Noncollagenous protein content was also increased by 13%. Table 1 shows the results obtained one month after injury.

Pospisilova et al (1976) have also studied changes in collagen synthesis following ultrasonic irradiation of experimental granulomata in rats. Ultrasonic exposure conditions are given as 0.8MHz, $1Wcm^{-2}$ continuous wave, for 5 minutes. This exposure does not raise the tissue temperature by more than $2.5^{o}C$. They found that total protein content in tissue was increased if treatment was in the acute inflammatory phase, but there was less new collagen formed. If treatment was withheld until the chronic inflammatory phase, then collagen synthesis was increased. This was thought to be due to ultrasonic stimulation of a resting cell population.

3. Remodelling Phase

The third phase in soft tissue healing is one of remodelling. In this phase, granulation tissue is gradually replaced by scar tissue. Normal connective tissue derives its elasticity from the arrangement of the collagen fibre network, which allows the tissue to tense and relax without undue strain. In scar tissue, the fibres are often laid down in an irregular, matted fashion, that does not allow stretch without tearing. This means that scar tissue is less elastic, and mechanically weaker than the normal tissue surrounding it.

There is some evidence that scars that have been irradiated with ultrasound are stronger, and more elastic than "normal" unirradiated scar tissue. This indicates that ultrasound may influence the fashion in which the new collagen is laid down, and this may aid the remodelling process.

Drastichova et al (1973) have studied the effect of ultrasound ($0.85Wcm^{-2}$) on the strength of sutured incisions on the backs of guinea pigs. The lesions were treated on the third and fourth days after incision. In one series, the breaking strength of scars was 189% of that of the controls, and 271% in the other. These investigators felt that ultrasound acted chiefly on the fibroblasts and collagen in the extracellular spaces, allowing more mature collagen fibres to develop in a given time interval. Other factors must surely also play a part. For example, ultrasound may improve the blood supply to the damaged region (Hogan et al, 1982).

Dyson et al (1979) have undertaken a study similar to
that of Drastichova et al to investigate the effect of pulsed
ultrasound (3MHz, 2ms:8ms, 0.5Wcm^{-2}) on the healing of cryosurgical lesions in rats. Ultrasonically treated scar
tissue was found to have a breaking strength of 109% of that
of mock-irradiated scars after 1 month, and 126% after 2
months. After 2 months, the breaking strength of untreated
scars was 42% of that of normal uninjured skin at the same
site. In another similar study (Dyson, 1982) the tensile
strength, extensibility and collagen content one month after
injury were compared for treated and untreated scars. The
results are shown in Table 1.

In this work, the extension of the scar until its breaking
point was measured as a function of load. The curves obtained
are shown in Fig.3.

The plots show that although the load that the treated
scar can bear is only slightly more than that of the untreated
scar, the elasticity, as shown by the area under the load/
extension curve (representing the stored energy in the tissue)
is considerably greater.

4. Scientific Evidence for Stimulation of tissue regeneration by ultrasound

Despite the widespread use of ultrasound in physiotherapy
over a number of years, there are very few published reports
of clinical trials, good or bad. Much of the evidence for
therapeutic benefit comes from animal studies.

An early tissue regeneration study was performed on the
rabbit ear by Dyson et al (1970). A 1cm^2 area of tissue was
removed from the full thickness of both ears. Pulsed 3.5MHz
ultrasound at a range of intensities was used to treat one
ear. The other ear on each rabbit was used as a contralateral control. It was found that the treated ear healed
more rapidly than the control ear, and the most effective

Table 1.   Mechanical properties of scar tissue, one month
after injury[*]. Expressed as percentages of the
value for normal uninjured skin.

	Tensile Strength	Extensibility (Load/Extension)	New Collagen Content
Normal, uninjured skin	100%	100%	100%
Ultrasonically treated experimental wounds	17.5%	34.6%	645%
Mock irradiated experimental wounds	15.7%	39.5%	827%

[*]Taken from Dyson, 1982.

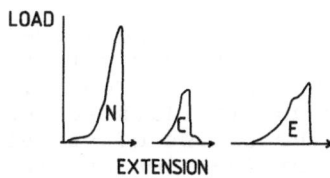

Fig. 3.   Load/extension curves for tissue 1 month after injury.
The wounds had received 5 ultrasound treatments
during the week following injury.   N: normal uninjured skin;   C: control, mock irradiated scar
tissue;   E: ultrasonically treated experimental wound.
(Adapted from Dyson, 1982).

treatment was $0.5Wcm^{-2}$ pulsed 2ms on, 8ms off.   Growth stimulation was a maximum at 21 days after injury.   Intensities
greater than $1.0Wcm^{-2}$ pulsed in the same way were less effective in stimulating regeneration.

Clinical studies of the effectiveness of ultrasound for
healing human soft tissue lesions are sparse.   Paul et al
(1960) used ultrasound to promote the healing of pressure
sores, and Galitsky and Levina (1964) found that 900 kHz pulsed
ultrasound applied pre-operatively improved the "take" of skin
grafts for trophic ulcers.   In a more precise trial, Dyson
et al (1976) studied the healing of chronic varicose ulcers
when treated with 3MHz ultrasound pulsed 2ms on:8ms off at a
spatial average intensity during the pulse of $1.0Wcm^{-2}$.   The
results obtained are shown in Fig.4.

There was a significant decrease in the surface area of
ulcers treated with ultrasound, as compared with the control
"mock" irradiated group.   After twelve treatments (thrice
weekly for four weeks) treated ulcers had an average surface
area of $66.4 \pm 8.8\%$ of their initial area, whereas control
ulcers had an area $91.6 \pm 8.9\%$ of their initial area.   Temperature rises in the treated area were measured, and found
to be less than $1^{\circ}C$.   This temperature rise on its own would
be insufficient to account for the observed stimulation of
regrowth.

Ultrasound has also been used with some success to
increase the elasticity of scar tissue and contractures.
Bierman (1954) reported that he had used ultrasonic therapy
successfully on patients with burns and lacerations of the
hand.   Markham and Wood (1980) and Pospisilova et al (1980)
have also reported successes in treating hands.   Markham and
Wood used 1MHz and 3MHz continuous wave ultrasound at intensities between 0.25 and $0.5Wcm^{-2}$ with good results on
Dupuytren's contractures.   Pospisilova et al used 0.8MHz

sound and intensities in the range 0.05-3.0Wcm^{-2}. They have
reported results from 84 patients with a range of connective
tissue disorders of the hand. Their findings included the
facts that (i) ultrasound facilitated rehabilitation exercises
by relieving pain in the course of exercise and improving
muscle tone, (ii) flexor function was influenced more than
extensor function, (iii) if injury was complicated by irreversible changes, the ultrasound effect was temporary, (iv) ultrasound was most effective immediately after injury, the effectiveness decreasing with lapsed time, and (v) that ultrasound
was more effective in men than in women. Interestingly,
Dyson et al (1976) found that the ulcers on female patients
responded better than those on men.

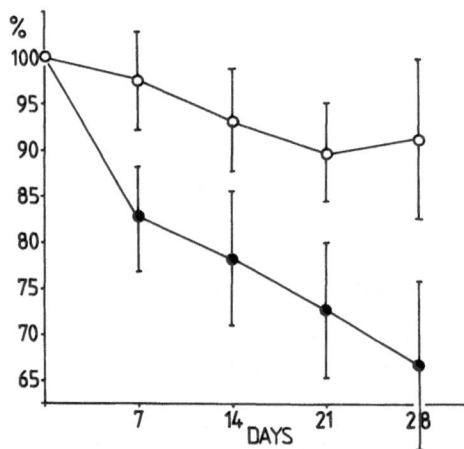

Fig. 4. The effect of ultrasound on the healing of varicose
ulcers. Time after beginning of treatment is plotted
against ulcer area expressed as a percentage of the
initial area. O Control "mock" irradiated ulcers;
O Ultrasonically irradiated ulcers. Adapted from
Dyson et al (1976).

It is thought that ultrasound may be used to reduce the
oedema associated with soft tissue injuries. Fyfe and Chahl
(1980) treated experimentally induced oedema in rats with
0.5Wcm^{-2} pulsed ultrasound at a range of frequencies (0.75MHz,
1.5MHz and 3.0MHz). A frequency dependent effect was found,
only 0.75MHz being effective. The mechanism involved in
producing this resolution was not known. In a subsequent
study (Fyfe and Chahl, 1985), they found that the wrong choice
of ultrasound treatment regime could increase the amount of
oedema and inhibit healing. It was found that oedema was less

than that in controls if only one treatment was given, or if it was only repeated once, 24 hours later. Further treatments were found to increase the length of the oedematous phase. Elhag et al (1985) have found that 3MHz ultrasound, pulsed 2ms on:8ms off at a space average, pulse average intensity of $0.5Wcm^{-2}$ reduces facial swelling in patients following removal of impacted teeth.

5. Summary

In summary then, there is evidence from the laboratory that ultrasound can stimulate the regeneration of soft tissue. The biophysical mechanisms involved have not been clearly elucidated, and until they have, treatment regimes are likely to be decided on a purely empirical basis. There is evidence, however, that many of the effects produced have a non-thermal origin. Ultrasound has been shown to interact with the different stages in the regenerative process in a number of ways.

1. Inflammatory Phase   Ultrasound stimulates histamine release from mast cells. It may also affect the release of other wound factors, thus accelerating the inflammatory phase.

2. Proliferative Phase   Ultrasound has been shown to increase the amount of collagen synthesized by fibroblasts both in vivo and in vitro.

3. Remodelling Phase   The mechanical properties of scar tissue have been shown to be improved by ultrasonic therapy. It is possible that ultrasound affects the way in which the new collagen fibres are laid down.

Ultrasound is widely used for the treatment of soft tissue injuries by physical therapists. Despite this, good scientific evidence for its benefits is sparse in the literature. However, there is both sufficient published and anecdotal information to indicate that, when used correctly, it has a useful role to play in the stimulation of tissue regeneration.

Acknowledgement

I should like to thank my colleague Dr. Mary Dyson for her help and advice in preparing this manuscript and the accompanying lecture.

REFERENCES

Bierman, W., 1954, Ultrasound in the treatment of scars. Arch. Phys. Med. Rehab. 35:209.
Crowell, J.A., Kusserow, B.K., Nyborg, W.L., 1977, Functional changes in white blood cells after microsonation. Ultrasound Med. & Biol. 3:185.
Drastichova, V., Samohyl, J., Slavetinska, A., 1973, Strengthening of sutured skin wound with ultrasound in experiments on animals. Acta Chir. Plast. (Praha) 15:114.
Dyson, M., 1982, Stimulation of tissue repair by therapeutic ultrasound. Surgery (Sept.) 37-44.
Dyson, M., Franks, C., Suckling, J., 1976) Stimulation of healing of varicose ulcers by ultrasound. Ultrasonics, 14:232.

Dyson, M., Pond, J.B., Joseph, J., Warwick, R., 1970, Stimulation of tissue regeneration by pulsed plane wave ultrasound. IEEE Trans. Sonics and Ultrasonics SU-17: 133.

Dyson, M., Webster, D.F., Pell, R., Crowder, M., 1979, Improvement in the mechanical properties of scar tissue following treatment with therapeutic levels of ultrasound in vivo. Proc. 4th Eur. Symp. Ultrasound in Biology & Medicine. Ed. P. Greguss, Vol.1, pp.129-134.

Elhag, M., Coghlan, K., Christmas, P., Harvey, W., Harris, M., 1985, The anti-inflammatory effects of dexamethasone and therapeutic ultrasound in oral surgery. Brit. J. Oral Max. Surgery, 23:17.

Fyfe, M., Chahl, L.A., 1980, The effect of ultrasound on experimental oedema in rats. Ultrasound Med. Biol. 6: 107.

Fyfe, M.C., Chahl, L.A., 1984, Mast cell degranulation and increased vascular permeability induced by therapeutic ultrasound in the rat ankle joint. Br. J. Exp. Path. 65:671.

Fyfe, M.C., Chahl, L.A., 1985, The effect of single or repeated applications of "therapeutic" ultrasound on plasma extravasation during silver nitrate induced inflammation of the rat hindpaw ankle joint in vivo. Ultrasound Med. Biol. 11:273.

Galitsky, A.B., Levina, S.I., 1964, Vascular origin of trophic ulcers and application of ultrasound as pre-operative treatment to plastic surgery. Acta Chir. Plast. (Praha) 6:271.

Harvey, W., Dyson, M., Pond, J.B., Grahame, R. 1975, The in vitro stimulation of protein synthesis in human fibroblasts by therapeutic levels of ultrasound. Proc. 2nd Europ. Congress Ultrasonics Medicine. Excerpta Medica International Congress, Series No.363:10.

Hogan, R.D., Burke, K.M., Franklin, T.D., 1982, The effect of ultrasound on microvascular hemodynamics in skeletal muscle effects during ischemia. Microvasc. Res. 23:370.

Markham, D.E., Wood, M.R., 1980, Ultrasound for Dupuytren's contracture. Physiotherapy,66:55.

Middlemast, S., Chatterjee, D.S., 1978, Comparison of ultrasound and thermotherapy for soft tissue injuries. Physiotherapy, 64:331.

Oakley, E.M., 1982, Evidence for effectiveness of ultrasound treatment in physical medicine. Br. J. Cancer, Suppl. V:45.

Paul, B.J., Lafratta, C.W., Dawson, A.R., Baab, E., Bullock, F., 1960, Use of ultrasound in the treatment of pressure sores in patients with spinal cord injury. Arch. Phys. Med. Rehab., 41:438.

Pizzarello, D.J., Wolsky, A., Becker, M.H., Keegan, A.F., 1975, A new approach to testing the effect of ultrasound on tissue growth and differentiation. Oncology, 31:226.

Pospisilova, J., 1976, Effect of ultrasound on collagen synthesis and deposition in experimental granuloma tissue. Acta Chir. Plast. (Praha) 18:176.

Pospisilova, J., Samohyl, J., Koprivova, M., Jelinkova, A., 1980, Our experience with the use of ultrasound in rehabilitation of hand. Acta Chir. Plast. (Praha) 22: 191.

Shamberger, R.C., Talbot, T.L., Tipton, H.W., Thibault, L.E., Brennan, M.F., 1981, The effect of ultrasonic and thermal treatment on wounds. Plast. Reconstr. Surg. 68:860.

Webster, D.F., Dyson, M., Harvey, W., 1979, Ultrasonically
        induced stimulation of collagen synthesis "in vivo".
        Proc. 4th Eur. Symp. on Ultrasound in Biology and
        Medicine. Ed. P. Greguss. 1:135.
Webster, D.F., Harvey, W., Dyson, M., Pond, J.B., 1980,
        The role of ultrasound-induced cavitation in the "in
        vitro" stimulation of collagen synthesis in human fibro-
        blasts. Ultrasonics, 18:33.
Webster, D.F., Pond, J.B., Dyson, M., Harvey, W., 1978, The
        role of cavitation in the in vitro stimulation of
        protein synthesis in human fibroblasts by ultrasound.
        Ultrasound in Med. & Biol. 4:343.

EFFECTS OF ULTRASOUND ON "SOLID" MAMMALIAN TISSUES AND TUMORS IN VIVO*

Padmakar P. Lele

Professor of Experimental Medicine
& Director, Laboratory for Medical Ultrasonics
Massachusetts Institute of Technology
Cambridge, MA   02139   U.S.A.

INTRODUCTION

Over the last decade, the main thrust of research on bio-effects of ultrasound has been directed towards prevention of the occurrence of any effects that may potentially be injurious to the fetus or the genetic material during diagnostic ultrasonic examination of the pregnancy. Several investigators in their studies on the mechanisms of ultrasound-tissue interactions have utilized various innovative approaches to maximize the occurrence of one or the other phenomenon to determine "the threshold" for biological effect. For example, introduction of stabilized resonant bubbles in the insonation system

---

*Supported in part by USPHS Grant # CA 31303

to maximize acoustic streaming[1], or induction of cavitation by inoculation of the medium with micron-sized metal particles, or by the use of Drosophila larvae containing resonant size air cavities[2] have dramatically illustrated the potential for biological injury through these phenomena at very low ultrasonic intensities. It is well known, however, that the nature and magnitude of the ultrasonically induced phenomena are dependent on the physical characteristics of the medium. It is also possible that the thresholds for biological damage may be different for different tissues and different species. Thus, the data on thresholds for biological damage obtained in these experiments are of little relevance to the problem of ultrasonic safety or hazard in clinical medicine[3]. For this purpose, the magnitude of these phenomena, their biological consequences and the ultrasonic dosage levels at which they first become apparent must be determined under conditions simulating clinical use, using insonation regimens typically employed in clinical practice and in structurally 'organized' ("solid") tissues and/or in fluid tissues in vivo. Studies in vitro on plant and animal tissues, and in vivo on small rodents, flies and plants do not meet these requirements, because their size, presence of chitinous exoskeleton, and morphological differences e.g. presence of air cavities or thick cellulose walls etc., are not representative of mammalian tissues. Scaling for differences in size by using appropriately small wavelengths is untenable because most of the acoustical properties of tissues are related to wavelength. Of the data on ultrasonic thresholds for bioeffects only those obtained in mammals in vivo (and in situ) would appear to be valid for extrapolation to clinical situations.

Adequate assessment of the potential hazards associated with clinical use of ultrasound requires knowledge at least of:
(a) the nature and magnitude of the physical events occurring in the mammalian tissues as a result of ultrasonic perturbation,
(b) the biological consequences of each of these phenomena over the range of their amplitudes, in each relevant tissue under different physiological and pathological states, and
(c) whether the effects summate or potentiate one another since many, if not all, of the physical events occur concurrently in the tissues.

This knowledge may point to the manner in which damage may occur and the site where it may become manifest, and thus may enable the right questions to be asked in prospective or retrospective studies on the safety/hazard of diagnostic ultrasound. This information is also essential for rational application of ultrasound for therapy, since ideally the desired biological effects should be maximized in and restricted to the treatment volume in the tissue and be non-existent elsewhere.

For studies of bioeffects and their mechanisms, it is useful to classify the interactions into two broad categories, although there may be some overlap between the two:
(a) those related to the mechanics of wave propagation, e.g. "direct" effects, radiation pressure, acoustic streaming, cavitation, and other non-linear phenomena;
(b) those related to the absorption of acoustical energy leading to heat generation and temperature rise and thus dependent on the acoustical absorption coefficient of the medium in addition to the acoustical field parameters and variables.

Quantitative studies on the magnitude of these phenomena during insonation of solid tissues in vivo in mammals and their biological consequences have been pursued in the author's laboratory since 1960 in order to develop scientific and rational dosimetry for surgical therapeutic and diagnostic applications. To place these studies in the proper context, it must be pointed out that at the initiation of these studies - and in the decade following - the prevailing doctrine held that purely mechanical mechanisms were responsible for ultrasonically induced tissue damage, without special regard to ultrasonic dosage or biologic conditions[4-11]. It was not until 1971 when a thermal hypothesis of the mechanism of ultrasonic focal destruction in organized tissues was formally presented[12] that heat generation was given serious attention as a factor in tissue destruction in surgery by focused ultrasound. It was only in 1973 that heat generation was considered as a possible factor in teratological effects produced by diagnostic ultrasound[13]. The salient features of the studies relating to heat generation and cavitation are presented below since these appear to be of crucial significance in insonation of human tissues for diagnostic[13] or therapeutic purposes[14].

MATERIALS AND METHODS

The studies were conducted _in vitro_ in air-saturated tap water, degassed deionized water, bovine blood-plasma, and fresh calf liver, and _in vivo_ in the liver and the brain of anesthetized cats and squirrel monkeys, and in tranquilized pregnant mice, in numbers large enough to permit analyses of statistical significance, over a range of ultrasonic field conditions (0.9 to 5.4 MHz frequency, 10^{-1} to 3 x 10^3 W.cm^{-2} intensity in the tissue, 10^{-5} to 10^5 sec burst duration, 1 to 100 bursts, 0-10 sec interburst interval etc.), and tissue state conditions (normothermia or hypothermia, normobaric or hyperbaric

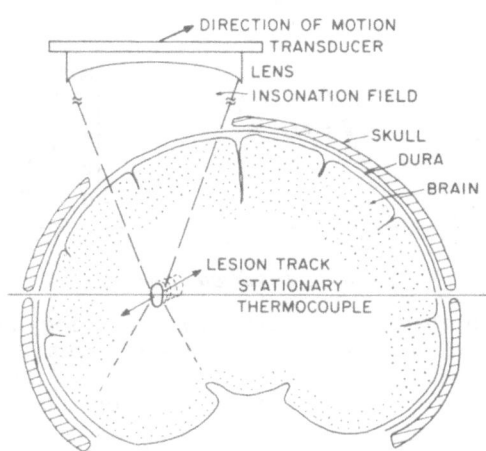

Fig. 1. Experimental set-up for studies on heat generation. Single burst lesions (shown in Figs. 2,3,16 and 17) were made with transducer held stationary. The array of lesions, shown as dotted lines, was made to determine the lesion boundary temperature (T_{LB}). The brain was allowed to cool down to pre-insonation temperature, before advancing the focus in steps of 0.1 mm.

pressures, alone or in combination). The volume of histologically detectable damage, being quantifiable, was used as the response criterion and dose-response relationships were obtained under the different experimental conditions varying the field or state conditions one at a time. Insonation of the brain was performed transdurally through a craniotomy adequate enough to transmit the beam of focused ultrasound without hindrance. The methods used for measurement of temperature and for detection of cavitation will be presented in the appropriate sections. Only a brief summary is given of the data published elsewhere.

STUDIES OF HEAT GENERATION

Supra-threshold insonation of the brain of the cat with focused ultrasound (Fig. 1) results in a trackless, circumscribed lesion at the focus in the brain. The dimensions of the lesions (Fig. 2) are found to be highly reproducible and are a linear function of the duration and of the intensity of insonation[15]. On gross examination and histologically (Fig. 3), as well as ultrastructurally, the lesions

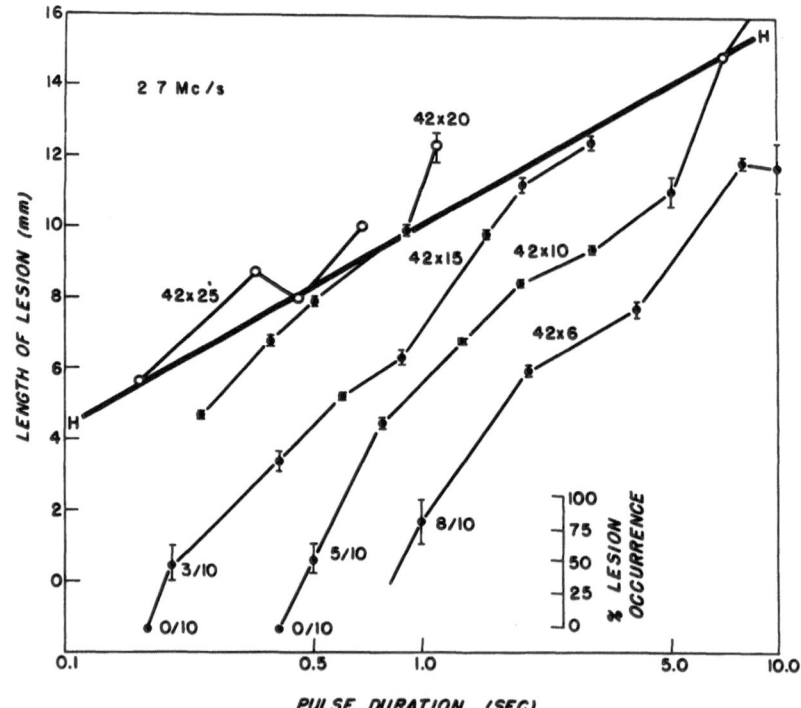

Fig. 2. Relation between burst duration (log scale) and the length of lesions with a single burst at average focal intensities of (42x) 6, 10, 15, 20 and 25 W/cm^2 respectively. The number 42 represents the gain of the focusing system at the frequency of 2.7 MHz. Peak focal intensity was x3 higher. Each point indicates mean of 10 lesions and the standard deviation. Probability of lesion occurrence when not shown is 100%. Hollow circles indicate hemorrhage distending the lesion and spreading intracerebrally when severe. Line H-H shows the safe limit below which hemorrhage (and as discussed later, collapse cavitation) was never encountered. The data on the diameters of these lesions are shown in Fig. 5.

below the line H-H in Fig. 2 show coagulation pan-necrosis without any evidence of mechanical damage to any component of the cellular structure, which is invariably present in lesions (Fig. 16) above line H-H. *The studies in this section deal with lesions below line H-H.* Lesions in the grey matter, the blood perfusion in which

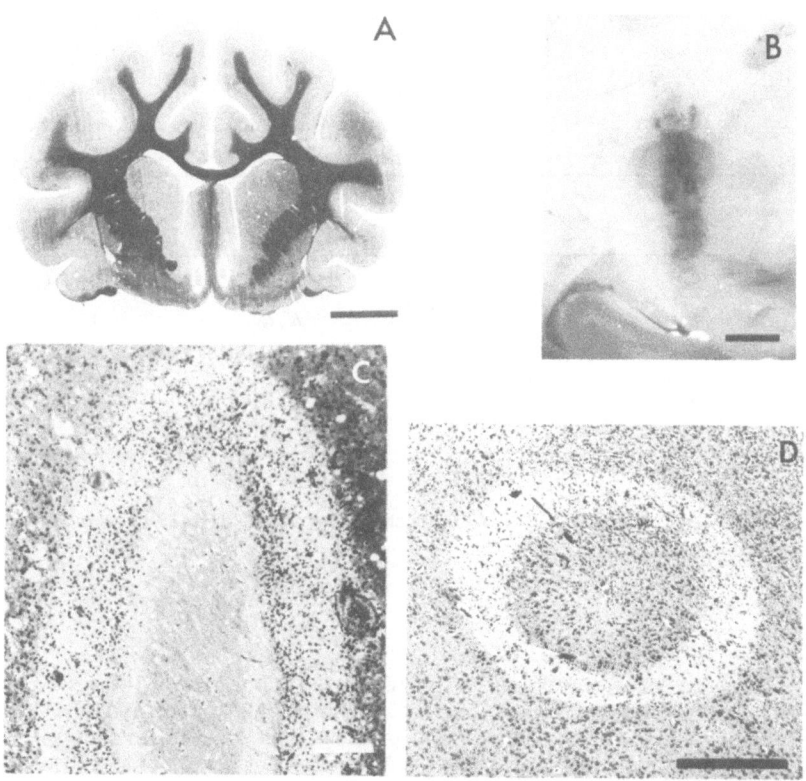

Fig. 3. Typical ultrasonic lesions in the brain below line H-H in Fig. 2. A, B and C are coronal sections through the length of the lesion in the brain of the cat, stained with Loyez myelin, Supravital Trypan Blue and Cresyl Violet stains respectively. D shows a lesion in the brain of the rabbit cut horizontally through the lesion diameter and stained with Hematoxylin & Eosin. The bars represent 5, 2, 1 and 0.5 mm respectively. Specimens A, B and D were obtained 20 min. after insonation; C, from the upper part of the lesion, obtained 6 days after insonation shows phagocytic and vascular capillary infiltration indicative of reparative process and a central core of coagulation necrosis, resistant to lysis. Note the island and moat pattern, sharp boundaries, and absence of any tissue fragmentation. In B, also note that the lesion is narrower and has taken up more Trypan Blue in the grey matter than in the white matter.

is generally about three-times that in the white matter, are smaller than those in the white matter (Fig. 3B). But if the intracranial blood circulation was transiently arrested during insonation, the lesions in grey matter were approximately of the same size as those in the white matter. The dose-lesion size relationship, in both the grey and white matter, is markedly influenced by the temperature of the brain prior to insonation: lowering of the temperature reduces the size of the lesion - a sufficient lowering completely prevents lesion formation (Table 1). This suggests that heat and ultrasound are additive and the lesion formation may depend upon a certain threshold temperature

Table 1. Relation between Lesion Length (l) and Tissue Temperature (T)

T,°C	n	l,mm	c
37	5	6.7	.099
31	5	4.4	.1
24	5	1.2	.098
22	10	0.0	

n = Number of Replicates; C = Coefficient of variation

Insonation: 2.7 MHz, 420 W.cm^{-2} average focal intensity,

1.3 sec burst

being reached in the tissue as a result of insonation. The temperatures within the lesion in different parts of the brain (grey and white matter) were measured during its formation by implanting a thermocouple 50 μm in diameter and making an array of lesions across it (Figs.1, 4A). The lesion diameter, measured from histological preparations of the brain (Fig.3), was superimposed on the plot of peak temperatures measured at each site (Fig. 5) to determine the temperature at the lesion boundary (T_{LB}), i.e. the threshold temperature for irreversible tissue damage, in different regions in the brain[16,17]. Considering the steepness of the spatial temperature gradient, and the uncertainty, however small, in the measurement of the lesion diameter in histological preparations, the T_{LB} was found to be remarkably constant, regardless of the type of the tissue - grey or white -, and sufficiently high to cause heat damage. To determine if thermal mechanisms alone can account for the development of lesions and all of their measurable characteristics, a purely thermal model of ultrasonic effects and of tissue destruction was assumed and an analytical prediction of lesion development, lesion size and lesion shape, for varying values of ultrasonic and thermal constants and controllable variables (frequency, focusing, dosage, target depth, etc.), was attempted. An empirical equation to describe the axial and radial ultrasonic energy distribution at the focus in water was derived. Appropriate heat transfer equations were developed for temperature distributions resulting from insonation. The computed temperature profiles were plotted against non-dimensionalized parameters.

Lesion dimensions read off the computed temperature profiles at the T_{LB} measured experimentally, as described above, were compared with the experimental data on lesion dimensions obtained previously[15]. The agreement between the analytically predicted results and the experimental data was close (Fig.6), indicating that within the range

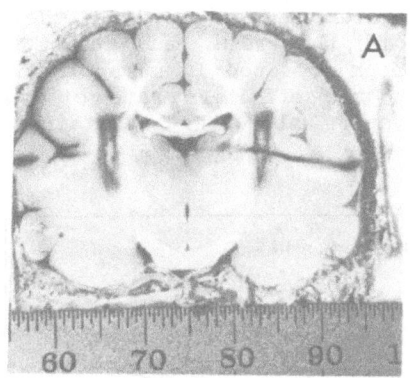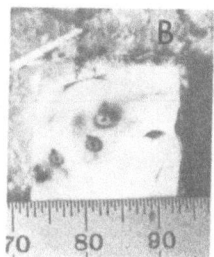

Fig. 4. Measurement of Lesion Boundary Temperature (T_{LB}).
Brain of the cat. Supravital Trypan Blue stain.
A: Ultrasonic lesions, brain cut coronally in the plane of the thermocouple; B: Heated Wire lesions, brain cut horizontally across the lesion. In each lesion, the central dot represents the heating wire, the peripheral, the thermocouple.

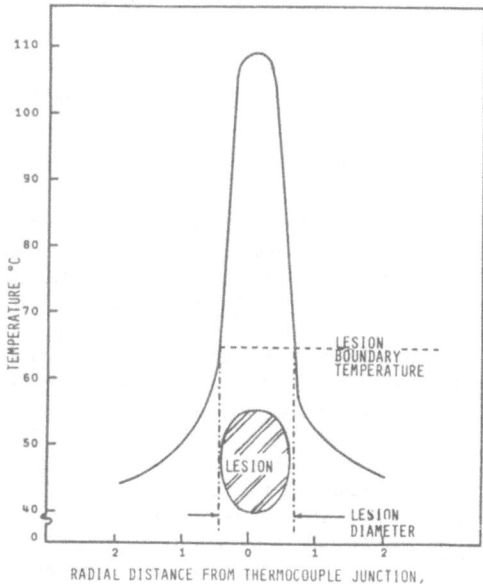

Fig. 5. Determination of the lesion boundary temperature by superimposing lesion diameter on the plot of peak temperatures recorded at each location of the focus. The symmetry of the plot indicates that reinsonation of a preinsonated region did not alter the ultrasonic characteristics of the tissue.

of ultrasonic parameters studied, the development of the lesions in the brain could be explained by purely thermal mechanisms.

The power of the analytical model to predict temperature distributions in the brain was amply confirmed by meticulous and extensive measurements of temperature distributions, and it is gratifying to find that Nyborg[18] has adopted the same approach for unfocused transducers. Caution should however be exercised in the application of the model to tissues other than the brain, particularly for heating durations of more than a few seconds, since in most other tissues the local blood perfusion, and thus the effective rate of heat transfer increases with temperature elevation above 43°C sustained for 5 sec or longer.

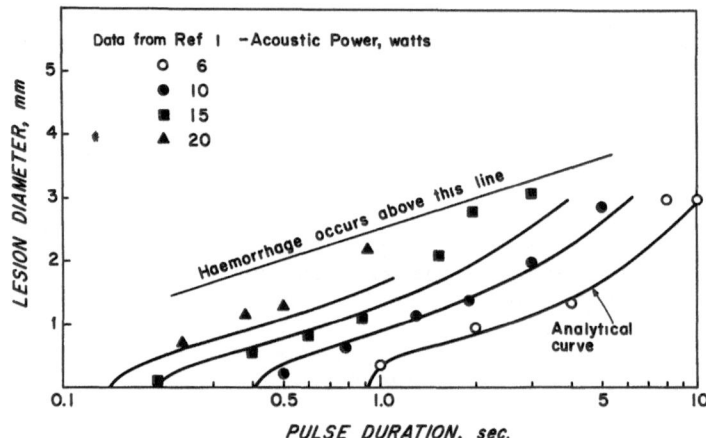

Fig. 6.   Comparison of experimental data and analytical results for lesion diameters in cat brain at various intensities and burst durations using the purely thermal model. (From Ref.17)

In order to determine the range of ultrasonic field and tissue state conditions under which ultrasonic tissue destruction could be explained by a purely thermal mechanism, T_{LB} was measured at different frequencies between 0.9 and 5.4 MHz [19], and over a range of insonation durations between 1 and 50 sec, adjusting the intensity to produce a histologically measurable lesion. The magnitude of ultrasonic non-thermal effects is known to be frequency dependent and their contribution to tissue injury, by summation or synergism with heat damage, should not be affected by the cooling of the tissue by perfusion and heat conduction over the extended insonation durations. If non-thermal effects contribute to tissue destruction, T_{LB} should exhibit some dependence on insonation frequency and duration of insonation. However, if the T_{LB} is found to be constant, the direct contribution of non-thermal effects to tissue injury could be deemed to be negligible. To assess the contribution of periodic forces, such as the radiation pressure, T_{LB} was measured using both single and multiple burst insonations with equivalent ON times. Experiments were also conducted in animals rendered hypothermic to a core temperature of 27°C. The T_{LB} was found to remain constant regardless of the frequency, insonation duration, single or multiple burst regime, tissue type and base temperature of the animal, indicating that non-thermal ultrasonic phenomena did not contribute to lesion formation measurably, and histologically detectable tissue destruction could be attributed entirely to heat generation by ultrasound. Previous studies by the author on the effects of focused ultrasound on nerve conduction in peripheral nerves[20] had also led to the same conclusion viz. the observed effects were mediated thermally and could be duplicated by application of graded amounts of heat. Since both ultrasonically induced irreversible tissue destruction and reversible physiological effects appeared to be mediated by heat generation, a thermal hypothesis was tentatively postulated[12] as follows:

"For a wide class of reversible and irreversible effects caused by the action of ultrasound on tissues, the same effects can equivalently be produced by non-acoustic localized heating of the tissue, provided the temperature history during heating and cooling duplicates the quasi-steady (averaged over a cycle) temperature history during insonation."

As a final test of the applicability of the Thermal Hypothesis to ultrasonic tissue destruction, T_{LB} was measured for lesions produced by non-ultrasonic sources of energy using hot water, microwave, focused infra-red, and focused CO_2 laser for superificial lesions, and implanted resistance wire heated by direct electric current for deep lesions. It was not possible to measure the T_{LB} for superficial lesions with any confidence, since their boundaries, even at a depth of a few millimeters, were not sharply defined, and measurements at the surface were vitiated by the ambient temperature. Electrically heated wire produced sharply circumscribed lesions (Fig.4B) provided that the temperature at the surface of the wire did not exceed the boiling point of the tissue fluid - approx. 100°C. This constraint imposed a limit of approx. 50 sec on the shortest heating duration which could be used to yield lesions comparable in size to the ultrasonic lesions studied. The T_{LB} for the heated wire was measured by an implanted thermocouple and the accuracy of the measurement was checked, and found to be precise, by calculations of the temperature field from the measured power dissipation assuming the wire to be a line source of heat[21]. Heating durations were varied between 5×10^{-1} and 5×10^3 sec. At the shorter durations, the T_{LB} was found to be the same for the heating wire lesions as for ultrasonic lesions but became consistently and progressively lower as the heating duration increased. The T_{LB} studies on ultrasonic lesions were therefore extended to cover insonation durations from 10^{-1} to 10^5 sec[22]. It was found that the T_{LB} for ultrasonic lesions also became consistently and progressively lower with increasing durations of insonation and at each duration of heating there was no statistically significant difference between the T_{LB} for ultrasonic and heating wire lesions. At tissue temperatures of 42°C or lower, no lesions were detected histologically even if insonation or wire heating was continued for 10^5 sec. It may, therefore, be concluded that:

1. Histologically detectable tissue destruction in the brain of the cat by ultrasound, below the Line H-H in Fig. 2, is due to heat generation, and the contribution of non-thermal phenomena is neglible.

2. There is no single, fixed, temperature threshold for tissue injury; the temperature threshold varies with duration of the temperature elevation.

3. On the basis of previous studies[20], the above two statements may also be true for reversible physiological effects on nerve conduction.

A Model for a Time-Dependent Temperature Threshold for Damage

A careful study of the literature on thresholds for heat necrosis of biological media using non-ultrasonic modalities, such as direct heat by waterbath, infrared, and lasers, revealed that their time-dependence had in fact been reported by several investigators[23-25] and was present, though neglected in the results of Peppers et al[26]. On the basis of these and our own observations shown in Fig. 7, a model for the temperature threshold for damage as a function of duration (time) was developed[19] and is summarized here briefly.

Many biological processes, especially biological inactivating reactions, can be described by a rate equation based on the theory of reaction kinetics[27,28]. From this theory the rate of reaction in any inactivating reaction can be given by

$$k' = \frac{kT}{h} \, e^{-\Delta F/RT} = \frac{kT}{h} \, e^{\Delta S/R} \, e^{-\Delta H/RT} \tag{1}$$

where

k' = overall reaction rate

k, h = Boltzmann's and Planck's constants

R = gas constant

T = temperature in ° absolute

$\Delta F, \Delta S, \Delta H$ = changes in free energy, entropy, and enthalpy of reactions

For a thermally mediated process the rate determining parameter is ΔF, the standard free energy of activation. Therefore the reaction rate, k', could be rapid even for a reaction with large heats of

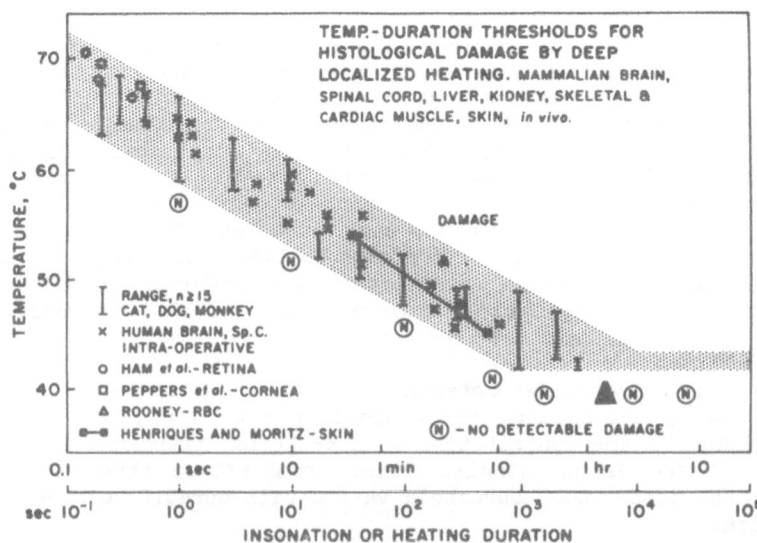

Fig. 7. Temperature-duration thresholds for histologically detectable damage by localized heating of mammalian tissues in vivo. The triangle indicates fetal damage.

formation, ΔH. For example, in highly structured molecules such as protein, the activation process is accompanied by a sizeable increase in the entropy, ΔS. The combination of the large ΔH and $T \Delta S$ gives a small value of ΔF which in turn gives a large reaction rate.

If one now considers q to be the surviving fraction of the cells being insonated or heated, then

$$\frac{dq}{dt} = k' \, q \tag{2}$$

where

$$q = \frac{n}{n_0} = \text{survival fraction}$$

$$n = \text{number of cells surviving}$$

$$n_0 = \text{number of cells originally present}$$

The reaction rate, k', is a function of the temperature, T, which is in turn a function of time. Therefore integrating Equation 2 with respect to time gives

$$q = \exp(-\int_0^t k' \, dt)$$

$$= \exp(-\int_0^t \frac{kT}{h} \, e^{\Delta S/R} \, e^{-\Delta H/RT} \, dt) \tag{3}$$

Thus, given the values of the energies of reaction and the temperature history, one can calculate the value of 'q' at any particular point. This value will then indicate whether that point lies in the area of necrotic or live tissue. The calculation of 'q' was done with the aid of a computer for temperature profiles generated during insonation. The value of ΔH (150,000 cal) was taken from Henriques[29] who used a similar analysis in an attempt to describe a thermal threshold for epidermal burns. The value of ΔS was also chosen from Henriques[29] but was varied slightly to optimize the fit of the data. The value used by Henriques was 219 cal/°C, whereas that used here was 216.7 cal/°C, a small difference considering the variation of ΔS reported by Wood[30] for various proteins and enzymes in suspension.

Since death is a discontinuous event whereas 'q' is continuous, a survival fraction less than 0.1 (or 10%) was defined to indicate total necrosis, and a fraction greater than 0.9 (or 90%) was defined to indicate survival. Intermediate values of 'q' fall into the threshold region. The values of 'q' were calculated for the temperature cycles generated by single and multiple burst insonations, and for heated wire lesions. These all fell within the stippled band shown in Fig. 7. The fact that the experimentally determined time-dependent temperature threshold for tissue damage correlates well with the theoretical predictions based on a thermodynamic model of first order reaction kinetics does reinforce the Thermal Hypothesis. The rather abrupt flattening of the slope at approximately 42°C for these mammalian tissues in vivo may represent a purely thermal threshold.

Table 2. Teratological Effects of Systemic Hyperthermia 2.5–5.0°C
for 1 Hour or Longer at the Stage of Organogenesis in the Fetus
(Guinea Pig, Sheep, Rat)[a]

General	Central Nervous System	Musculo-Skeletal System
Fetal resorption/ abortion	Reduction in brain weight	Talipes-like conditions
Growth retardation	Microencephaly	Arthrogryposis multiplex
Microphthalmia	Anencephaly	Amyoplasia
Cataract	Defects in the spinal cord	Hypoplasia of forefeet
Defects of the abdominal wall		Absence, defects or deformations of tibia, fibula
Renal agenesis		
Defects of the palate		Failure of incisor teeth to erupt, abnormal amelogenesis

[a]For details see Lele (13).

Effects on Embryonic Tissues

Since heat generation appears to be valid as a mechanism of tissue
destruction not only in the fixed, post-mitotic cell population in
the central nervous system, but also in tissues such as the liver,
which can regenerate, it is interesting to see if it also holds true
for the dividing and differentiating tissues of the embryo. These
cell populations, specially at the stage of organogenesis, are known
to be particularly susceptible to damage by a variety of agents including
thermal insults. Systemic hyperthermia of 2.5 to 5°C (above the normal
temperature for the species) for 1 hour or longer, occurring during
specific critical developmental stages of organogenesis, is known to
cause abortion or fetal malformations[13]. Table 2 lists the variety
of teratological effects that have been observed by exposure of pregnant
animals to elevated ambient temperatures and humidity. The effect
is directly on the embryo; the specific abnormality is related to the
developmental stage of the fetus and to the temperature elevation and
its duration. The effect is related not to the agent causing
hyperthermia, but to hyperthermia itself. Thus, in addition to
environmental chambers, water baths, radiant heat sources, microwave
diathermy[13], and ultrasound have all yielded comparable results. Lele[3]
lists twelve reports of deleterious effects of ultrasound on fetal
development in mammals in which hyperthermia of the embryo is almost
certainly the primary causative factor. Calculations based on insonation
parameters in these experiments predict temperature elevations of 5
to 15°C in the fetus and correlate rather well with the actual
measurements. In man, any infection such as rubella, influenza,
smallpox, occurring and giving rise to fever during early pregnancy,
is known to cause substantial numbers of abortions and fetal
malformations, as is induction of artificial fever or heat exposure
in sauna[31]. It thus appears that heat generation by ultrasound is
the prime mechanism involved in the production of teratological effects,

abortions and resorption of the embryo. As with ionizing radiations, all of these effects are related to the death or irreversible injury to one or more cells of the embryo during organogenesis. Consistent with the hypothesis of Bergonie and Tribondeau[32], the threshold for damage to the dividing cell population in the embryo, shown as a triangle in Fig. 7, is seen to be a little lower than that for mature or post-mitotic cells. Temperature duration thresholds for other dividing cell populations, as for example, in transplanted murine tumors[33], as well as in spontaneous canine tumors are found to be in the same range as those in the embryo. The slope of the Temperature-Duration relationships for "cell killing" in suspension cultures[34] appear to be slightly different and may be related to the different micro-environment of cells under these conditions.

STUDIES ON CAVITATION

Ultrasonically induced cavitation is known to have significant effects on cells and organisms in suspension. But no conclusive data on the occurrence of and/or damage by cavitation in "solid" tissues are available in the literature, except perhaps those of Fry et al[35] who invoked cavitation as an explanation for occurrence of lesion formation at points other than the location of beam focus at intensities above 2000 $W.cm^{-2}$. Although cavitation cannot be ruled out at these intensities, the demonstration of correlation between the location of such lesions and the distribution of cavitation nuclei, or a positive proof of the occurrence of cavitation within the tissue during its insonation would be more convincing. In contrast to the very high intensity required for cavitation postulated by Fry et al, Ter Haar et al[36] state that free gas bubbles could be induced within living mammalian tissue by insonation with 0.75 MHz ultrasound at 680 $mW.cm^{-2}$, though "no specific indications of associated hazard" were observed with 5 min. insonations. Carstensen and Flynn[37], on the other hand, have drawn attention to the possibility of transient cavitation from microsecond-length pulses of ultrasound with peak intensities of the order of as low as 10 $W.cm^{-2}$ if appropriate sub-micron sized gas bubbles are present in the tissues. In view of the paucity of published data on cavitation in vivo, the results of studies which were aimed at quantification of cavitation activity evoked in mammalian tissues during insonation under different field and tissue state conditions and its correlation with gross, histological and ultrastructural tissue alterations[38-40], are reported below in some detail. Some of the data were previously reported in 1973[41] and 1977[42] but are apparently not widely available.

The relative sensitivities of sound scattering and acoustic emission as reliable indices of the occurrence of cavitation were studied in air-saturated tap water and the latter was found to be preferable. Studies elsewhere[43-46] and in our laboratory have shown that half-harmonic (frequently accompanied by second and higher harmonic) acoustic emission from a liquid medium during insonation are a strong indication of the occurrence of cavitation and can be taken as a criterion of its occurrence. For monitoring acoustic emission, a wide-band (3 dB bandwidth 0.8 to 10 MHz), sensitive (200 picowatts.cm^{-2} = 20μV) receiver was acoustically coupled to the tissue in the focal plane of and perpendicular to the main axis of the insonating beam (Fig. 8). The output was analyzed both in time and frequency domains and also was integrated over the period of insonation to derive a measure of "total cavitation power". A bandwidth of 300 kHz was commonly used in frequency and time-domain studies. Half-harmonic (or subharmonic) and anharmonic emission were studied routinely as indicative of the occurrence of stable (bubble oscillation) and unstable (bubble collapse) cavitation respectively. The fundamental, second and higher harmonics and wide-band emission were also measured. At the insonation frequency of 2.7 MHz, for example, half-harmonic emission was measured at 1.35 MHz ± 150 KHz, subharmonic at 0.5 to 2.0 MHz, and anharmonic at 4.0 MHz ±150 KHz and 4.6 MHz ±150 KHz. Anharmonic emission was found to be quantitatively related to wide-band emission.

Equipment was fabricated for maintenance of surgically prepared and instrumented animals under anesthesia and in physiological condition (respiratory gas composition adjusted to prevent various types of toxicity) under an ambient pressure of 42 atmospheres absolute (atm) for the durations required for the studies including that for careful decompression and perfusion fixation to prevent formation of gas bubbles in the tissues[39].

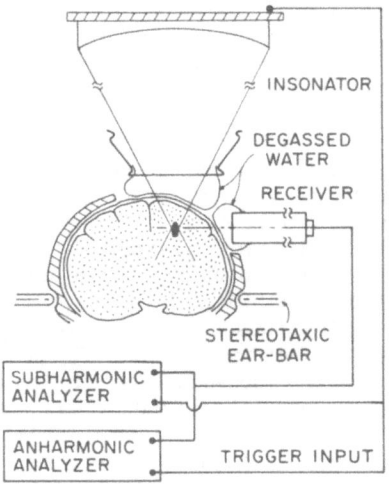

Fig. 8. System for monitoring acoustic emission from the brain of the cat _in vivo_. Studies on liquids were conducted in an anechoic vessel, utilizing similar geometric arrangement of the insonator and receiver.

Since the data available for decompression were restricted to 10 atm - pressures encountered within the diving range - schedules were developed for decompression after pressurization to 42 atm. The times required for successful decompression of the live animal from 42 atm to 1 atm were found to be prohibitively long, ranging from 35 hr. for a 5 min. exposure at 42 atm to 60 hr. for 60 min. exposure. The rate for successful decompression is highly non-linear, and for short exposures to pressure, over one half of the total pressure decrease occurs in the first 15 min. of decompression. The prohibitively long decompression times were therefore avoided by decompressing the live animal for a set time, sacrificing the animal with an overdose of the anesthetic and perfusing it for tissue fixation and then reducing the pressure to 1 atm. Histological and ultrastructural studies, in control animals, showed absence of any detectable damage.

The pressure vessel was built to the specifications of the American Society of Mechanical Engineers Boilers and Pressure Vessel Code to withstand 60 atm and was large enough to accomodate a stereotaxic head holder for the cat, the insonation head and a 3-axis transpositioning system to permit measurement of T_{LB}, local and systemic temperature monitoring subsystem, acoustic emission monitoring transducer, systemic (core) temperature control system to maintain the desired core temperature, various feed-throughs for electrical connections and hydraulic lines, and incorporated safety devices to protect against overpressurization. Tests were conducted on methyl-methacrylate phantoms[47] to ascertain that the output of the insonation system, and the characteristics of the coupling medium and temperature and acoustic emission measurement systems were not affected by cyclical pressure changes.

Measurements of acoustic emission were made for insonation at different intensities for each of several burst durations between 0.1 and 10.0 sec. for single or multiple bursts. Intensity or burst duration was increased or decreased progressively in consecutive insonations, or was varied in a random manner. The influence of ambient pressure and the base temperature of the animal under pressures of 1 and 42 atm on acoustic emission, as well as on the size of resultant lesions, was studied. In parallel experiments the T_{LB} and the peak temperatures in the tissue at the center of the insonation beam were measured with an implanted 50 μ thermocouple. At least 6, generally 10 and frequently up to 25 replicates were obtained for each data point and subjected to statistical analyses.

All tissues insonated in vivo and samples of tissues insonated in vitro were examined histologically for morphological alterations. The presence and nature of these were then correlated with that of acoustic emission measured previously. Modelling and analytical studies were also undertaken to understand the physical mechanisms by which insonation induced cavitation may damage mammalian tissues. These are not included in this paper; some of the early work was reported previously[41].

Acoustic Emissions

Representative recordings of the typical swept frequency spectra and the time course of acoustic emissions from air-saturated water, degassed deionized water, bovine plasma, and from cat brain in vivo during a burst of insonation are presented in Figs. 9 and 10. In the frequency domain the emission from air-saturated water (Fig. 9A) is characterized by a strong signal at the fundamental and the half-harmonic and relatively weaker signals at the second, third and higher harmonics. In all of the media the amplitude of the signal at the fundamental was found to be invariably proportional to the square root of the insonation power indicating that it was the result of the direct coupling between the insonation and receiver transducers, through the medium or its boundaries (glass, air or skull), and was not associated with cavitation activity. In the time-domain (Fig. 9B), the half-harmonic emission from air-saturated water is seen as sharp "spikes" or a burst of spikes, occurring only during insonation, but randomly with respect to its beginning or end. Though the half-harmonic emissions were thus random, both in occurrence and amplitude, it was obvious from an analysis of hundreds of records of integrated power output that their time-averaged energy content was statistically stable and constant at any particular insonation intensity. Below a certain threshold insonation intensity there was no emission at any anharmonic frequency,

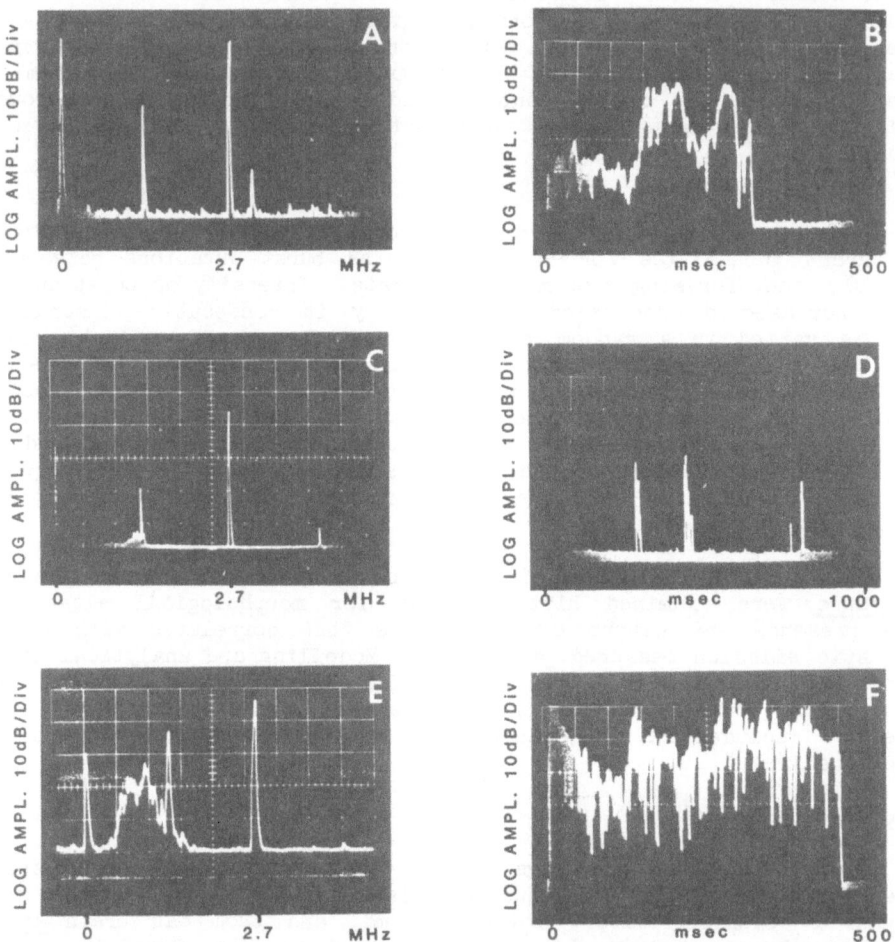

Fig. 9. Representative records of acoustic emission from
air-saturated water (A,B), degassed deionized water
(C,D), and bovine blood plasma (E,F) in frequency (Left)
and time (Right) domains. The vertical axis shows
the logarithmic amplitude (10 dB/div.) of the acoustic
emission with the average base line due to instrument
noise at -100dBm ($=10^{-13}$W). The scales for the
horizontal axes are as shown on each record.

that is, at frequencies other than the harmonics of the half-harmonic or the fundamental frequency. If, however, the peak focal insonation intensity exceeded a threshold value (which was dependent on the medium, as well as on the insonation frequency), then in addition to the harmonic and half-harmonic emissions and their harmonics, erratic, wideband emissions, with rise and fall times of the order of a microsecond, were observed. The frequency spectrum of these wide-band emissions encompassed the frequency bandwidth of the receiver, with an essentially flat power distribution. It was therefore concluded that the magnitude of the anharmonic emission at 4.6 MHz ± 150 kHz could be used for quantification of the wide-band emission, and the associated bubble collapse type of cavitation (unstable cavitation). Acoustic emission from degassed, deionized water (Figs. 9C,D) was found to be similar to that from air-saturated water, but of significantly lower magnitude (approx.-40 dB) at each insonation intensity, whereas that from bovine blood plasma (Figs. 9E,F) was consistently of greater magnitude (approx. +3dB) and of wider bandwith centered at a frequency below the

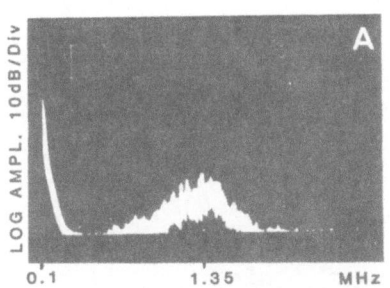
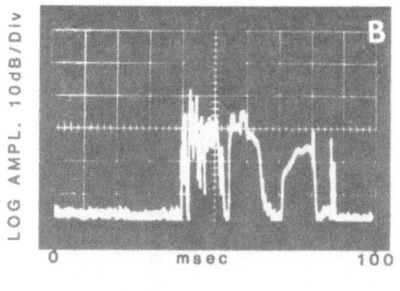

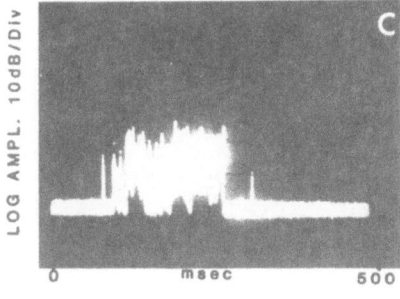
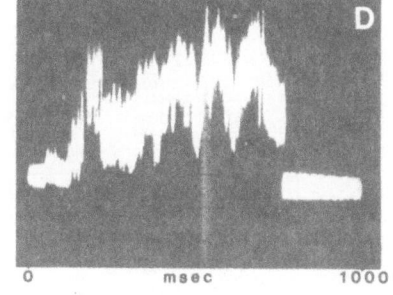

Fig. 10. Representative records of acoustic emission from the brain of the cat _in vivo_, in frequency (A) and time domains (B,C,D). Records B, C : Subharmonic emission: D: Anharmonic emission.

half-harmonic spike. The bandwidth of the comparable emission from the calf liver _in vitro_ and from the brain of the cat _in vivo_ (Fig. 10A) was found to be even wider and was centered around the half-harmonic frequency. This progressive increase in the bandwidth of acoustic emission from water to plasma to brain, on theoretical considerations, was believed to be due to the progressively higher viscous damping in the three media. This was confirmed in a study of acoustic emission from a series of progressively more viscous solutions of increasing concentrations of glycerol in water. Based on these considerations, the term 'subharmonic' is used hereafter in this article to include the half-harmonic 'spike' when present.

Intensity and Frequency Dependence of Acoustic Emission

Subharmonic and anharmonic emissions were measured for a burst 0.5 sec in duration, at insonation frequencies of 2.7 and 1.8 MHz, varying the peak focal intensity in the medium, in steps from 100 mW.cm^{-2} to 3,100 W.cm^{-2}. The averaged values for 10 or more replicates under each insonation condition showed a monotonic increase in subharmonic

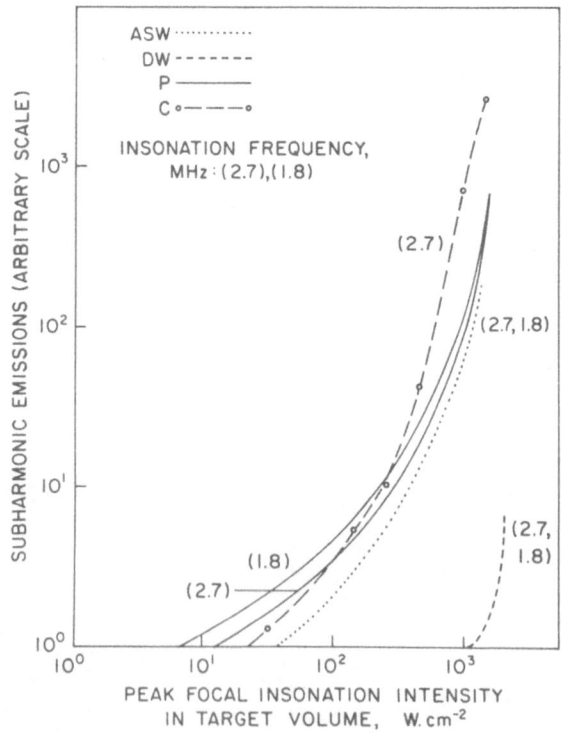

Fig. 11. Intensity and frequency dependence of subharmonic emission from air-saturated water (ASW), degassed deionized water (DW) and bovine blood plasma (P) and the brain of the cat _in vivo_ (C) for 0.5 sec burst at insonation frequencies of 1.8 and 2.7 MHz. Values for peak focal intensity are corrected for attenuation in each medium.

emission with intensity from 150 mW.cm^{-2} to 1,500 W.cm^{-2} (Fig. 11), although there was no distinct threshold intensity for the occurrence of the emission. Above the intensity of 1,500 W.cm^{-2}, there was a remarkably sharp increase, of many orders of magnitude, in the subharmonic emission (Fig. 12). The magnitude of the emission from plasma and from the brain of the cat in vivo was only slightly greater than that from air-saturated water, the emission from which was 2 to 3 orders of magnitude greater than that from degassed, deionized water. Comparison of data at insonation frequencies of 2.7 and 1.8 MHz (Fig. 11) showed no significant differences in the emission from water, but slightly higher levels of emission was evident from plasma at the lower insonation frequency.

No anharmonic emission was ever observed at peak focal intensities of 1,000 W.cm^{-2} in air-saturated water, calf liver in vitro or in brain of the cat in vivo even with burst durations of up to 10 sec. It occurred only sporadically at intensity levels between 1,000 W.cm^{-2} and 1,500 W.cm^{-2}. But above 1,500 W.cm^{-2} there was an abrupt and marked increase in anharmonic emission (Figs. 10D,13), as well as in subharmonic emission (Fig. 12) and both types of emission were detected at each insonation at intensities above 3000 W.cm^{-2}. Compared to that in air-saturated water, the 'threshold' for the onset of anharmonic emission from the tissues is lower, and at intensities above the threshold, the energy content of the emission from the tissues is found to be approximately two orders of magnitude higher than that from air-saturated water. This lower threshold and higher acoustic emission from biological tissues implies not only the presence of a larger number of cavitation sites and nuclei, but possibly also the higher probability of retaining the oscillating bubble(s) within the insonation focus for longer periods

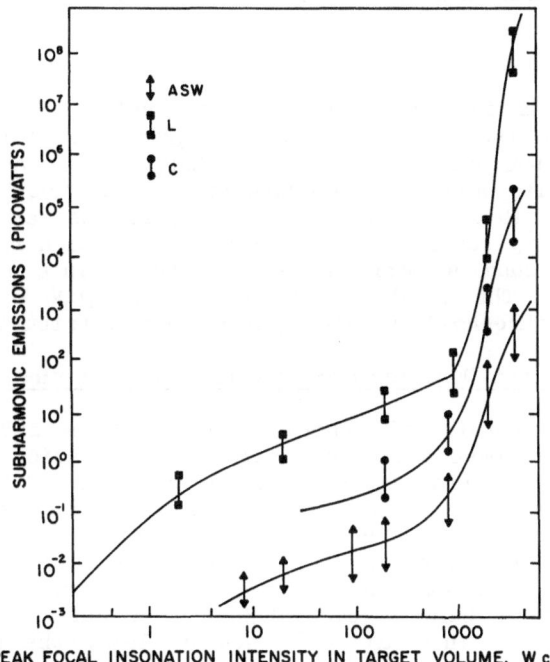

Fig. 12. Intensity dependence of subharmonic emission from air-saturated water (ASW), calf liver in vitro (L), and brain of the cat in vivo (C), for a 0.5 sec burst at insonation frequency of 2.7 MHz. The vertical lines indicate the spread in data.

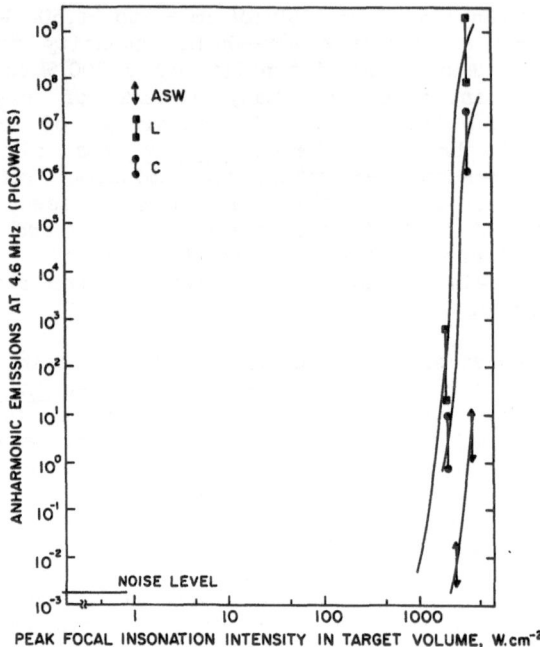

Fig. 13. Intensity dependence of anharmonic emission (4.6 MHz) from air-saturated water (ASW), calf liver in vitro (L), and brain of the cat in vivo (C), for a 0.5 sec burst at insonation frequency of 2.7 MHz. The vertical lines indicate the spread in data.

in the tissue matrix as compared to air-saturated water in which a bubble can move freely down a pressure gradient. Figure 14 shows the probability of the occurrence of any subharmonic and anharmonic emission regardless of its amplitude or duration, as a function of local peak intensity above 1000 $W.cm^{-2}$, in the brain of the cat in vivo. If the critical intensity required for the onset of emission followed a Gaussian distribution around a mean value, all the points should fall on a straight line. The break in the slope at 1,600 $W.cm^{-2}$ implies the existence of a threshold, resulting in a skew distribution.

Dependence on Burst Duration and Multiple Burst Insonation

For single bursts, the energy content of the subharmonic emission was found to increase with increasing burst durations between 0.1 and 10.0 sec, but the average power over the duration of the burst remained statistically constant; with burst durations shorter than 0.1 sec, the probability of the occurrence of acoustic emission was too low for statistically valid comparisons with 10 replicates. In studies on multiple burst insonations an interesting phenomenon was observed. If two insonation bursts, each 0.3 sec in duration, were delivered with an interburst interval of 15 sec or less, the energy content in the acoustic emission during the second burst was significantly higher than that during the first burst. With interburst intervals of 15 to 30 sec, the phenomena became progressively less pronounced and were not observed with interpulse intervals longer than 30 sec. This observation may imply that although acoustic emission ceases with the insonation burst, some of the effects in the tissues persist for periods up to 30 sec. Considering the mechanism(s) leading to cavitation and accompanying acoustic emission, it is plausible that some of the bubbles (gas or vapor) which were enucleated during the first burst (and did not grow to the size of instability and collapse) persist in the tissue until they are reabsorbed over a period of 30 sec, following insonation. Should this hypothesis be correct, once acoustic emission has been initiated from a target volume it should be possible to maintain it at progressively lower insonation intensities. To test this hypothesis, subharmonic acoustic emission from calf liver _in vitro_ was measured with paired insonation bursts of 0.3 sec, and interburst intervals of 30 sec and 2 sec respectively. The experiments were started with 30.0 sec interburst interval at a low level insonation intensity which was first raised successively to the higher limit and then the interpulse interval was reduced to 2.0 sec and the intensity level lowered in steps until no acoustic emission was recorded. The experiment was repeated five times and the pooled data are shown in Fig. 15. With 30 sec interburst interval, the magnitude and intensity dependence of the subharmonic acoustic emission was comparable to that for single bursts (Fig. 11), but note that with the interburst interval of 2 sec, there was significant increase in its magnitude. Furthermore, under these conditions there was significant lowering of the "threshold" for their occurrence.

Effect of Ambient Pressure on Acoustic Emission

In the 50 atm pressure vessel described previously, studies could be conducted safely under ambient pressures of up to 42 atm,

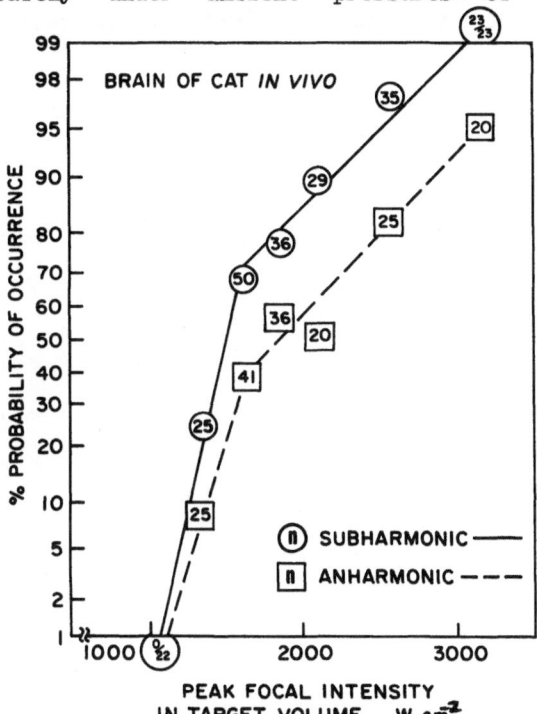

Fig. 14. Probability of the occurrence of acoustic emission from the brain of the cat _in vivo_ at peak intensities in the target volume from 1000 to 3100 $W.cm^2$. n = number of replicates. The fractions represent the proportion of positive results. Insonation frequency: 2.7 MHz; burst duration: 0.5 sec.

approximately equivalent to the peak acoustic pressure associated with an intensity of 525 W.cm^{-2} at the target volume in brain. Subharmonic acoustic emission from air-saturated water, blood plasma, calf-liver <u>in vitro</u> and the brain of the cat <u>in vivo</u> were completely suppressed during insonation with bursts up to the peak focal intensity of 525 W.cm^{-2}. Above this intensity, the subharmonic emission was seen to consist of discrete spikes, about 5 to 10 msec apart with the signal returning to the baseline between the spikes, rather than the steady level of emission with superimposition of spikes observed at ambient pressure of 1 atm (Fig. 9B,C). Quantitatively, the average delay in the first occurrence of subharmonic emission from the start of insonation was significantly longer than that at 1 atm. The number of anharmonic emissions also appeared to be reduced and the average delay in their occurrence was longer under the ambient pressure of 42 atm than at 1 atm.

Biological Studies

The Size, Shape and Characteristics of Lesions

The hypothesis that the negative pressure (tension) phase is a factor in tissue damage was experimentally tested by comparing the size and shape of lesions formed under normal atmospheric pressure and those under an ambient pressure of 42 atm under identical conditions in the same animal. Peak focal insonation intensity of 525 W.cm^{-2}, the peak acoustical pressure at which is less than 42 atm, was used. Following the procedure for insonation and measurement of lesion size described in detail previously[15,48,49], twelve pairs of lesions from

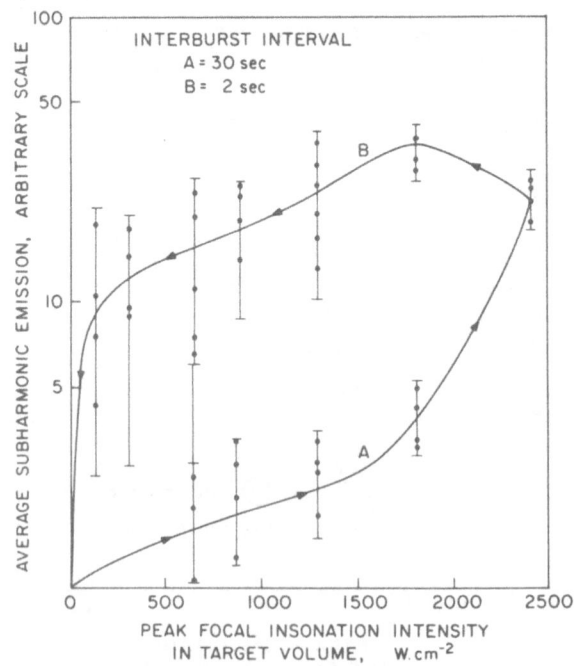

Fig. 15. Effect of interburst interval on subharmonic acoustic emission. Interburst interval was 30 sec for curve A and 2 sec for curve B. Arrowheads indicate the direction of stepwise change in the insonation intensity. Vertical lines indicate the spread in data.

5 animals were compared. Gross examination (Fig. 16) and blind reading of the histological preparations did not reveal any differences in the appearance of the lesions, nor was there any statistically significant difference between the size and shape of the lesions formed under the two conditions (Table 3). As stated previously (Fig. 12), at the insonation intensity used subharmonic acoustic emission from the brain occurs regularly and predictably at 1 atm, but no acoustic emission is detected at an ambient pressure of 42 atm. On the basis of these results, it appears that stable or bubble-oscillation type of acoustic cavitation does not contribute to histologically detectable tissue damage. In order to permit more time for cavitational or other mechanical phenomena to inflict tissue damage, the studies were repeated in hypothermic animals at a core temperature of 27°C and extending the burst duration by 100% to 8.0 sec. No differences were found between lesions made at 1 and 42 atm ambient pressures.

Studies on the effects of higher peak focal insonation intensities from 1,050 to 2,600 $W.cm^{-2}$ on the brain of the cat _in vivo_ were conducted at ambient pressure of 1 atm. Acoustic emission was recorded during insonation with 2.7 MHz focused ultrasound and correlated with the size, shape and characteristics of the lesion. Burst durations were selected to keep the size of the resultant lesions comparable to those in studies at the lower intensities. The results are presented in Table 4. At the peak focal intensity of 1,050 $W.cm^{-2}$, only subharmonic acoustic emission was recorded and the lesions appeared to be indistinguishable from those at 525 $W.cm^{-2}$. At the intensity of 1,600 $W.cm^{-2}$, anharmonic emission was also evident during approx. 50% of the insonation bursts and all of those lesions showed gross tissue fragmentation, including that of capillaries, expressed as hemorrhage, within the lesion volume. At the peak focal intensities of 1,840 and 2,600 $W.cm^{-2}$ anharmonic emission and hemorrhage were present in all instances (Fig. 17). The coincidence of the occurrence of anharmonic acoustic emission during insonation and the occurrence of hemorrhage and tissue fragmentation, as well as the coincidence of the absence of both of these, was so clear cut that no tests of statistical significance were necessary. It is interesting to note that these data on the intensity dependence of the occurrence of hemorrhage confirm the results obtained in 1960[15], shown in Fig. 2.

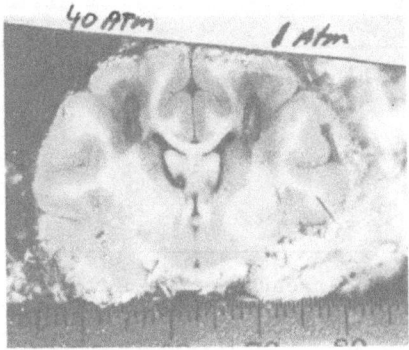

Fig. 16. Supravitally stained lesions in the brain of the cat insonated _in vivo_ under ambient pressures of 40 and 1 atm.

Table 3. Comparison of Lesion Size from Insonation of the Brain of the Cat _In Vivo_ under Atmospheric and Elevated Ambient Pressures and Normothermia and Hypothermia

T °C	AP ATM	IBD sec	n	$\overline{\overline{LD}}$ mm	s
37	1	4.0	12	1.62	.16
37	42	4.0	12	1.55	.21
27	1	8.0	8	1.35	.18
27	42	8.0	10	1.28	.18

T = Core Temperature; AP = Ambient Pressure; IBD = Isonation Burst Duration; n = Number of Replicates; $\overline{\overline{LD}}$ = Mean Lesion Diameter; s = Standard Deviation. Insonation: 2.7 MHz; Peak Focal Intensity: 525 W.cm^{-2} for T = 37°C and 420 W.cm^{-2} for T = 27°C.

Table 4. Occurrence of Acoustic Emission and Hemorrhage in the Brain of Cat _In Vivo_

I_{PF} W.cm^{-2}	IBD sec	n	Presence of Anhormonic Emission	Presence of Tissue Hemorrhage
1.050	1 & 2	6	0	0
1.600	1	24	13	14
1.840	0.5	12	12	12
2.600	0.1 & 0.2	6	6	6

I_{PF} = Peak Focal Insonation Intensity;
IBD = Burst Duration; n = Number of Replicates
2.7 MHz, 1 ATM Pressure

Lesion Boundary and Lesion Core Temperatures

A further test of the hypothesis that the negative pressures (tension phase) associated with bubble-oscillation type of cavitation do not contribute to tissue damage would be to determine if the T_{LB} was influenced by ambient pressure. Although the lesion size remained constant when occurrence of negative pressures (absolute) during insonation was precluded, it is possible that a second effect, such as a change in the acoustic or thermal properties of the tissue with pressure, counterbalanced the effects of cavitation. Any changes in the acoustic or thermal properties of tissues with pressure would be apparent as a change in the shape of temperature distribution across the lesion, and its contribution to tissue damage would be apparent as a change in the T_{LB}. Since, as previously stated, hypothermia does not affect the T_{LB} at ambient pressure of 1 atm, the studies were conducted in hypothermic animals at elevated ambient pressures and peak focal insonation intensity of 420 W.cm^{-2}. The T_{LB} in 3 animals, determined as described earlier in this paper, were statistically identical to those obtained at 1 atm (Fig. 7) confirming that the bubble-oscillation (stable) cavitation did not contribute to tissue damage, which was entirely related to heat generation. The peak temperatures in the core of the lesion, however, were found to be 245°C - very close to the boiling point (254°C) of normal saline at 42 atm absolute. Inspite of these high peak-core-temperatures, the lesions were grossly and histologically indistinguishable from those

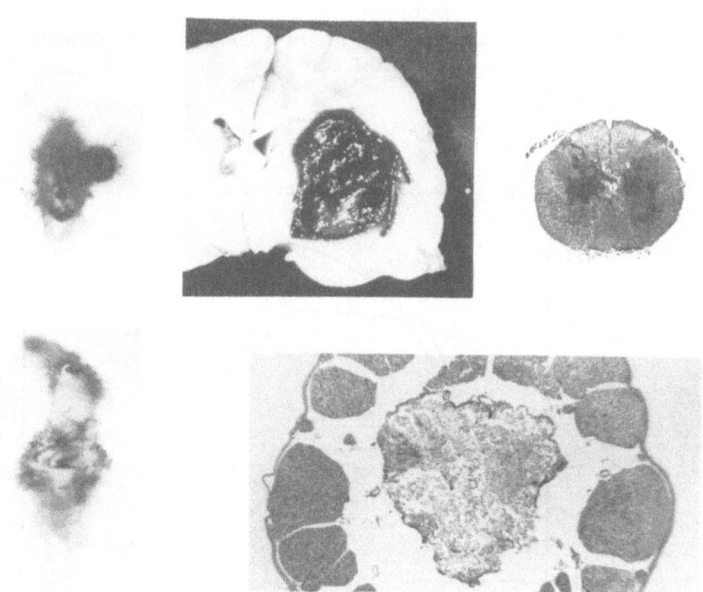

Fig. 17. Lesions in the brain and spinal cord of the cat insonated _in vivo_ at peak focal intensity of 1,840 W.cm^{-2}. Anharmonic emission was recorded during insonation. Supravital Trypan Blue and Hematoxylin & Eosin stains. Top: hemorrhage, Bottom: tissue fragmentation in brain (Left) and spinal cord (Right) respectively. Compare these lesions with those in Figs. 3,4 and 16.

produced at 1 atm in normothermic[17,48,49] and hypothermic[19] animals, in which the peak-core-temperatures were close to the boiling point of normal saline at 1 atm.

Typical temperature-time histories of peak focal temperatures recorded in fresh calf liver in vitro during insonation with a burst 0.3 sec at 2.7 MHz at 2 different intensities and ambient pressures are shown in Fig. 18. In Curve A, under normal atmospheric pressure and peak focal insonation intensity of 1,480 W.cm^{-2}, the temperature rises smoothly to approx. 61°C and is typical of the curves used for determination of ultrasonic absorption coefficient of tissues[50]. In Curve B, at 1 atm and the higher intensity of 2,200 W.cm^{-2}, the temperature is seen to rise rapidly to approx. 100°C (the approx. boiling point of normal saline under ambient pressure of 1 atm absolute) and is seen to fluctuate at that level for a prolonged period during insonation. However, if the insonation at 2,200 W.cm^{-2} is performed under an ambient pressure of 22 atm (Curve C), the temperature rises smoothly to 125°C (the approx. boiling point of normal saline under an ambient pressure of 22 atm). At higher ambient pressure of 42 atm and higher peak focal insonation intensity of 3,000 W.cm^{-2}, a temperature of 300°C was recorded.

The temperatures measured during insonation of tissues are thus restricted by the boiling point of the tissue fluid under the conditions of the experiment. It is thus possible that during insonation at 1 atm ambient pressure, the heat generation is, in fact, significantly larger than that calculated from the temperatures actually measured. Since ultrasonic absorption coefficients, used in calculations of heat generation, are themselves based on measurements of tissue temperature during insonation under ambient pressure of 1 atm, they might be fallaciously too low, specially under insonation conditions at which the peak temperatures approach 100°C.

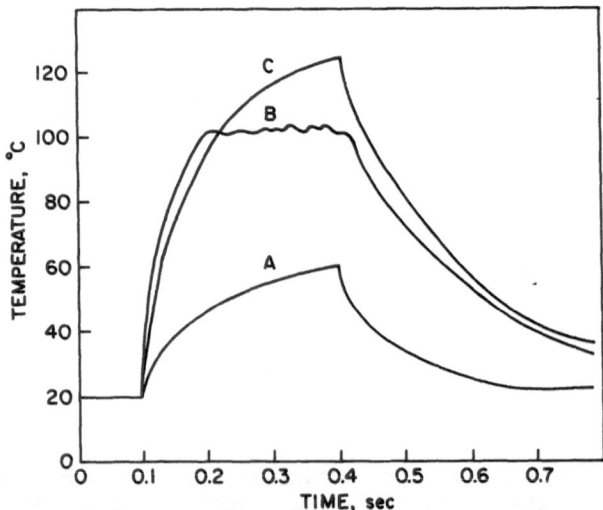

Fig. 18. Tracings of temperature-time histories of peak focal temperatures in calf liver in vitro at 20°C. A: 1,480 W.cm^{-2}, 1 atm; B: 2,200 W.cm^{-2}, 1 atm; C: 2,200 W.cm^{-2}, 22 atm.

Intensity Dependence of Ultrasonic Absorption Coefficient

Ultrasonic absorption coefficient of fresh calf liver _in vitro_ at 20°C was measured using a 50μ m thermocouple, 0.2 and 0.3 sec bursts of focused 2.7 MHz ultrasound, at peak focal intensities up to 2,500 W.cm^{-2}. Acoustic emission was measured concurrently with the temperature. At intensities up to approx. 500 W.cm^{-2}, the intensity absorption coefficient was found to be approx. 1.3 dB.cm^{-1} and no acoustic emission was observed (Fig. 19). Between intensity levels of 500 and 1,000 W.cm^{-2}, the absorption coefficient increased monotonically, reaching 1.74 dB.cm^{-1} at 1,000 W.cm^{-2}, and was accompanied by subharmonic acoustic emission. At intensities above 1,000 W.cm^{-2}, there was a large scatter in the values of the absorption coefficient i.e. the temperature rises measured, with the peak temperatures approaching 100°C. The studies at intensities above 1000 W.cm^{-2} were therefore conducted under an ambient pressure of 24 atm to raise the boiling point of the tissue fluid and enable measurement of true peak temperatures. Some of the values were found to be as high as 4.35 dB.cm^{-1} and were invariably accompanied by violent anharmonic emission, in addition to high levels of subharmonic emission. The lower values remained between 1.74 to 2.0 dB.cm^{-1} and remarkably showed an absence of anharmonic emission. These data indicate that bubble-oscillation (stable) cavitation increases the heat generation to a small but measurable extent and that bubble-collapse (unstable) cavitation, in addition to producing mechanical effects in the tissues, simultaneously produces very high temperatures in them.

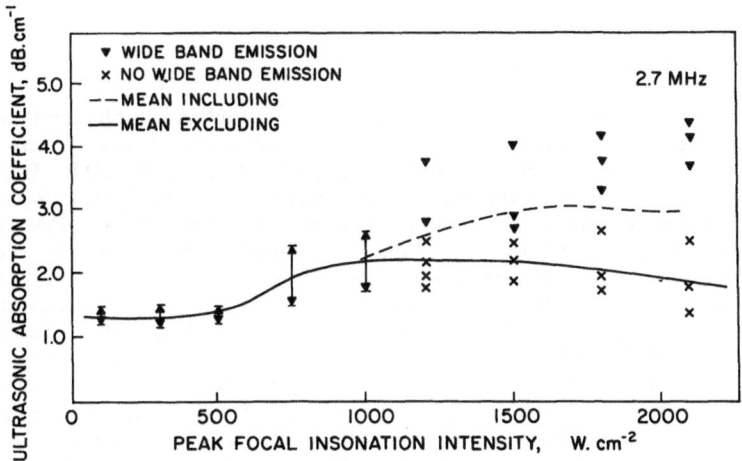

Fig. 19. Intensity dependence of ultrasonic absorption of coefficient at 2.7 MHz in fresh calf liver _in vitro_ at 20°C. Ambient pressure was raised to 24 atm at intensities above 1,000 W.cm^{-2} to raise the boiling point of tissue fluid and permit measurement of true temperatures.

ULTRASONIC ABSORPTION COEFFICIENTS OF TISSUES AND CELLS

The ultrasonic absorption coefficient of tissues is extensively used for calculating expected temperature elevations by insonation under different conditions. It is traditionally determined, as in the study described above, from the temperature rise measured with an implanted fine wire thermocouple during insonation with a short burst of ultrasound. The thermocouple is typically 50μm or more in diameter, i.e. an order of magnitude larger than the size of a typical mammalian cell. In these measurements the tissue is tacitly assumed to be homogeneous with respect to its ultrasonic and thermal properties and injury thresholds, notwithstanding the fact that all 'soft' tissues consist of a matrix of cells rich in protein, bathed in an extracellular fluid consisting primarily of water and electrolytes. Since ultrasonic absorption is known to be high in the large biomolecules, especially proteins, and low in water, it is plausible that most of the ultrasonic absorption is intracellular and the values normally measured are "diluted" by the low absorption in extracellular fluids. Should this be true, the temperature elevations within the cells could be higher than those calculated from the bulk absorption coefficients of the tissue.

The bulk ultrasonic absorption coefficients of tissue and the intracellular absorption coefficient of its constituent cells were therefore measured in the ovary and ova of the sea-urchin (approx. 100μm in diameter), using a 50μ m thermocouple and a microthermocouple probe with a tip diameter of 10μ m respectively[51]. The absorption coefficients at 2.7 MHz were found to be 0.35± 0.09dB.cm^{-1} in the ovary and 1.22± 0.17dB.cm^{-1} in the ova. The heat generation within the cells thus is $3\frac{1}{2}$ times greater than that in the ovary as a whole. This intracellularly generated heat must diffuse through the cell wall into the surrounding extracellular space where it is normally measured. During insonation the cell constituents and bounding membranes would thus be subjected to significantly higher temperatures than those measured extracellularly or predicted on the basis of bulk tissue absorption coefficients.

DISCUSSION AND CONCLUSIONS

From the data presented it is obvious that both heat generation and cavitation occur in solid tissues during insonation at any intensity level. Heat generation increases almost linearly with intensity up to approximately 1,500 W.cm^{-2}; at intensities higher than 1,500 W.cm^{-2}, transient (bubble-collapse) cavitation can add greatly to heat generation at the site of cavitation. Stable (bubble-oscillation) cavitation is a probabilistic phenomenon with no definite intensity threshold, whereas at the frequency of 2 to 3 MHz, transient cavitation does not occur below 1,000 W.cm^{-2}, and occurs only sporadically between 1,000 and 1,500 W.cm^{-2}, beyond which intensity level the probability of its occurrence is very high. The threshold for the occurrence of cavitation in tissues, both in solid and liquid, is lower, and the magnitude of both types of cavitation activity, as well as heat generation is higher than that in air-saturated water. This is not surprising in view of the presence of greater numbers of cavitation sites and nuclei in tissues as compared to water, both of which are saturated with dissolved gases, and the higher viscocity and ultrasonic absorption coefficient of tissues.

As to the biological effects of these phenomena, within the constraint of the end point in these studies - namely the occurrence of histologically detectable, irreversible tissue injury and reversible functional alterations - heat generation has a time dependent temperature threshold which is linked to the state of the tissue (stable versus dividing cells). Stable cavitation has no direct discernible effect on solid tissues, but adds to heat generation to a small, but measurable extent. Transient (collapse) cavitation not only produces mechanical fragmentation of the tissue, including that of capillaries expressed as hemorrhage, but also greatly augments local heat generation. However since transient (collapse) cavitation does not occur below the intensity of 1,000 W.cm^{-2} in solid tissues, no biological damage can be attributed to "cavitation" at lower intensities. These findings thus confirm and extend the observation of Carstensen and Gates[52] who after a very thorough and painstaking examination of the literature conclude "If we are looking for a clear sign that cavitation affects the fetus it is evident that it is not provided in the studies which have been conducted up to the present time". Enucleation and oscillation of gas or vapor bubbles in the tissues could augment acoustic streaming. But in careful and extensive studies[53], summarized previously[42], no evidence for the occurrence of any biological effects attributable to acoustic streaming could be obtained.

Occurrence of transient cavitation and associated tissue fragmentation would militate against the use of intensities above 1,500 W.cm^{-2}. Extreme caution is indicated in the use of intensities between 1,000 W.cm^{2} and 1,500 W.cm^{-2} at a frequency of 2 to 3 MHz, even for cancer therapy by hyperthermia[54] because of the randomness of the occurrence of collapse cavitation and damage to tissue vasculature which may lead to uncontrollable internal hemorrhage and, at the least, promote metastases. Furthermore, there is evidence that cavitation, once induced, can perpetuate at lower insonation intensities.

Heat generation by ultrasonic absorption occurs principally intracellularly i.e. within the cells. Enucleation of bubbles and their oscillation and eventual collapse are most likely to occur in the interstitial fluid because of their higher dissolved gas content and lower viscosity. The heat generated interstitially by bubble oscillation and collapse is additive to that generated intracellularly. Similarly, any other forms of heating, such as water bath, environmental chambers (including sauna), microwaves (which generate heat interstitially by coupling to the polar water molecules), infrared, CO_2 laser and infections which raise the tissue temperature would be additive to ultrasound. Tissue temperature elevation by ultrasonic absorption, on the other hand, may be synergistic with transient (collapse) cavitation, since the threshold of biological membranes to mechanical damage seems to be lower at elevated temperatures[25]. Any other agents which lower the threshold of cells and tissues for thermal or mechanical damage would be expected to potentiate the effects of ultrasound. Conversely ultrasound, by raising the tissue temperature, may potentiate the effects of other agents directly if those effects are temperature dependent, or indirectly through changes induced in the tissue, such as increased blood and/or lymphatic circulation.

REFERENCES

1. W. L. Nyborg, D. L. Miller, and C. C. Whitcomb, Sensitive tests for bio-effects of ultrasound, Reflections, 4:205 (1978).
2. S. Z. Child, E. L. Carstensen, and K. Smachlo, Effects of Ultrasound on Drosophila: III. Exposure of larvae to low-temporal-average-intensity, pulsed irradiation, Ultrasound Med. Biol., 7:167 (1981).
3. P. P. Lele, Ultrasound bioeffects and human reproduction, Ultrasound Annual 1985, R. C. Sanders and M. C. Hill, eds., Raven Press, New York (1985).
4. F. Dunn, Physical mechanisms of the action of intense ultrasound on tissue, Amer. J. Phys. Med., 37:148 (1958).
5. W. J. Fry, V. J. Wulff, D. Tucker, and F. J. Fry, Physical factors involved in ultrasonically induced changes in living systems: I. Identification of non-temperature effects, J. Acoust. Soc. Amer., 22:867 (1950).
6. J. W. Barnard, W. J. Fry, F. J. Fry, and R. E. Krumins, Effects of high intensity ultrasound on the central nervous system of the cat, J. Comp. Neurol. 103:459 (1955).
7. F. J. Fry, G. Kossoff, R. C. Eggleton and F. Dunn, Threshold ultrasonic dosages for structural changes in the mammalian brain, J. Acoust. Soc. Amer., 48:1413 (1970).
8. J. B. Pond, A study of the biological action of focused mechanical waves (focused ultrasound), Doctoral Thesis, University of London (1968).
9. F. Dunn, Summary paper for session on "Effects on tissues and organs" of the workshop on interaction of ultrasound with biological tissues, in: "Interactions of ultrasound and biological tissues - workshop proceedings", p. 103, J. M. Reid and M. R. Sikov, eds., U.S.D.H.E.W. Publication (FDA) 73-8008 BRH/DBE 73-1 (1972).
10. C. R. Hill, Interaction of ultrasound with cells, in: "Interactions of ultrasound and biological tissues - workshop proceedings", p. 57, J. M. Reid and M. R. Sikov, eds., U.S.D.H.E.W. Publication (FDA) 73-8008 BRH/DBE 73-1 (1972).
11. W. L. Nyborg, Mechanisms for nonthermal effects of sound, J. Acoust. Soc. Amer., 44:1302 (1968).
12. P. P. Lele and A. D. Pierce, The thermal hypothesis of the mechanism of ultrasonic focal destruction in organized tissues, in: "Interactions of ultrasound and biological tissues - workshop proceedings", p. 121, J. M. Reid and M. R. Sikov, eds., U.S.D.H.E.W. Publication (FDA) 73-8008 BRH/DBE 73-1 (1972).
13. P. P. Lele, Ultrasonic teratology in mouse and man, in: "Excerpta Medica International Congress Series No. 363 (ISBN 90 219 02974) Ultrasonics in Medicine", Proceedings of the 2nd European Congress on Ultrasonics in Medicine, Munich, 12-16 May 1975, pg. 22, M. de Vlieger, D. N. White, and V. R. McCready, eds., Excerpta Medica, Amsterdam (1975).
14. P. P. Lele, Physical aspects and clinical studies with ultrasonic hyperthermia, Chapter 16, p. 333, in: "Hyperthermia in Cancer Therapy", F. K. Storm, ed., G. K. Hall and Co. (1983).
15. L. Basauri and P. P. Lele, A simple method for production of trackless focal lesions with focused ultrasound: statistical evaluation of the effects of irradiation on the central nervous system of the cat, J. Physiol. 160:513 (1962).
16. T. C. Robinson, An analysis of lesion development in plexiglas and nervous tissue using focused ultrasound, Doctoral Thesis, Massachusetts Institute of Technology (1968).

17. T. C. Robinson and P. P. Lele, An analysis of lesion development in the brain and in plastics by high-intensity focused ultrasound at low-megahertz frequencies, $\underline{J}$. Acoust. Soc. Amer. 51: 1333 (1972).

18. W. L. Nyborg, Interaction mechanisms: heating, in: "Ultrasound: Medical Applications, Biological Effects and Hazard Potential", M. H. Repacholi, M. Grandolfo and A. Rindi, eds., Plenum Pub. Corp., New York (1986).

19. W. L. Hsu, Thermal factors in the ultrasonic destruction of mammalian tissue, Sc.D. Thesis, Massachusetts Institute of Technology (1974).

20. P. P. Lele, Effects of focused ultrasound radiation on peripheral nerve, with observations on local heating, Exper. Neurol. 8:47 (1963).

21. H. S. Carslaw and J. E. Jaeger, "Conduction of Heat in Solids", 2nd Ed., Oxford University Press, London (1959).

22. J. L. Stein, A study of the time-dependent temperature threshold of ultrasonic damage in mammalian tissue, M.S. Thesis, Massachusetts Institute of Technology (1976).

23. F. C. Henriques, Jr. and A. R. Moritz, Studies of thermal injury; conduction of heat to and through skin and temperatures attained therein; theoretical and experimental investigation, Am. J. Path. 23:531 (1947).

24. W. T. Ham, Jr., R. C. Williams, H. A. Mueller, D. Guerry, III, A. M. Clarke, and W. J. Geeraets, Effects of laser radiation on the mammalian eye, Trans. N.Y. Acad. Sci. 28:517 (1966).

25. J. A. Rooney, Shear as a mechanism for sonically induced biological effects, J. Acoust. Soc. Am. 52:1718 (1972).

26. N. A. Peppers, A. Vassiliadis, K. G. Dedrick, H. Chang, R. R. Peabody, H. Rose, and H. C. Zweng, Corneal damage thresholds for CO_2 laser radiation, Appl. Optics 8:377 (1969).

27. S. Glasstone, K. J. Laidler, and H. Eyring, "The Theory of Rate Processes", McGraw-Hill Book Co., Inc., N.Y. (1941).

28. F. H. Johnson, H. Eyring, and M. J. Polissar, "The Kinetic Basis of Molecular Biology", John Wiley and Sons, Inc., N.Y. (1954).

29. F. C. Henriques, Studies of thermal injury, V. The predictability and the significance of thermally induced rate processes leading to irreversible epidermal injury, Arch. Path., 43:489 (1947).

30. T. H. Wood, Lethal effects of high and low temperatures on unimolecular organisms, Adv. Biol. Med. Physics, IV:119 (1956).

31. P. Miller, D. W. Smith and T. Shepard, Maternal hyperthermia as a possible cause of anencephaly, Lancet, March 11, 519 (1978).

32. J. Bergonie and L. Tribondeau, De quelques resultats de la radiotherapie et essai de fixation d'ue technique rationelle, C. R. Acad. Sci. (Paris) 143: 983 (1906), English translation Radiat. Res. 11: 587 (1959).

33. P. P. Lele, Temperature-duration thresholds for irreversible. histologic and/or ultrastructural damage to normal mammalian tissues and tumors in vivo, in: "Symposium on Tumour Biology and Therapy", p. D6-30, J. J. Broerse, G. W. Barendsen, H. B. Kal, A. J. Van Der Kogel, eds., Proc. of the Seventh Int. Congress of Rad. Res., Amsterdam, July 3-8, 1983, Martinus Nijhoff Publishers (1983).

34. S. A. Sapareto and W. C. Dewey, Thermal dose determination in cancer therapy, Int. J. Radiat. Oncol. Biol. Phys. 10: 6: 787 (1984).

35. F. J. Fry, G. Kossoff, R. C. Eggleton, and F. Dunn, Threshold ultrasonic dosages for structural changes in the mammalian brain, J. Acoust. Soc. Amer. 48: 1413 (1970).

36. G. Ter Haar, S. Daniels, K. C. Eastaugh, and C. R. Hill, Ultrasonically induced cavitation in vivo, Br. J. Cancer 45: Suppl. V, 151 (1982).

37. E. L. Carstensen and H. G. Flynn, The potential for transient cavitation with micro-second pulses of ultrasound, Ultras. Med. Biol. 8:L720 (1982).

38. N. Senapati, A study of ultrasonic cavitation in biological tissues and its possible damaging effects, Sc.D. Thesis, Massachusetts Institute of Technology (1973).

39. J. M. Veranth, The use of elevated pressure and acoustical emission to study ultrasonic cavitation in tissue, M.S. Thesis, Massachusetts Institute of Technology (1974).

40. R. A. Handler, Nonlinear absorption of ultrasound in biological media, M.S. Thesis, Massachusetts Institute of Technology (1976).

41. P. P. Lele, N. Senapati, and W. L. Hsu, Mechanisms of Tissue Ultrasound Interaction", p. 345, in: "Ultrasound in Medicine", Excerpta Medica Int. Cong. Series No. 309 (ISBN 90 219 0187 0), Proc. of the 2nd World Cong. on Ultras. in Med., Rotterdam, The Netherlands, 4-8 June 1973, M. de Vlieger, D. N. White, and V. R. McCready, eds., Excerpta Medica, Amsterdam (1973).

42. P. P. Lele, Thresholds and mechanisms of ultrasonic damage to 'organized' animal tissues, in: "Symposium on Biological Effects and Characterization of Ultrasound Sources", p. 224, DeWitt G. Hazzard and M. L. Litz, eds., Proc. of a Conf. held in Rockville, MD, June 2-3, 1977, HEW Pub. (FDA) 78-8048 (1977).

43. E. A. Neppiras, Subharmonic and other low-frequency emissions from bubbles in sound-irradiated liquids, J. Acoust. Soc. Am. 46: 587, (1969).

44. A. Eller and H. G. Flynn, Generation of subharmonics of order one-half by bubbles in a sound field, J. Acoust. Soc. Amer. 46: 722 (1969).

45. W. T. Coakley, Acoustic detection of single cavitation events in a focused field in water at 1 MHz, J. Acoust. Soc. Amer. 49: 792 (1971).

46. K. I. Morton, G. R. Ter Haar, I. J. Stratford and C. R. Hill, The role of cavitation in the interaction of ultrasound with V79 chinese hamster cells in vitro, Br. J. Cancer 45: Suppl. V, 147 (1982).

47. P. P. Lele, Irradiation of plastics with focused ultrasound: a simple method for evaluation of dosage factors for neurological applications, J. Acoust. Soc. Amer. 34: 412 (1962).

48. G. F. Young and P. P. Lele, Focal lesions in the brain of growing rabbits produced by focused ultrasound, Exper. Neurol. 9: 502 (1964).

49. K. E. Astrom, E. Bell, H. T. Ballantine, Jr. and E. Heidensleben, An experimental neuropathological study of the effects of high-frequency focused ultrasound on the brain of the cat, J. of Neuropath. and Exper. Neurol. 20: 484 (1961).

50. W. J. Fry and R. B. Fry, Determination of absolute sound levels and acoustic absorption coefficients by thermocouple probes, J. Acoust. Soc. Am. 26: 294 (1954).

51. K. M. Mason, A method for measurement of intracellular ultrasonic absorption, M.S. Thesis, Massachusetts Institute of Technology (1976).

52. E. L. Carstensen and A. H. Gates, The effects of ultrasound on the fetus, Univ. of Rochester, Electrical Engng. Tech. Report No. GM 09933-21R (1983).

53. R. S. Mecca, The effects of acoustic streaming from a resonant bubble on the action potential characteristics of a nerve, B.S., M.S. Thesis, Massachusetts Institute of Technology (1973).

54. W. Swindell, A theoretical study of nonlinear effects with focused ultrasound in tissues: an "acoustic bragg peak", Ultrasound in Med. & Biol. 11: No. 1, 121 (1985).

ULTRASOUND : SYNERGISTIC EFFECTS AND APPLICATION IN

CANCER THERAPY BY HYPERTHERMIA*

Padmakar P. Lele

Professor of Experimental Medicine

& Director, Harvard-M.I.T. Hyperthermia Center

Massachusetts Institute of Technology

Cambridge, MA   02139   U.S.A.

INTRODUCTION

In a previous paper[1], it was shown that heat generation is the principal mechanism for the occurrence of histologically detectable irreversible injury, as well as reversible functional alterations, in solid, mammalian tissues from insonation with 2 to 3 MHz ultrasound at intensities up to at least 1,000 W.cm^{-2} and probably up to 1,500 W.cm^{-2}. A well defined time-dependent temperature threshold, linked to the state of the tissue, governs the occurrence of tissue damage. Thus, any other modality or agent leading to heat generation and/or temperature elevation in the tissues will be additive to ultrasound and reduce the amount of ultrasonically generated heat needed to reach the threshold for tissue damage or for functional alteration. Water bath, environmental chambers, sauna, infra-red,

* Support in parts by USPHS Grants CA30944, CA31303, and Georgiana and Frank Massa, Jr. Memorial Fund, the help of numerous colleagues, staff, and students is gratefully acknowledged.

307

CO_2 laser, fever from systemic infection or induced artificially by injection of pyrogens (e.g. Cooley's Toxin), local tissue inflammation from local infection, etc. may thus act additively with ultrasound. On the other hand, some agents may act directly or indirectly on the biological system and alter its functional, ultrastructural and/or histological state in such a manner that its threshold for ultrasonic thermal damage is lowered or its ability to recover from sublethal damage by biological repair is compromised. In this instance, it is not essential that the cellular site of action of the other modality or agent be the same as that of ultrasound. Ultrasound may also enhance or potentiate the effects of an agent, such as a drug or a toxin, directly at the target site, if its activity is temperature dependent, or indirectly through changes induced in the tissue, such as increased blood or lymphatic circulation. Thus, ultrasonic heat generation can be used either alone, additively, or synergistically with other modalities for therapeutic purposes.

SYNERGISM WITH X-RADIATION AND DRUGS

Localized heating of tissues in mammals in vivo to approx. 42°C or higher for a certain duration leads to coagulation pan-necrosis of the tissue volume involved, and can be used for non-invasive surgery of tumors. Temperatures below 42°C apparently do not produce irreversible histological damage in tissues consisting of mature, post-mitotic cells, but can affect dividing cell populations as in the embryo (Fig. 1). Although the time-dependent temperature thresholds for many post-mitotic and mature-cell organs fall within the same range, no data are available for the dividing cell populations in different

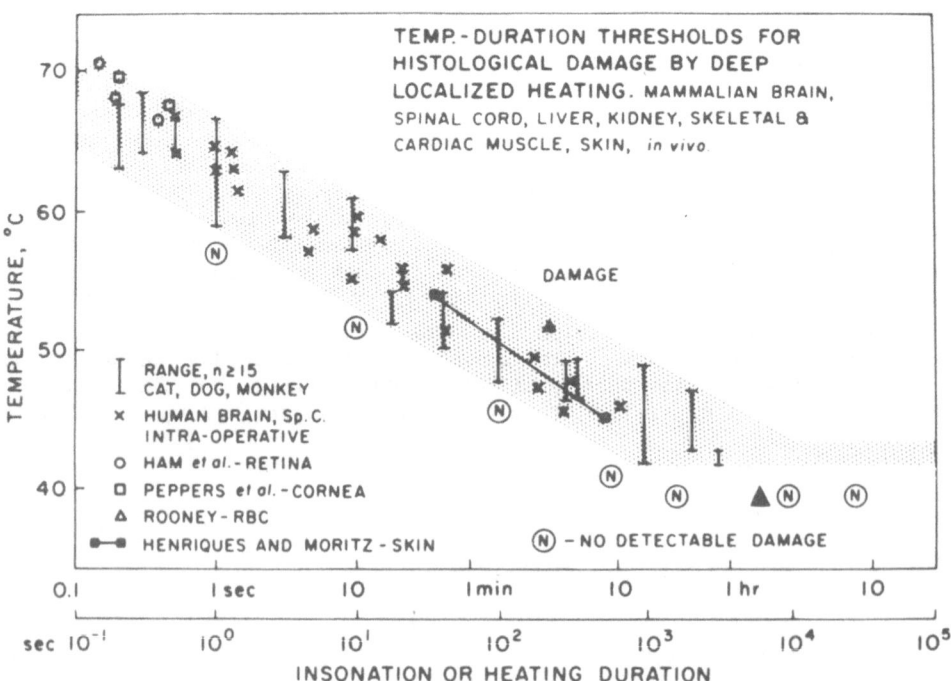

Fig. 1. Temperature-duration thresholds for histologic damage to mammalian tissues in vivo by LHT by different modalities. For details see Lele[1].

organs in the fetus. However, the sensitivity of various different cell lines to heat, radiation or both has been intensively studied in cell cultures <u>in vitro</u>. It is well recognized that effects of various agents on cells in culture <u>in vitro</u> are highly dependent on a number of factors, such as the local pH, oxygenation, nutrient levels, types and amount of sera in the medium, etc. and the results may be somewhat different on cells in tumors <u>in vivo</u>. However, certain general conclusions, which may be applicable to clinical cancer therapy, may be drawn[2]. The heat sensitivity of different mammalian cell lines is found to vary over a wide range. The data on the relative sensitivities of transformed and untransformed cells are contradictory and thus there is little firm evidence to support the conjecture that malignant cells are inherently more sensitive to heat than normal cells. In addition to killing the cells, heat also sensitizes the surviving cells to X-radiation. The rate of cell-killing and of radiosensitization by heat varies greatly with temperature – a change of only a 0.5°C produced a difference of an order of magnitude in the number of cells killed. Hyperthermia selectively kills and radiosensitizes cells that are relatively resistant to ionizing radiation – that is those which are hypoxic, malnourished and at a low pH. Hyperthermia has been shown to substantially inhibit recovery from potentially lethal radiation damage. Cells in S phase of the cell cycle, which are generally resistant to radiation the most, are sensitive to heat injury. Hyperthermia and X-rays given within an hour or two of each other can enhance the tumoricidal effects of either by 100%. Hyperthermia also greatly enhances the cytotoxic activity of certain classes of chemotherapeutic agents used in cancer therapy, such as alkylating agents (e.g. HN_2), antimetabolites (e.g. 5-FU) and antibiotics (e.g. Bleomycin). A rudimentary model of the steps involved in chemotherapeutic cytoxicity is presented in Fig. 2. Note that almost

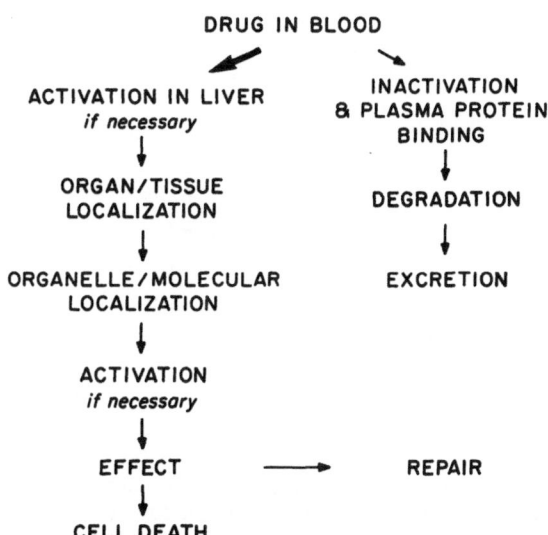

Fig. 2. A simplified, generalized model of chemotherapeutic action. Note that almost all of the processes are temperature dependent.

all of the processes are temperature dependent, though the coefficients of enhancement of the different steps and thus the final therapeutic enhancement may differ from one drug to another. Furthermore, in addition to thermal enhancement of cytotoxic effects, other synergistic effects may also exist. Heat can thus greatly enhance the effects of X-radiation and of chemotherapy.

Data obtained in murine, canine and human tumors as discussed by Hahn[3], in general, support the results in cell cultures in vitro, inspite of the fact that the tumors in vivo almost invariably were heated, non-uniformly, and frequently inadequately. Thus, hyperthermia indeed would appear to have a strong potential in cancer therapy. Unfortunately however, there appears to be little difference, if any, between malignant and normal tissues as regards their sensitivity to heat or the potentiation of radio or chemo-toxicity by heat. Thus unless the heating can be localized to the tumor (or the treatment) volume, little therapeutic gain is likely to accrue. The ability to heat a tumor selectively, specially at its proliferative, well-perfused margin (Fig. 3), regardless of its location in the body is thus crucial for durable, local control of tumor without unacceptable tissue toxicity (Fig. 4). It is also imperative that such local control be obtained without increasing local and metastatic dissemination of the disease. In the long run it is thus essential that the local tumor hyperthermia (LHT) be produced non-invasively. We shall, therefore, briefly examine the available modalities for their potential for LHT before discussing the various ways in which ultrasound (US) is used.

MODALITIES CURRENTLY USED FOR PRODUCTION OF LHT

The principal modalities in clinical use of LHT are microwave (MW) and radio-frequency (RF) electromagnetic energy (EM) and US. Theoretical predictions of their capabilities for controlled localized heating of deep or superficial tumors have been based on considerations of their propagation characteristics in biological tissues and the

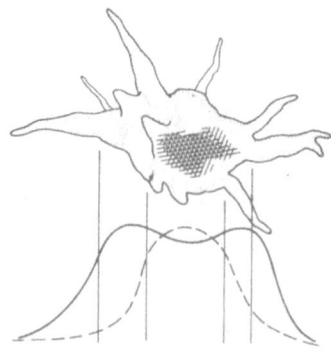

Fig. 3. Diagram of a tumor with a central necrotic core. Solid curve shows the heat-dose distribution essential for local control. Dashed line shows overheating of central necrotic core with subthreshold heating at the well vascularized margin, characteristic of many heating devices. (From Lele[4])

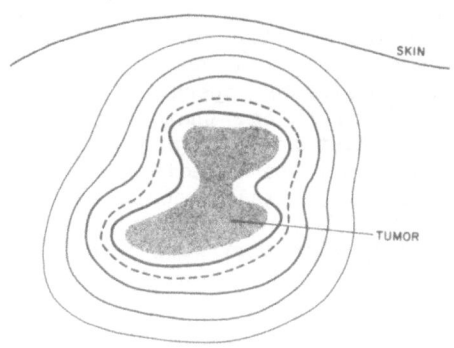

SKIN

TUMOR

Fig. 4. Diagram of a subcutaneous tumor showing ideal hyperthermia temperature distributions. The volume between the tumor edge and the solid or dashed line must be treated with adequate heat-dose to control malignant cells infiltrating the tumor bed which cannot be visualized. The temperature should then drop off radially outwards in all directions to minimize normal tissue toxicity. (From Lele[4])

at transfer phenomena, including blood perfusion. These are confirmed measurements in intercomparison studies in patients and experimental imals being conducted in the author's laboratory and elsewhere. summarizing the heating characteristics of deep heating techniques le[4,5] rated the depth-dose distribution and flexibility of heating stribution of US as being far superior to those of MW and RF. The periority of US is now generally accepted and is entirely due to e fact that for comparable tissue penetration depths the wavelength US is at least 500 times shorter than that of EM. Let us suppose at we want to heat a tumor 4 cm in diameter, situated at a depth 4 cm as in Fig 4. From Fig 5, which shows the attenuation curves r various frequencies of EM and US in muscle, we note that for the lf-power penetration depth of 4 cm, the frequency cannot be higher an 40.68 MHz for EM and 1.5 MHz for US. The corresponding wavelengths e 513 mm and 1 mm respectively. The dimension of the wavelength termines the smallest area over which the energy can be focused and us the smallest area which can be heated. Thus with EM even for rather short half power penetration depth of 4 cm, the wavelength so large that heating cannot be localized to the target volume - situation which has been aptly described as "dump (the energy) and ay (that it will selectively heat the target and not some critical rmal tissue)". On the other hand, with US it is possible, both in eory and in practice, to deposit the energy over a 1 mm area at a pth of 4 cm or more.

The dimension of the wavelength also governs the radiation pattern a source. The aperture of a radiative EM hyperthermia applicator erating in the low RF range typically is 15 x 20 cm since larger eas cannot be effectively coupled to curved contours of the body rface. The largest dimension of the antenna is thus typically only quarter of a wavelength. The emanating radiation pattern is widely vergent - the energy being literally broadcast. Consequently, the

EM field intensity is maximal at the surface of the body, which tends to heat excessively, and falls off as it reaches the target. An ultrasonic hyperthermia applicator operating at a frequency of 0.3 to 6.0 MHz is typically 4 to 10 cm, that is 50 to 70 wavelengths, in diameter. The emanating radiation is highly directional and collimated in the near field and can be precisely aimed at the target. Significantly lower levels of total absorbed power are required for LHT of a target volume with US than with EM and the risk of systemic temperature elevation is thus also very much lower.

ULTRASONIC HEATING

Single Planar Transducer

Single, planar, disc-shaped, piezoelectric transducers 0.3 to 6.0 MHz in frequency, and up to 12 cm in diameter, coupled to the body through an integral water column 10 to 25 cm long as shown in Fig 6 have been used clinically for LHT. In most designs cooled, degassed water can be circulated through the coupling chamber. Fig 7 depicts the radiation pattern of such transducers. Note that in the near field, which extends to r^2/λ (typically 50 to 250 cm in case of transducers used for hyperthermia), the field is uneven as shown in the ring diagram in Fig 7. The relative amplitude and location of the peaks depends on whether the transducer is driven at or slightly off resonance, on its mounting etc.[8], but their amplitude can be 3 times as high as the spatial average intensity. If such a peak is located on the skin, heating from it can frequently be dose-limiting, even with cooling of the skin.

Let us suppose that the energy distribution at the surface of the body was uniform and see what the heating pattern would be at depth. As seen in Fig 8 the intensity will be highest at the surface and due to attenuation will decay exponentially with increasing depth of penetration. Since heat generation is proportional to local intensity, it will be maximal at the surface and underlying tissues and decay exponentially at depth. Cooling of the skin will shift the 'hot spot' to subcutaneous, fatty tissue which has little blood perfusion and cannot readily dissipate heat. In a very large tumor the temperature in its necrotic/ischemic core may be higher than other tumor or normal

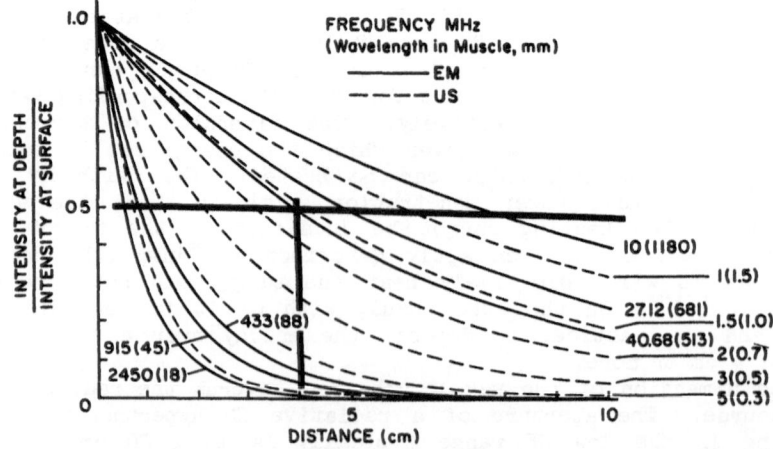

Fig. 5. Attenuation curves for different frequencies of EM and US in muscle. The horizontal and vertical straight lines indicate the half-power level and 4 cm depth respectively. (From Lele[4])

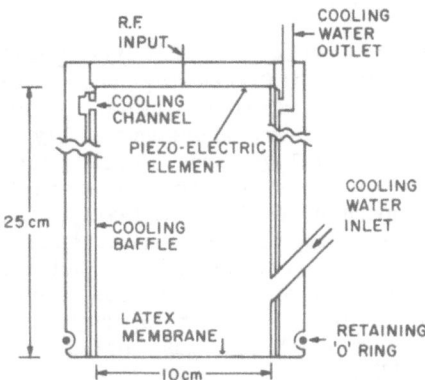

Fig. 6.   Cross-sectional diagram of a typical, single element
           hyperthermia applicator. The chamber between the
           piezo-electric element and the latex or plastic membrane
           is filled with degassed water. During therapy, the
           compliant membrane is coupled to the body with
           ultrasound conducting gel (After Corry et al[6]).

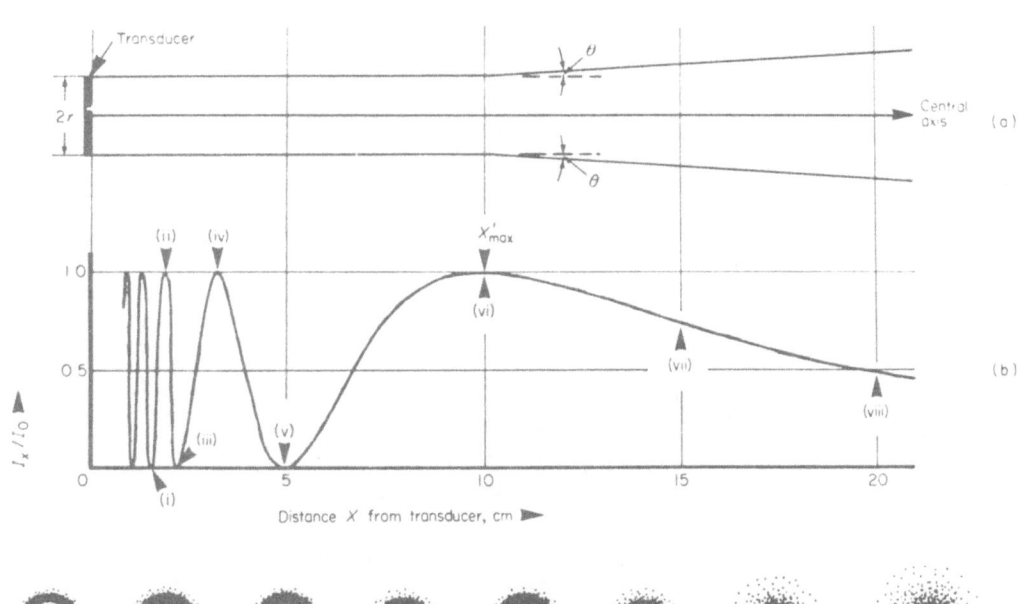

Fig. 7.   The ultrasonic field of a planar transducer operating
           in continuous wave mode. (a) the envelope containing
           almost all of the ultrasonic energy; (b) relative
           intensity distribution along the central axis of the
           beam; (c) ring diagrams showing the energy
           distribution of beam sections at positions indicated
           in (b). (After Wells[7]).

tissue at the same depth (Fig 9). But the proliferating cells in the well-perfused tumor margin infiltrating the tumor bed, will be cooler than the surrounding or superficial tissues. Clearly it is this region which must be heated to higher, therapeutically adequate, temperatures. Thus, on elementary physical grounds, with planar sources, it is not possible to heat a tumor at depth to a therapeutic temperature without producing higher temperatures in overlying tissues in spite of the fact that the tumor may be within the so-called "penetration depth", whether it be half-power, 1/e, or 1/e². Note in Fig 5 that tissues superficial to the half-power penetration depth line will bear the brunt of the energy flux. Penetration depth is not synonymous with safe therapeutic heating depth and must not be confused with it whether US or EM is used for LHT.

Extensive studies of steady state temperature distributions measured in vivo in anesthetized dogs using an array of thermocouples for scanning ("thermal mapping") confirmed these intuitively obvious theoretical conclusions. Salient results have been published previously[10-14]. The laboratory data are substantiated clinically by non-uniformity of tumor heating, dose-limiting local pain and extensive central tumor necrosis (shelling out), blistering and ulceration with the use of planar ultrasonic transducers (Table 1), as well as with EM applicators.

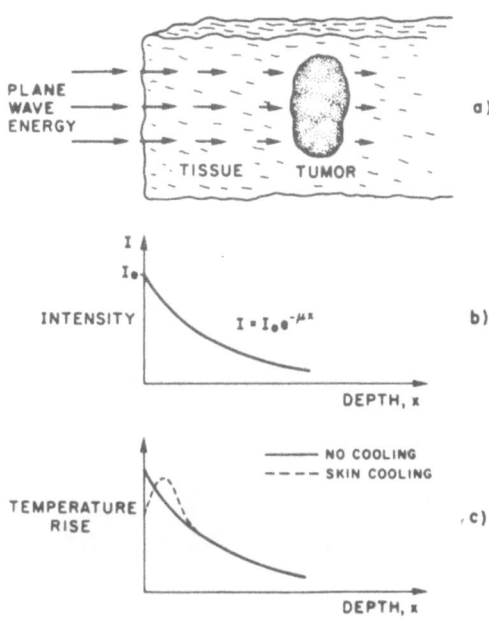

Fig. 8. Intensity and temperature distribution patterns in a homogenous medium with plane wave radiation (from Lele[9]).

TABLE 1.   Toxicity to HT by Planar, Stationary US

	Marmor et al[15]	Corry et al[6]
Moderate Pain		45%
Severe Pain	40%	34%
Erythema		45%
Desquamation		23%
Blister	19%	27%
Ulcer	15%	5%

Multiple, Planar Transducer Systems

In the process of heating a deep tumor, toxicity to overlying tissues could possibly be avoided by aiming multiple beams of ultrasound through different portals at the target, as was done by Fry and Fry[16] for trackless neurosurgery over a quarter of a century ago. A comparable system is used for LHT at Stanford by Fessenden et al[17] and is shown in Fig 10A. This "iso-centric" system has 6 planar 350 kHz transducers whose last axial maxima can be confocal. For heating deep tumors, the transducer axes are rotated a few degrees outwards, yielding the intensity profile shown in Fig 10B. A temperature profile from one treatment is shown in Fig 10C. Note that although the heating in the

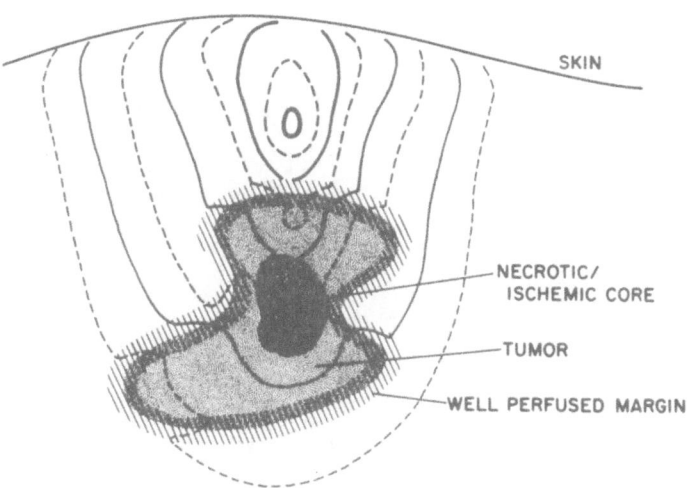

Fig. 9.   Temperature distributions in a subcutaneous tumor from plane wave energy deposition. Compare this temperature distribution with that ideally required as shown in Fig 4. (From Lele[4])

315

target volume is non-uniform, it is maximal at a depth of approx. 7 cm. The system has been used in 57 trials in 15 patients. Local discomfort was reported in 50% of the trials and was dose-limiting in 30%.

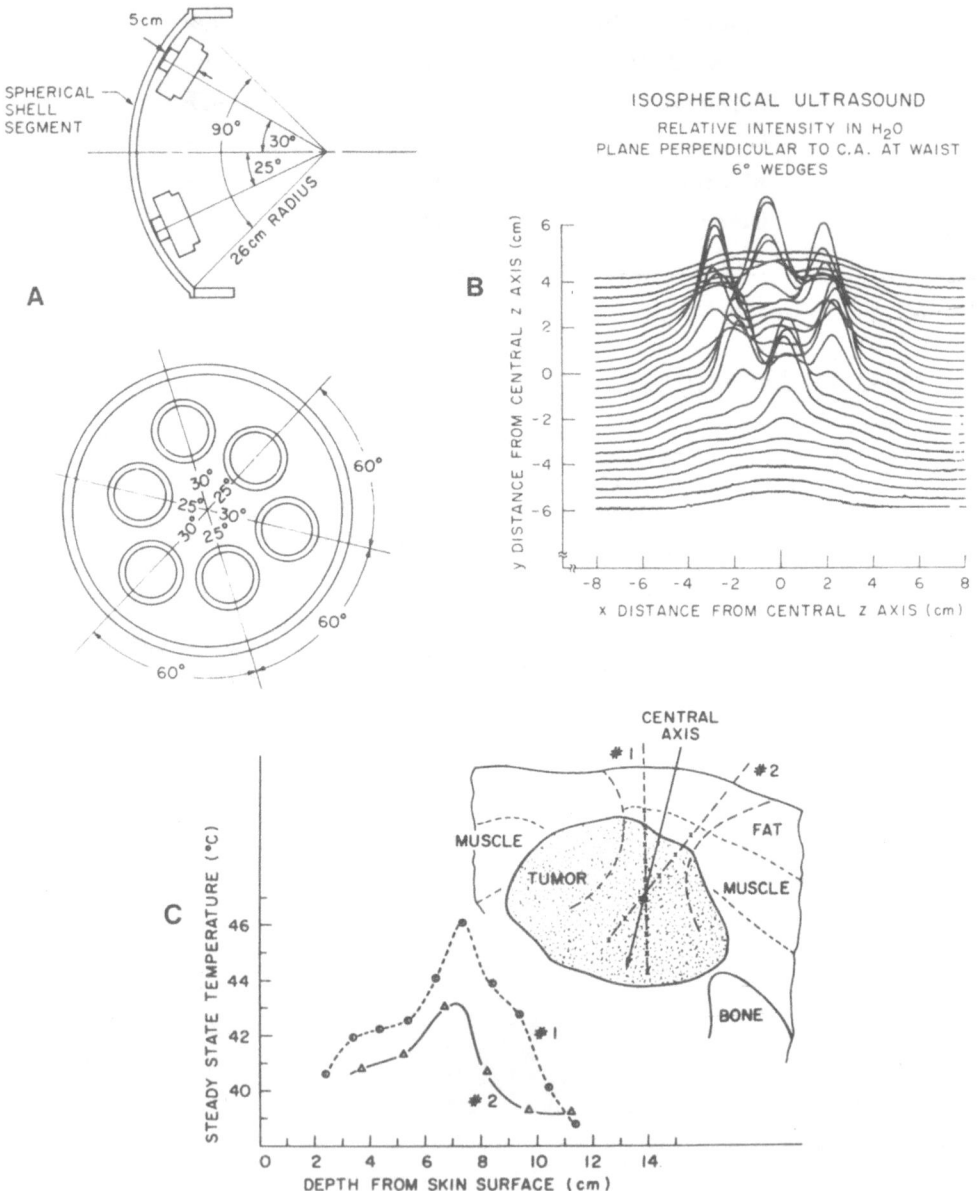

Fig. 10. (Reproduced by courtesy of Dr. Fessenden[17]) A. Schematic of the geometry of six power transducers mounted on 90° spherical shell sector.
B. Intensity scans in a plane perpendicular to system central axis.
C. Two temperature profiles obtained from thermocouple measurements in the pelvis of a patient heated with the system. The insert shows the location of the catheters containing the temperature sensors.

Dose-limiting nerve pain occurred in 20% of the trials and bone pain was also frequently encountered. These deserve attention since they may portend development of neuropathies and bone necrosis, especially if X-radiation is combined with HT. The probable cause for the occurrence of deep pain is shown in Fig 11 which shows the attenuation of US at different frequencies in muscle. Note that at the frequency of 0.3 MHz only 30% of the energy is attenuated at a depth of 15 cm representing the distal margin of HT volume. Thus 70% of the energy passes to deeper tissues where bones and nerves are located. Since, once launched into body tissues by proper coupling, US cannot normally leave the body, it will "bounce around" inside until it is totally absorbed, heating the interfaces - periosteum and the nerves - in the process. The obvious solution for minimizing the power required and for protection of deeper structures is to optimize the frequency so that maximum absorption occurs in the tumor.

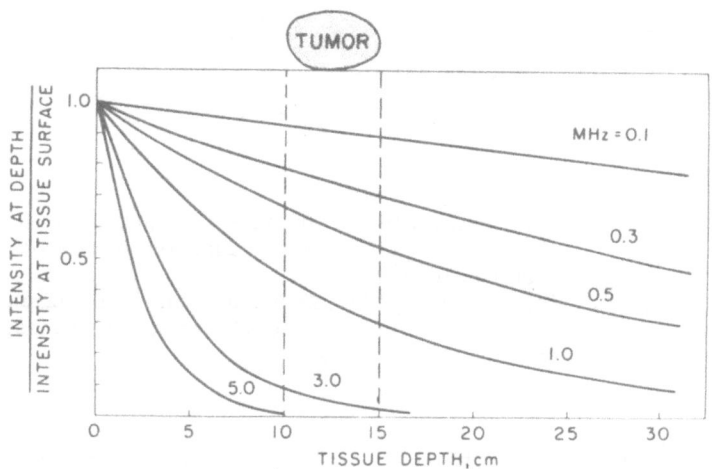

Fig. 11. Attenuation of ultrasound at different frequencies in soft tissues. See text. (From Lele[4])

A multiple transducer, adjustable beam system[13,14] using 6 therapeutic transducers and 1 diagnostic transducer Fig 12 was also evaluated at MIT. Each therapeutic transducer can be tilted at any angle, can be planar or focused and can be operated at any of 9 frequencies between 600 kHz and 6 MHz to obtain maximum absorption within the particular tumor. The frequency of the diagnostic transducer is chosen to minimize any coupling between it and the therapeutic transducers. The temperature distribution along the plane of any two transducers Fig 13 showed a 'hot spot' near the proximal point of intersection of the 2 beams and progressively lower temperatures due to attenuation distally within the tissue volume in which the beams overlapped. These 'hot spots' resulted from the intensity distribution in the field which was comparable to that of the Stanford system shown in Fig 10B.

Stationary and Scanning Focused Transducer Systems

Superposition of multiple beams, whether EM or US, may yield unexpected and unpredictable intensity distributions due to phase reinforcement and phase cancellation. Focusing within and restricted to a deep target, which is practicable with US but not with EM, as

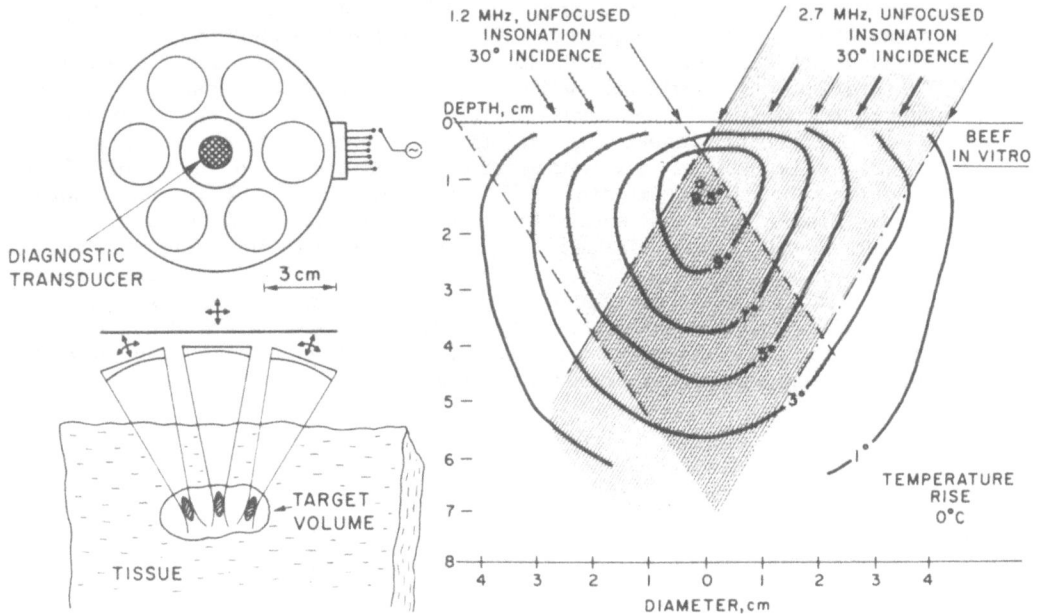

Fig. 12, (Left).   MIT, multiple transducer, adjustable beam
ultrasonic system for planar or focused transducers.
(From Lele[13])

Fig. 13, (Right). Temperature distributions in the plane through
the diagnostic and two therapeutic transducers.
(From Lele & Parker[14])

discussed earlier, eliminates most of the problems of field
inhomogeneity, and higher intensities can be achieved at the desired
target at depth (Fig 14) with resultant higher temperatures.   The
temperature rise at the integument of the portal and in the relatively
poorly perfused subcutaneous tissues can be held to a negligible value.
Beam divergence and attenuation rapidly lower the intensity in tissues
beyond the focus, thus sparing underlying tumor-bed tissues and bone.
Note also that if the ultrasonic absorption coefficient of the tumor
is higher than that of normal tissue or displays some intensity-dependent
non-linearity, the heat generation in the focal region in the tumor
would be even higher as shown by dashed line in Fig 14.   Absorption
coefficients of some transplanted murine tumors and spontaneous canine
tumors were found to be higher than those of normal soft tissues[14]
and a similar trend is seen in human tumors.   With a focused transducer
the maximum depth to which selective heating can be achieved is a
function both of the frequency and the aperture.   Note in Fig 14, that
while there is gain in intensity with progressive convergence towards
the focus following the inverse square law, energy is lost by attenuation
following an exponential function.   Therefore, with a beam of a given
angle of convergence and for a given attenuation in the tissue, there
is no effective gain in intensity beyond a certain depth (Fig 15).
This depth can be increased by increasing the angle of convergence
(use of a larger aperture).   It can also be increased by the use of
a lower frequency to reduce attenuation in the tissues superficial
to the focus (Figs 5,11), but this would also reduce heat generation
within the tumor, requiring proportionately higher intensities to achieve
therapeutic temperature levels.   Furthermore, it will permit
proportionately higher intensities to be transmitted to tissues beyond

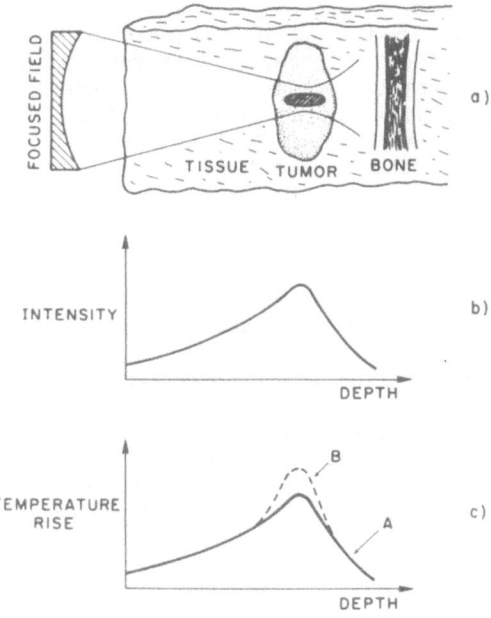

Fig. 14. Intensity and temperature distribution patterns with a focused field. See text, (From Lele[9]).

the tumor as was discussed previously (Fig 11 and related text). The choice of the proper frequency, which is crucial to localization of hyperthermia and of the aperture, is thus an exercise in optimization of these conflicting requirements for the size and depth of each specific tumor and the ultrasonic attenuation/absorption properties of the tumor and overlying tissues. These computations, followed by calculation

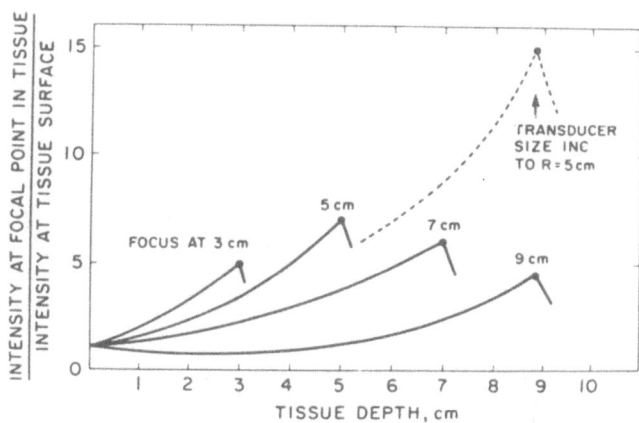

Fig. 15. Variation of intensity gain with the depth of placement of the focus of a transducer, 3 cm in radius and 10 cm focal length, in a tissue with an absorption coefficient of 0.3 dB/cm (solid lines). Note the increase in gain with an increase in the aperture of the transducer (dotted line). (From Lele[12])

of heat generation in the tumor and heat loss by conduction and blood flow, are an essential component of therapy planning and are routinely performed on our system computer. Transducers of 3 different diameters up to 20 cm, at 9 frequencies between 600 kHz and 6 MHz, and a number of interchangeable lenses from "ultra-wide angle" to "extreme telephoto" focal length are used experimentally to optimize the insonation conditions for each specific tumor. Fewer transducers and lenses adequately serve the clinical needs.

Focusing concentrates the energy emanating from the transducer into a small focal region typically between 0.5 to 5.0 mm in diameter and 2.5 to 25 mm in length (Fig 16) that serves as a heat source, the intensity of which can be controlled externally to generate the amount of heat required to produce and sustain hyperthermia in the tissue within and surrounding the focal volume. Thus it functionally resembles an implanted MW antenna or an RF electrode, but can be placed in the deep target non-invasively and will produce a hot spot with rapid fall-off of temperature, particularly in the radial direction. Multiple, stationary, focused beams (MIT multiple transducer, adjustable beam ultrasonic system Fig 12) produce multiple hot spots with low

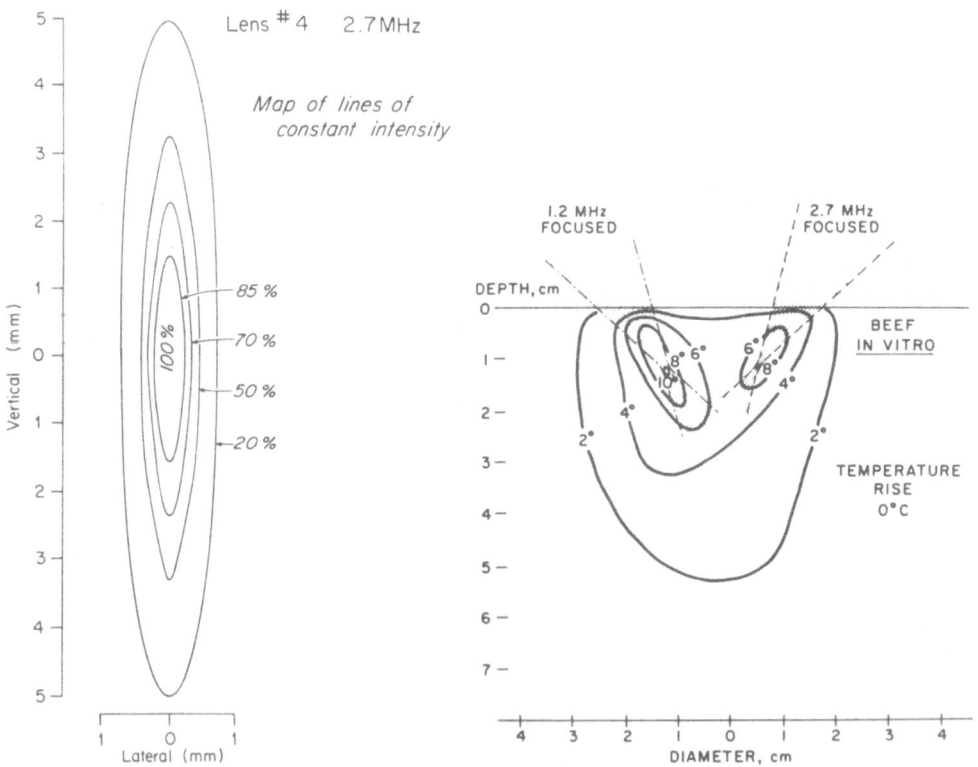

Fig.16,(Left). Intensity distribution in the focus of an ultrasonic transducer. The diameter and the length are a function of the frequency and aperture. The lower the frequency the larger is the diameter, and the smaller the aperture the longer the focal region. (After Lele[18], Robinson & Lele[19]).

Fig.17,(Right). Temperature distribution in the plane of two focused beams aimed at the margin of a treatment volume. (From Lele & Parker[14])

temperatures in intervening tissue as seen in Fig 17 similar to those by arrays of implanted MW antennae[20]. Such thermal inhomogeneity - hot spots and cool troughs - is inevitable with any stationary heating system - invasive or non-invasive. However, unlike the MW antenna, the ultrasonic focus can be moved about within the tissue non-invasively - without repeated or multiple insertions - and such scanning leads to merging of the hot spots, yielding uniform temperature distribution over the desired trajectory. The small size and the sharp definition of the ultrasonic focus, the ability to change its location in tissue continuously and non-invasively, and the ability to control the intensity and thus the heat generation rate at each location, enable full utilization of tissue heat transfer models[21] for production of desired temperature distributions. The focal trajectories and intensity modulation regimens for uniform HT of simple geometric shapes such as circles, cylinders, ovals, etc. have been analyzed theoretically and confirmed experimentally[22,12,13,23]. Shapes of most of the human tumors can be described in terms of combinations of simple geometrical patterns. The results of these studies substantiate the intuitively simple argument that since heat from a hyperthermic volume of tissue must leave the region through its surface, by conduction and through perfusion, the surface will always be cooler than the center (Fig 18A). For this reason, the energy needs to be deposited preferentially at the surface of a tumor to achieve uniform hyperthermia therein (Fig 18B), and particularly so if higher temperatures are desired at the proliferative margin. Such heating of spherical/cylindrical tumors can be accomplished by rotating a focused ultrasound transducer in a circular trajectory by a motor or by the use of a stationary annular-focus lens as discussed by Lele[11], Beard et al[24] and Higgins et al[25]. All these groups concluded that a simple annular-focus lens yields uniform tissue temperature distributions over 20 to 25 mm diameter tumors with sharp fall off in surrounding tissues. This is not possible with planar or other stationary systems. But in practice, very few tumors are spherical, cylindrical or oval, and more complex trajectories are required. These are best implemented by microprocessor/minicomputer-controlled stepping motors. The MIT system

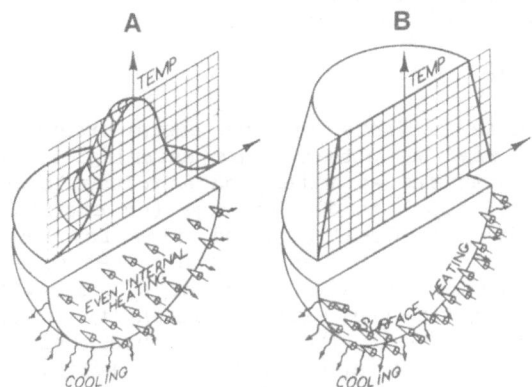

Fig. 18. Temperature distribution in a tissue volume resulting from deposition of energy (A) uniformly through its volume and (B) preferentiallly on its surface. (From Lele[13]).

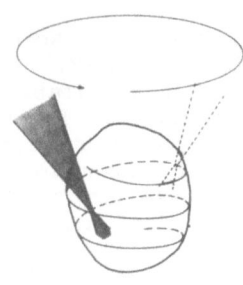

Fig. 19. A typical, simple scan pattern with intensity
modulation. (From Lele[4])

provides 6 degrees of freedom of motion, with flexibility to vary the
trajectories or their dimensions as needed, and modulation of intensity
is possible at every location of the transducer[26]. A sophisticated
power modulation program permits automatic control of tumor
temperature[27]. A simple typical trajectory is shown in Fig 19. Note
that little motion is required along the axis of radiation and that
intensity is raised when the focus is deeper in the tissue to compensate
for greater attenuation in the path. For small tumors up to 5 cm,
deposition of energy on the surface is adequate for uniform HT across
its diameter. More complex scanning patterns are needed for vascular
or larger tumors.

For uniform or controllable distribution of HT with sparing of
surrounding tissues (LHT) (1) Focusing, (2) Scanning, (3) Optimization
of Frequency and Aperture, and (4) Spatial and Temporal Intensity
Modulation are essential. This fact is being recognized by an increasing
number of hyperthermia investigators who are incorporating focusing,
scanning and computer controlled intensity modulation in their HT
production equipment[6,8,17,24,28-40].

Energy Requirements

An approximate estimate of the energy requirements for heating
a given target may be obtained by assuming it to have the same
thermophysical properties as water and a volume larger than the target
by a factor proportional to the average (or estimated) blood flow for
the target tissue. Typically, blood flow may impose an additional
heat load equivalent to 70 percent of the target volume. The ultrasonic
power needed to raise the temperature of a tumor with "typical" blood
flow, 6 cm in diameter and with an intensity absorption coefficient
of 0.3 dB/cm/MHz[14,41,42] by 7°C in 10 minutes using 1 MHz ultrasound,
can be calculated to be approximately 10 watts. If the tumor was
situated at a depth of 6 cm, and the overlying tissue had the same
ultrasonic absorption (attenuation) characteristics as the tumor,
approximately 15 watts of power will be needed at the portal. If a
1 MHz, 6 cm diameter transducer focused at 12 cm was used for heating
this tumor, the spatial average intensity would be approximately 20 W/cm^2
with a spatial peak intensity of approximately 60 W/cm^2.

322

Avoidance of Collapse Cavitation

Such acoustic power requirements for induction of hyperthermia might lead to cavitation damage because of the high peak intensities if sharp focusing were used. Special "smeared focus" lenses, in which peak intensities are lowered without compromising the angle of beam convergence, were therefore designed. The peak intensities employed for production of hyperthermia are always well below the threshold for cavitation-induced damage in organized mammalian tissues[1]. Extensive theoretical and experimental research on ultrasonically induced cavitation and damage thresholds in mammalian tissues _in vitro_ and _in vivo_ conducted in this laboratory shows that although stable bubble-oscillation type of cavitation occurs even at intensity levels associated with diagnostic ultrasound, transient collapse-cavitation resulting in structural damage does not occur in organized tissues until peak focal intensity is higher than 1,500 W/cm^2 at 2 to 3 MHz frequency. Occurrence of transient cavitation was invariably associated with occurrence of tissue damage but no damage was ever found to occur with bubble-oscillation type of cavitation unless it was induced by temeprature elevation. Thresholds for both types of cavitation are known to be lower at lower frequencies in liquid media, and in the absence of definitive information are presumed to be similarly lower in organized tissues.

Temperature Distributions

Figure 20 shows the steady state temperature distributions obtained in the gluteal muscle mass of dog _in vivo_ from 1.8 MHz ultrasound applied in (A) stationary, planar and (B) scanned, focused (SFUS) modes.

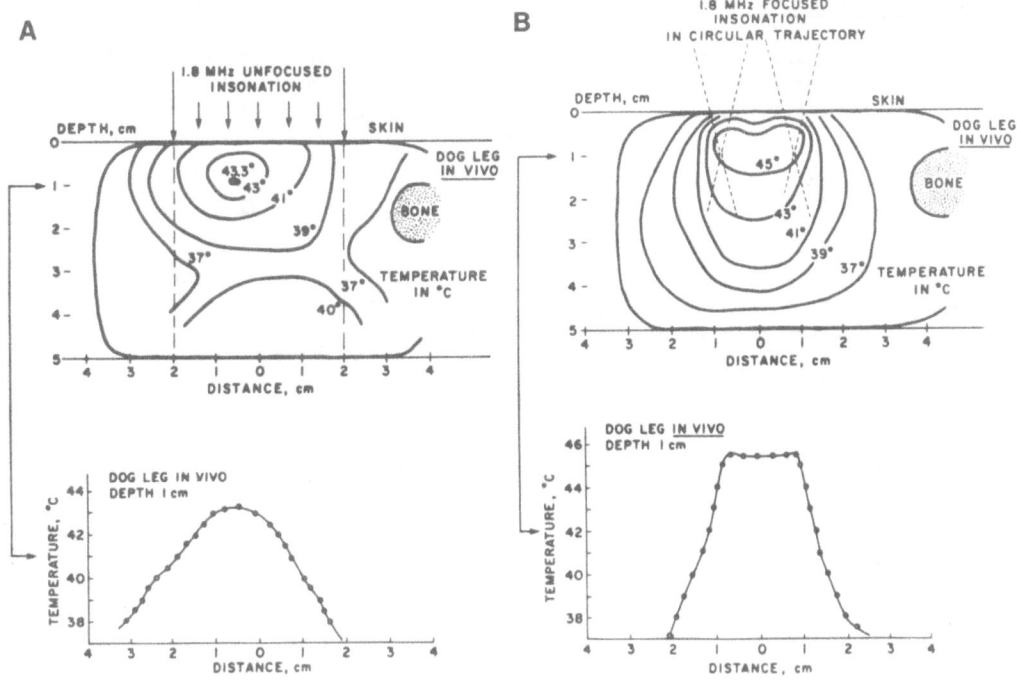

Fig. 20.   Temperature distributions in gluteal muscle mass of dog _in vivo_. A. Stationary, planar ultrasound.
B.   Scanned, focused ultrasound (SFUS). For details see Lele and Parker[14].

Isotherms were plotted from temperatures measured at 1 mm spacing along 9 tracks. Temperature distributions at the depth of 1 cm are shown at the bottom. Details are presented elsewhere[14] but note in B the uniformity of temperature distribution within the HT field, the sharp drop off at its edges, the absence of distortion by bone and of reflective heating at the bottom. Spatially uniform LHT, restricted to different target volumes at different depths, can be achieved to a depth of 12 to 15 cm with the equipment available. Two examples, in pieces of meat larger than those obtainable in experimental animals, are shown in Figure 21. The ability to heat deep-seated tumors _in vivo_ with sparing of overlying and surrounding tissues was evaluated in anesthetized rats bearing large tumors placed deep in the peritoneal cavity of anesthetized dogs. For details, see Lele[13,14].

Temperature distributions measured in deep seated tumors such as pelvic chondrosarcoma, transitional cell carcinoma in urinary bladder, retroperitoneal sarcoma, rectal carcinoma, etc. in patients tend to confirm these results, though it is generally not possible to plot isotherms from the few tracks of measurement permissible clinically due to invasiveness of thermometry. The CT scan in Fig 22A shows the track of a triple-junction thermocouple probe in a lesion in the rectum. One of the junctions was placed at a depth of 11 cm to continuously monitor temperature at that depth as the reference. Another thermocouple was used to scan the temperatures from 8 to 14 cm depth. Hyperthermia was induced through the greater sciatic foramen using scanned, focused ultrasound at 0.6 MHz. Temperatures measured during two thermocouple scans are shown in Fig 22B. Note the sharp fall off both proximally and distally. These data are similar to those obtained in other patients and in deep tumor simulations _in vivo_ described earlier.

Clinical Results

The clinical results of such HT are remarkable in significantly high response rates at rather low doses of LHT (42.5° to 43.0°C for 20 min., once weekly for 6 weeks) in tumors that had failed conventional

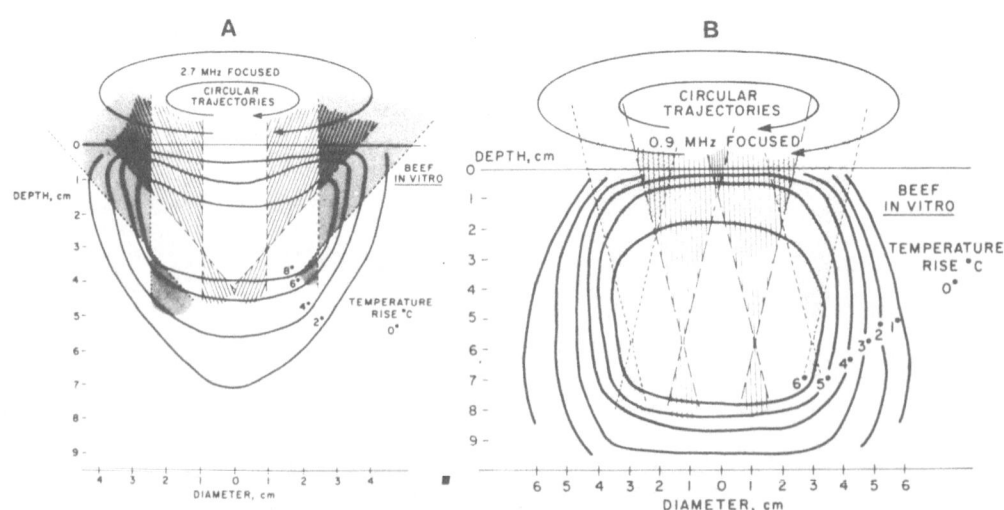

Fig. 21. Temperature distribution in beef _in vitro_.
    A. Two scanning beams, 2.7 MHz, focused at 3 cm depth
    B. Two scanning beams, 0.9 MHz, focused at 6 cm depth.
    For details see Lele[13], Lele and Parker[14].

therapy, especially with respect to the durability of the response, and enhancement of local chemotherapeutic effects. Details are presented in references 13, 43 and 44. These results could be attributed to the fact that in contrast to other HT studies, in this study margins of the tumor were invariably heated to the preselected temperature, although data are insufficient to draw firm conclusions. More significant in the present context is the relative absence of toxicity in this series (Table 2) as compared with that of stationary, planar systems (Table 1). The burning and stinging pain, noted only once, were evoked while the skin temperature was 26° to 28°C and were found to be related to the rate of rise of skin temperature and were immediately controlled by lowering the power level. The sensation of pressure was traced to the applicator bag resting on the thermocouple probe and was relieved by repositioning the applicator.

Rapid Hyperthermia and *In Situ* Cytoreduction

The selection of the heat-dose in our protocols is based on our data on temperature-duration relationships for thermal damage to mammalian tissues, <u>in vivo</u>, including several intra-operative

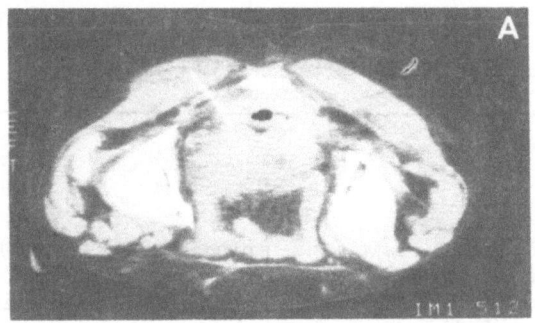

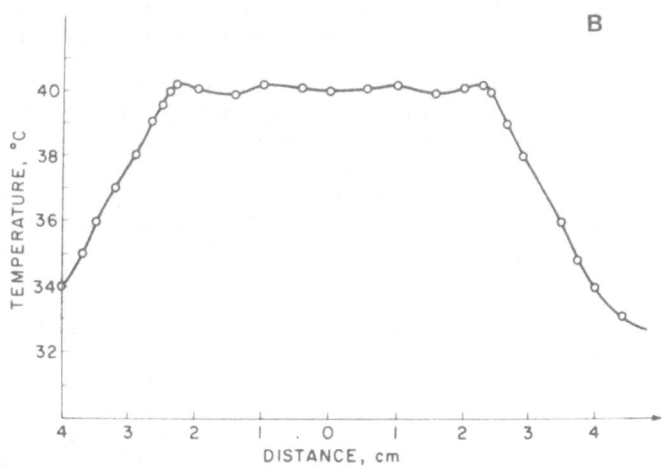

Fig. 22. A: CT scan of a patient with rectal carcinoma with a thermocouple probe implanted to a depth of 14 cm. In this section the probe-tip is at 11 cm.

B: Temperature distribution at 8 to 14 cm depth during ultrasonic HT.

TABLE 2.   Incidence of Toxicity of Scanned Focused
Ultrasound

		Patients	Sessions
Total		35	176
Toxicity			
Subjective			
Burning pain		1	1
Stinging pain		1	1
Pressure		2	2
Objective			
Erythema		1	1
Desquamation		1	1
Blister		0	0
Ulceration		0	0
No Toxicity		29	170 (97%)
Dose Limiting Toxicity		0	0

measurements on human brain and spinal cord (Fig 1). The different temperature-duration combinations along the slope of the stippled band represent equivalent "heat-doses", and LHT doses are selected from the bottom edge of the band representing absence of damage to normal tissues. Thus, HT for 20 min at 42.5°C should be biologically equivalent to that for 10 sec at 55°C or 1 sec at approx. 60°C. The very short duration at high temperature has an obvious advantage that delivery of the prescribed heat dose to the target volume can be assured regardless of any differences in local blood flow at different sites in that volume, since blood flow has no effect on the local temperature in such a short time. The late Dr. Britt had aptly coined the term 'Rapid Hyperthermia' to describe this strategy.

Tissues subjected to heat doses in the stippled band or above undergo coagulation pan-necrosis[1]. The focused ultrasound system used for LHT can be used to produce discrete, trackless focal lesions (Fig 23) of controllable and predictable size at predetermined locations and has been successfully used in neurosurgery for over a quarter of a century because of absence of any damage to tissues overlying the target. For therapy of bulky tumors, one can, in a single session, perform graded cytoreduction or controlled debulking (Fig 24) of the solid tumor mass at the higher heat-dose levels, and deliver LHT to tumor-bed tissues at lower dose levels to ensure sparing of the normal tissue components therein. This strategy has successfully been utilized in the therapy of spontaneous tumors in dogs[47,48].

The MIT SFUS system incorporates a confocal diagnostic ultrasound transducer[49]. This enables continuous monitoring of the location of the focus relative to blood vessels, bone, air interface etc., as well as of the morphology of the tissue (tumor or non-tumor) in the focal region, and the inception of its coagulation using tissue characterization techniques[50,51].

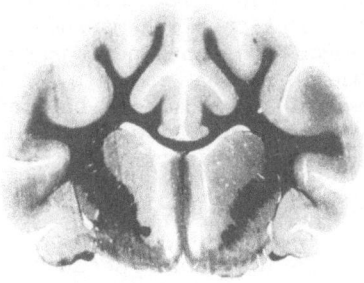

Fig. 23. Discrete, trackless focal lesions of coagulation pan-necrosis at the base of the brain. For details see Basauri and Lele[45], Lele[46].

The discreteness of the focal region and the small size (approx. 0.25 mm) of the thermocouple probe normally used for monitoring tumor temperature permit measurement of effective thermal diffusivity of the tumor at different stages of HT from which local blood flow can be estimated with reasonable accuracy[52-54]. The importance of these data to rational sequencing of HT in relation to radiation or chemotherapy is obvious. It may be germane to point out here that measurement of tissue temperature can be performed accurately during USHT with simple thermocouples which are much smaller in size and expense than specialized non-perturbing probes needed during hyperthermia by EM energy[55].

Unlike EM energy, in which leakage fields can pose problems of the safety of non-target tissues (for example of eyes, in HT of head & neck lesions), the directionality of US propagation, and the tight coupling through a non-gaseous path needed for its transmission to body tissues, virtually ensure their safety. For safety of the tissue in the focal region, the maximum spatial intensity must be held below the threshold for collapse or unstable cavitation at the frequency

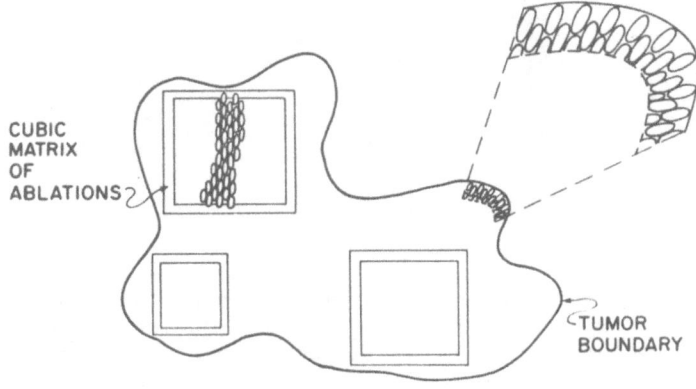

CUBIC
MATRIX
OF
ABLATIONS

TUMOR
BOUNDARY

Fig. 24. Use of SFUS LHT system for graded cytoreduction (From Lele[4]).

used, since intensities above that level are invariably associated with the occurrence of unpredictable hemorrhages[1]. Non-linear phenomena such as these are analogous to non-linear phenomena such as dielectric saturation, pearl chain formation etc. in EM fields which also must be avoided. The threshold for collapse cavitation in solid mammalian tissues _in vivo_ is approximately 1500 W/cm^2 at 2 to 3 MHz frequency, and drops at lower frequencies.

Mosaic and Phased Array Applicators

The current generation of scanned US systems utilizes electro-mechanical devices (stepping motors, DC servo-motors) for steering the transducer(s). Work on mosaic of transducers with or without electronic steering is being pursued at many laboratories. Dickinson[56] has developed a non-rigid, mosaic applicator for hyperthermia of extensive, superficial lesions and Ocheltree et al[38] presented a novel concept for a "stacked linear phased array applicator". The design requirements of a US phased array, with performance comparable to that of MIT SFUS system, have been critically examined also in the author's laboratory. It is concluded that stacked linear phased arrays cannot provide adequate resolution to heat small, deep tumors, and would need to be excessively large to heat large, deep tumors. In order to eliminate overheating of tissues superficial to a deep tumor, the ultrasonic hyperthermia scanning system must allow for lateral displacement of the ultrasonic beam[57].

DISCUSSION

Scanned, intensity-modulated, focused ultrasound presently is the only non-invasive technique for LHT of deep (or superficial) tumors, including their well-perfused, proliferative margins. Tumors which are enclosed by air or/and thick bone, such as those in the mediastinum or deep in the lung are inaccessible. Large retroperitoneal tumors,

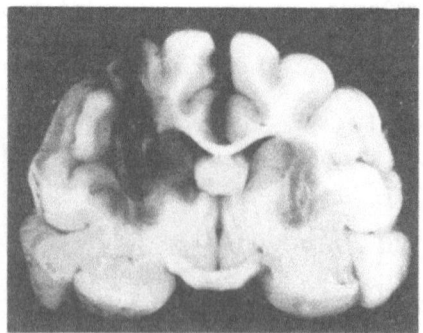

Fig. 25. A coronal section through a brain stained supravitally with trypan blue. _In situ_ ablation of equal focal volumes of tissue at depth was attempted using an RF electrode (Left) and Focused Ultrasound (Right). Note the extensive trauma to overlying tissues by the invasive probe in contrast to the absence of any damage to suprafocal tissue by focused ultrasound, Lele[4].

as well as those in the pelvis, abdomen, head and neck, and extremities have been heated satisfactorily with proper therapy planning, and selection of the portal(s), with the aid of scanned A-mode diagnostic ultrasonic examination to ensure an unimpeded path for the therapeutic beam(s) to the target. Loops of the bowel can generally be moved out of the ultrasonic path for the duration of HT session by suitable positioning of the patient,or the energy can be delivered through a posterior (for example as in Fig 22A) or perineal approach. Good localization of the HT volume ensures safety to surrounding normal tissues whether HT is used alone or with radiation or chemotherapy. Heating of critical normal tissues in the path of ultrasound propagation can be totally avoided by turning the ultrasonic power off in the appropriate segment(s) of the trajectory of the transducers. The trajectory, in which the focus of each transducer can be moved, is flexible and continuously adjustable. This can be varied to encompass the variations in the size and shape of any tumor, due to growth or regression. Intensity modulation enables the intensity to be specified at any location of the focus in the trajectory, and a sophisticated feed-back control maintains the temperature at the preset level, without droop or overshoot. Thus, in contrast to interstitial hyperthermia with implanted MW antennae or RF electrodes[4,5], both the treatment field and the heat-dose can be tailored to the specific needs of any tumor at the time of the treatment. Patients are treated on an outpatient basis and do not need hospitalization. The interval between consecutive LHT sessions therefore can be optimized to avoid development of significant thermotolerance. Since the progress of the lesion can be followed at suitable intervals, overtreatment with possible toxicity can be avoided. In addition to non-invasiveness, in-situ cytoreduction and "rapid HT", which are unique to scanned, focused ultrasound, greatly enhance its potential clinical usefulness. Interstitial hyperthermia with implanted MW antennae or RF electrodes, on the other hand, not only lacks the uniformity of heating and flexibility in changing the loci of heating, but also inflicts considerable amounts of trauma to the tissues superficial and deep to the target volume (Fig 25).

REFERENCES

1. P. P. Lele, Effects of ultrasound on "Solid" mammalian tissues and tumors in vivo, in: Ultrasound: Medical Applications, Biological Effects and Hazard Potential, M. H. Repacholi, M. Grondolfo and A. Rindi, eds., Plenum Pub. Corp., New York (1986).
2. W. C. Dewey, M. L. Freeman, G. P. Raaphorst, E. P. Clark, R. S. L. Wong, D. P. Highfield, I. J. Spiro, S. P. Tomasovic, D. L. Denman and R. A. Coss, Cell biology of hyperthermia and radiation, in: Radiation Biology in Cancer Research, R. E. Meyn and H. R. Withers, eds., Raven Press, New York (1980).
3. G. M. Hahn, "Hyperthermia and Cancer", Plenum Press, New York (1982).
4. P. P. Lele, Ultrasound: Is it the modality of choice for controlled, localized heating of deep tumors? in: Hyperthermic Oncology 1984 2: 129, J. Overgaard, ed., Taylor & Francis Publishers, London and Philadelphia (1985).
5. P. P. Lele, Scanned, focused, ultrasound for controlled, localized heating of deep tumors, in: Hyperthermia in Cancer Treatment, L. J. Anghileri and J. Robert, eds., CRC Press, Inc., Boca Raton, FL (1986).
6. P. M. Corry, K. Jabboury, E. P. Armour, and J. S. Kong, Human cancer treatment with ultrasound, in: IEEE Trans. on Sonics and Ultras., SU-31, 44 (1984).
7. P. N. T. Wells, "Physical Principles of Ultrasonic Diagnosis", Academic Press, New York (1969).

8. P. Munro, R. P. Hill, and J. W. Hunt, The development of improved ultrasound heaters suitable for superficial tissue heating, Medical Physics 9:888 (1982).

9. P. P. Lele, Induction of deep, local hyperthermia by ultrasound and electromagnetic fields, Radiat. Environ. Biophysics 17 (1980).

10. P. P. Lele, Hyperthermia by ultrasound, Proc. of the Int. Symp. on Cancer Therapy by Hyperthermia and Radiation, Amer. Coll. of Radiology, Wash., D.C. 168 (1975).

11. P. P. Lele, An annular-focus ultrasonic lens for production of uniform hyperthermia in cancer therapy, Ultras. in Med. and Biol., 7: 191 (1981).

12. P. P. Lele, Local hyperthermia by ultrasound, in: Physical Aspects of Hyperthermia, G. H. Nussbaum, ed., published for American Assoc. of Physicists in Med. by the Amer. Instit. of Physics, Inc., New York, NY (1982).

13. P. P. Lele, Physical aspects and clinical studies with ultrasonic hyperthermia, in: Hyperthermia in Cancer Therapy, F. K. Storm, ed., G. K. Hall and Co., Boston, Chap. 16 (1983).

14. P. P. Lele and K. J. Parker, Temperature distributions in tissues during local hyperthermia by unfocused, focused and steered, focused ultrasound, British J. of Cancer 45: Suppl. V, 108 (1982).

15. J. B. Marmor, D. Pounds, T. B. Postic, and G. M. Hahn, Treatment of superficial human neoplasms by local hyperthermia induced by ultrasound, Cancer 43: 188 (1979).

16. W. J. Fry and F. J. Fry, Fundamental neurological research and human neurosurgery using intense ultrasound, IRE Trans. on Medical Electronics, ME-7 166 (1960).

17. P. Fessenden, E. R. Lee, T. L. Anderson, J. W. Strohbehn, J. L. Meyer, T. V. Samulski, and J. B. Marmor, Experience with a multitransducer ultrasound system for localized hyperthermia of deep tissues, IEEE Trans. on Biomed. Engng., BME-31: 126 (1984).

18. P. P. Lele, A simple method for production of trackless focal lesions with focused ultrasound: physical factors, J. Physiol. 160: 494 (1962).

19. T. C. Robinson and P. P. Lele, An analysis of lesion development in the brain and in plastics by high-intensity focused ultrasound at low-megahertz frequencies, J. of the Acoust. Soc. of Amer. 51: 1333 (1972).

20. W. H. Houston, M. S. Coffee, S. F. Wahid, and P. P. Lele, Temperature distributions produced in animal tissues and tumor in vitro and in vivo by implanted microwave antennas, RF electrodes and by scanned focused ultrasound, presented at the 4th Int. Symp. Hyperthermic Oncol., Aarhus, Denmark, 2-6 July 1984, Abstract # I-1.

21. H. F. Bowman, Heat transfer mechanisms and thermal dosimetry, "Third Int. Symp.: Cancer Therapy by Hyperthermia, Drugs, and Radiation", L. A. Dethlefsen and W. C. Dewey, eds., N.I.H. Pub. No. 82-2437, NCI Monograph 61: 437 (1982).

22. K. J. Parker and P. P. Lele, The effect of blood flow on temperature distributions during localized hyperthermia, Annals New York Academy of Sciences 335: 60 (1980).

23. M. G. Curley and P. P. Lele, Power requirements using steered focused ultrasound in elliptical patterns, presented at the 4th Int. Symp. Hyperthermic Oncology, Aarhus, Denmark 2-6 July 1984, Abstract # M-21.

24. R. E. Beard, R. L. Magin, L. A. Frizzell, and C. A. Cain, An annular focus ultrasonic lens for local hyperthermia treatment of small tumors, Ultras. in Med. and Biol. 8: 177 (1982).

25. P. D. Higgins, X. W. Zeng, J. A. Zagzebski, B. R. Paliwal, and R. A. Steeves, Versatility of distributed focus ultrasound in treatment of superficial lesions, Int. Journal of Radiat. Oncol. Biol. Physics 1923 (1984).

26. P. P. Lele, E. Blanco, H. Das, R. O. Keough, P. S. Hamilton and G. E. Sleefe, Scanned focused ultrasound system for hyperthermia of deep tumors, in: Hyperthermic Oncology 1984 1:625, J. Overgaard, ed., Taylor & Francis, London (1984).

27. H. Das and P. P. Lele, Design of a power modulator for control of tumor temperature, in: Hyperthermic Oncology 1984 1:707, J. Overgaard, ed., Taylor & Francis, London (1984).

28. R. H. Britt, Personal Communication (1984).

29. D. M. Cooper, J. J. Butler, F. D. Ketterer, A scanning, focused ultrasound hyperthermia delivery system, in: Proc. of the Tenth Annual Northeast Bioengng. Conf., E. W. Hansen, ed., 97 (1982).

30. R. J. Dickinson, An ultrasound system for local hyperthermia using scanned focused transducers, IEEE Trans. on Biomedical Engng. BME-31: 120 (1984).

31. R. J. Dickinson, J. W. Hand, and S. Leeman, The design of focused transducers for ultrasound hyperthermia, Proc. IEEE Ultrasound Symp. 739 (1982).

32. H. Gerhardt and U. Brinn, Personal Communication (1984).

33. S. A. Goss and F. J. Fry, High intensity ultrasonic treatment of tumors, IEEE 1982 Ultras. Symp. 743 (1982).

34. J. W. Hand and G. Ter Haar, Heating techniques in hyperthermia. 1. Introduction and assessment of techniques, Brit. J. Rad. 443 (1981).

35. J. W. Hunt, R. P. Hill and A. Worthington, High-powered ultrasound sources using conical geometries used for hyperthermic studies, Rad. Res. 94: 580 (1983).

36. K. Hynynen, D. J. Watmough, J. R. Mallard, and M. Fuller, Local hyperthermia induced by focused and overlapping ultrasonic fields-an in vivo demonstration, Ultras. in Med. and Biol. 621 (1983).

37. I. Kindlein and S. Kindlein, Experimental system for induction of hyperthermia by focused ultrasound, in: Hyperthermic Oncology 1984 1:727, J. Overgaard, ed., Taylor & Francis, London (1984).

38. K. B. Ocheltree, P. J. Benkeser, S. G. Foster, L. A. Frizzell, and C. A. Cain, An ultrasonic phased array applicator for deep localized hyperthermia, presented at the 4th North Amer. Hyperthermia Group Meeting in Orlando, Fla. (1984).

39. W. Swindell, R. B. Roemer and S. T. Clegg, Temperature distributions caused by dynamic scanning of focused ultrasound transducers, IEEE 1982 Ultrasonics Symp. 750 (1982).

40. G. R. Ter Haar and J. W. Hopewell, Ultrasonic heating of mammalian tissues in vivo, Brit. J. of Cancer 45: 65 Suppl.V.

41. K. J. Parker and P. P. Lele, The thermal pulse-decay method for determining ultrasound absorption coefficients, in: IEEE Ultras. Symp. B. R. McAvoy, ed., IEEE Press, Piscataway, NJ, 754 (1982).

42. S. A. Goss, L. A. Frizzell, and F. Dunn, Ultrasonic absorption and attenuation in mammalian tissues, Ultra. in Med. Biol. 5: 181 (1979).

43. P. P. Lele, Local hyperthermia for advanced squamous carcinoma of the head and neck, in: Head and Neck Oncology, Chap. 11, G. T. Wolf, ed., Martinus Nijhoff Publishers, Boston/Dordrecht/Lancaster (1984).

44. P. P. Lele, Local hyperthermia by ultrasound for cancer therapy, in: Biological Effects of Ultrasound, Chap. 12: 135, W. L. Nyborg and M. Ziskin, eds., Churchill/Livingstone, Inc., Medical Pubs., New York (1985).

45. L. Basauri and P. P. Lele, A simple method for production of trackless focal lesions with focused ultrasound: statistical evaluation of the effects of irradiation on the central nervous system of the cat, J. Physiol. 160: 513 (1962).

46. P. P. Lele, Production of deep focal lesions by focused ultrasound-current status, Ultrasonics 5: 105 (1967).

47. P. P. Lele, R. J. Frere, K. J. Parker, R. C. Greenwald, M. Shalev and K. E. Greene, Local hyperthermia by focused ultrasound: technique and results in spontaneous tumors in dogs, Third Int. Symp.: Cancer Therapy by Hyperthermia, Drugs, and Radiation, June 22-26, 1980, Fort Collins, Colorado, Abstract TIII30.

48. M. Shalev, K. J. Parker, K. E. Greene and P. P. Lele, Local tumor hyperthermia by focused ultrasound: technique and results in spontaneous tumors in dogs, J. of Ultrasound in Med. 3: Suppl., 154 (1984).

49. P. P. Lele, Concurrent detection of the production of ultrasonic lesions, Medical and Biological Engng.4: 451 (1966).

50. P. P. Lele and N. Senapati, The frequency spectra of energy backscattered and attenuated by normal and abnormal tissue, in: Recent Advances in Ultrasound in Biomedicine, D.N. White, ed., Research Studies Press, Oregon, 55 (1977).

51. G. E. Sleefe and P. P. Lele, A non-invasive tissue characterization technique for use in hyperthermia studies, in: Hyperthermic Oncology 1984 1:851, J. Overgaard, ed., Taylor & Francis, London (1984).

52. P. P. Lele, A transient thermal pulse technique for measurement of tissue thermal diffusivity in vivo, Annals New York Academy of Sciences 335: 83 (1980).

53. W. H. Newman and P. P. Lele, Tissue thermal property measurements with an ultrasonic heating technique, in: Hyperthermic Oncology 1984 1:531, J. Overgaard, ed., Taylor & Francis, London (1984).

54. W. H. Newman and P. P. Lele, A transient heating technique for the measurement of thermal properties of perfused biological tissue, ASME Advances in Bioengng. (1985).

55. M. G. Curley and P. P. Lele, Some potential errors in measurement of temperatures in vivo during hyperthermia by ultrasound and electromagnetic energy, in: Hyperthermic Oncology 1984 1:561, J. Overgaard, ed., Taylor & Francis, London (1984).

56. R. J. Dickinson, A non-rigid mosaic applicator for local ultrasound hyperthermia, in: Hyperthermic Oncology 1984 1:671, J. Overgaard, ed., Taylor & Francis, London (1984).

57. G. E. Sleefe and P. P. Lele, The limitations of an ultrasonic phased array for the induction of local hyperthermia, IEEE Ultras. Symp., Oct. 16-18, 1985, San Fran., CA, Abstract # GG-4.

RECENT ADVANCES AND TECHNIQUES IN THERAPEUTIC ULTRASOUND

Gail ter Haar

Physics Department
Institute of Cancer Research
Sutton, Surrey, U.K.

INTRODUCTION

Therapeutic ultrasound has for a long time been the poor relation, in terms of research effort, of diagnostic ultrasound, although its use predates that of diagnosis by more than a decade.

The uses of ultrasound for therapy can broadly be divided into three types: physical therapy, beam surgery and ultrasound hyperthermia.

The use of ultrasound for cancer therapy is discussed in detail elsewhere in this volume (see chapter by Lele). Ultrasound is used in this context for the controlled description of energy to give predetermined temperature distributions for hyperthermic treatment of tumours, often in conjunction with radiotherapy or chemotherapy.

Ultrasound in physical therapy has been used mainly for the treatment of soft tissue injuries, but recently it has been used successfully for enhancing bone repair (Dyson and Brookes, 1983). This aspect of ultrasound therapy will be discussed in some detail in this chapter.

Focussed ultrasound can be used for the local destruction of soft tissues, especially in the brain where good localization is essential. Techniques making use of focussed ultrasound are also discussed in this chapter.

ULTRASOUND IN PHYSICAL MEDICINE

In many countries of the world, ultrasound is used very widely by physiotherapists for the treatment of soft tissue problems. Although the use is widespread, almost all treatment regimes are decided empirically, and knowledge of the mechanisms of interaction that give the beneficial effects seen and of the best way to deliver the ultrasonic energy, is scant. In the past, a thermal effect was usually sought as it is known that mild tissue heating may lead amongst other things to increased extensibility of collagenous tissues, decreased joint stiffness, changes in blood flow and pain reduction. More recently, the trend has been towards the use of lower intensities for treatment, and it is thought that benefit has been derived from non-thermal interaction mechanisms.

There is a wide variety of ultrasound therapy machines available commercially. Most are small, light and designed to be portable. Spatial average intensities up to 3Wcm^{-2} are usually available, often with a choice of two or three transducers giving discrete frequencies in the range 0.75-5 MHz. The choice of frequency is determined by the depth of lesion to be treated. The acoustic energy may be delivered either in a continuous, or a pulsed (tone burst) mode. Pulsed exposures are often chosen when non-thermal effects are sought. Typical pulsing regimes are 2ms on: 2ms off, or 2ms on: 8ms off. Transducer design for therapy use has been described in detail elsewhere (see chapter by D. Benwell in this book).

Ultrasonic energy is introduced to the treatment site either by a "contact" technique, or via a water immersion method. When a contact method is used, the skin surface is coated with a thin layer of a coupling medium that has acoustic impedance well matched to skin. The coupling medium is often liquid paraffin or a light mineral oil. Water immersion is used when an awkward geometry is to be treated and maintenance of contact is difficult, such as the elbow or ankle. The transducer is usually kept moving throughout treatment. A stationary head method runs the risk of setting up standing waves (see chapter by ter Haar, "Interaction mechanisms:non thermal non-cavitational effects", this volume), and also there is a possibility of unwanted effects being caused by local "hot" spots in the ultrasonic field, the effects of which may be smeared out if the transducer is kept in motion.

In a recent survey (1985)·of the use of ultrasound therapy both in hospitals (204 replies), and in private practice (191 replies) in England and Wales some interesting facts came to light. It was found that over 20% of all treatments in hospital physiotherapy departments and 54% of all treatments performed by private practitioners involved ultrasound. The frequencies used by hospital departments were 0.75 MHz (18%), 1.0 MHz (32%), 1.5 MHz (25%), and 3.0 MHz (25%). In response to the question, "What intensities do you use ?" 15% of hospital users claimed to use intensities in the range 0.1-0.25Wcm^{-2}, 36% used 0.25-0.5Wcm^{-2}, 36% 0.5-1.0Wcm^{-2} and 12% used 1.0-3.0Wcm^{-2}. 14% used continuous wave ultrasound only, 19% used pulsed beams only, and 67% used both. Figure 1 shows results from the survey. The frequency and intensity histograms on the left show the results from hospital departments, those on the right show those from private practice. The conditions treated include acute soft tissue injuries, inflammatory conditions, sports injuries, and joint problems. The most commonly treated injuries are listed in Table 1.

An exciting recent development on the therapeutic ultrasound front has been a systematic scientific study of the effect of pulsed ultrasonic exposures on the different stages of bone repair. (Dyson and Brookes, 1983). The phases involved in bone repair following, for example, fracture have some similarities with those found in soft tissue regeneration (see

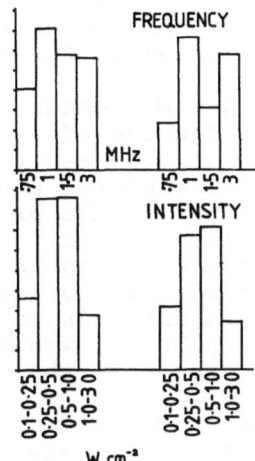

Fig. 1. Results from a survey of therapeutic ultrasound use
by physiotherapists in hospitals and in private
practice in England and Wales.   Left hand histograms
represent replies from hospital, right hand histograms
represent those from private practice.   The top histograms show the frequencies used, the lower histograms
show the intensity ranges.

Table 1. Some conditions treated by therapeutic ultrasound

Contusions
Local oedema
Varicose ulcers
Scar tissue
Dupuytren's contracture
Torn ligaments
Torn tendons
Strained tendons
Strained ligaments
Tendinitis
Tenosynovitis
Bursitis
Torn muscles
Chondromalacia patellae
Low back pain
Carpal tunnel syndrome
Post herpetic neuralgia
Torn joint capsules
Adhesive capsulitis

(ter Haar, Dyson, Oakley, in preparation).

ter Haar, G.R. "Tissue Regeneration" in this volume).   There
are overlapping stages of inflammation, proliferation and remodelling.   In the first, inflammatory and early proliferative
stages, the fracture site is cleared of debris, repair stimulating factors are released, a blastema and soft callus is
formed, and the bone fragments are united.   In the late proliferative phase, hard callus is formed.

     In this study, Dyson and Brookes made bilateral fractures
in the upper part of the fibulae of adult rats.   The rats
remained mobile.   One fracture was treated with ultrasound
(0.5Wcm^{-2} spatial average, temporal peak, pulsed 2ms on: 8ms
off, for 5 minutes at either 1.5MHz or 3.0MHz) in degassed
water, and the other, contralateral fracture was mock irradiated using the same method, but with the sound off.   Repair
was assessed using microradiography and histology.   The
results obtained are represented in Table 2.   The percentages
shown are those for the number of fractures that have responded
better, as well as, or worse than their control.

     It can be seen that 1.5MHz was more effective than 3.0MHz,
and that the treatment was most useful if given during the
first two weeks following injury (inflammatory and early
proliferative phases).   Bone repair was found to be of a
juvenile type - ossification with little cartilege formation.
Ultrasonic exposure at 3-4 weeks however (late proliferative
phase) seemed to be disadvantageous, cartilege growth being
accelerated with delay to firm bony union.

     Thus, it seems that ultrasound can be a useful therapy
for bone fractures if used in the early stages of repair.   It
appears to accelerate whichever natural process is going on
at the time of exposure.   Thus, if unwanted cartilege is
being formed, ultrasonic treatment at this time can accelerate
the process.

     Dyson and Brookes postulate a non thermal mechanism of
action as 1.5MHz has proved more useful than 3.0MHz.   This
hypothesis awaits proof.

     The idea that ultrasound accelerates whatever process is
going on at the time, is a useful one, and should be investigated for soft tissue injuries.   When mechanisms of action
are more fully understood it will no doubt become clear that
there are times at which it will be beneficial to treat with
ultrasound, but equally well there may be times when the situation may be made worse.   Most ultrasound users agree that
it is most effective when used as soon as possible after an
injury has occurred.

APPLICATIONS OF ULTRASOUND IN SURGERY

     Ultrasound can be used in one of two ways in surgery.
It can either be used as a highly focussed beam to produce
local tissue destruction (focussed beam surgery) or it can be
used to provide mechanical vibrations that drive a blade, saw,
metal tip or other instrument.

Table 2.   Effect of ultrasound on fracture repair

	Percentage Responses		
	Ultrasound treated better than mock treated	Ultrasound treated same as mock treated	Mock treated better than ultrasound treated
Treatment at 1.5 MHz			
Treatment weeks			
1 + 2	78.6	14.3	7.1
1 +̲ 2 + 3	68.4	15.8	15.8
3 +̲ 4 +̲	50.0	12.5	37.5
4 +̲ 5 +̲ 6	50.0	16.7	33.3
Treatment at 3.0 MHz			
Treatment weeks			
1 + 2	56.2	12.5	31.3
1 +̲ 2 + 3	50.0	18.2	31.8
3 +̲ 4 +̲	62.5	12.5	25.0
4 +̲ 5 +̲ 6	20.0	40.0	40.0

+̲ denotes and/or

(adapted from Dyson and Brookes, 1983).

i. Focussed beam surgery

If a new surgical technique is to become widely accepted, and to replace more conventional knife techniques, it must be reproducible and controllable in its ability to destroy tissue, it should only affect the required region, and where possible should be rapid and give minimum blood loss. In theory highly focussed ultrasound beams can fulfil most of these criteria. Typically, focal spots 1-2mm in width, and 3-4mm in length may be achieved.

Techniques for producing surgery beams have been discussed elsewhere in this book (see chapter by D. Benwell). Focussing may be achieved by a variety of methods (ter Haar and Hand, 1981). Focussed bowl transducers or the combination of plane transducer and acoustic lens are the most commonly used techniques.

Ultrasonically induced focal lesions have mainly been studied in the brain, although the liver, spinal cord, kidney and eye have also been studied.

There have been various attempts to collate available data providing threshold intensities for lesion production. It has been suggested that on a log-log plot of intensity as a function of exposure time three colinear regions can be identified.   This is a purely empirical observation.   It has been proposed that the relationship between intensity and exposure time to produce a lesion is

$$It^{\frac{1}{2}} = c(f,T) \qquad\qquad\qquad 1$$

where c is a weak function of frequency, f, and possibly the base temperature of the tissue, T, (Dunn et al, 1975).

It has been suggested that for intensities greater than 2.10^3 Wcm^{-2}, and exposure times less than 4.10^{-2} secs, cavitation mechanisms are involved (Fry et al, 1970), for exposure times greater than 1 sec, and intensities less than 200 Wcm^{-2} thermal mechanisms are invoked (Frizzell et al, 1977).   In the region between, the mechanism of lesion production is unclear.   A threshold intensity in the region 30-40 Wcm^{-2} seems to exist for exposure times of 10^2-10^3s (Johnston and Dunn, 1981).

Microscopy of these focussed lesions shows "island" and "moat" structures (Warwick and Pond, 1968) similar to those seen when a fine heated wire is embedded in tissue (Pond, 1970).   In the brain the "island" is a coagulated core, and the "moat" shows liquefaction of nerve cells with some intact blood vessels.   Mitochondria are amongst the first organelles to show damage, although in the brain, synapses show early damage (Fallon et al, 1973; Borrelli et al, 1981).

Ultrasonic beam surgery has been used experimentally in neurosurgery for the investigation of brain function (Fry et al, 1978) and for behavioural studies (Lee et al, 1979). There is a limitation on the use of this technique in adult humans as a portion of the skull must be removed to provide an

acoustic window.   Beam surgery has, however, been used ·in
the eye (Coleman et al, 1980, 1985a,b; Lizzi et al, 1978) and
in the kidney (Linke et al, 1973).

Menière's disease is a disorder of the inner ear which
leads to attacks of vertigo.   Successful treatment entails
relieving the vertigo while preserving the existing level of
hearing.   A fine ultrasonic beam may be directed into the
lateral semicircular canal of the ear, and the sensory neuro-
epithelium of the cristae and maculae in the labyrinth are
destroyed using high intensities.   Accurate dosimetry is
essential as the facial nerve is close to the semicircular
canal, and may be damaged, causing facial paralysis.   The
most commonly used irradiation method is one devised by Arslan
(1953).   A groove is made by removing mastoid cells, and the
transducer is put into the groove.   Kossoff et al (1966, 1967)
have devised another technique (the round window technique)
that reduces the risk of damage to the facial nerve.

ii.   Ultrasonically driven tools

Ultrasonically driven tools are usually comprised of a
half wavelength rod of magnetostrictive or piezoceramic transducer, coupled to a waveguide and terminated in a working end
that has a shape relevant for specific jobs.   The vibration
amplitude is usually in the range 15-350µm, with working frequencies in the range 20-30 kHz.

It appears that ultrasonically driven knives have some
advantages over conventional knives.   The friction between
two surfaces is reduced if one surface is vibrating, and so
less force is needed to achieve a cut (Goliamina, 1974).   High
temperatures may be reached at the tip of an ultrasonic scalpel,
and this may cauterize vessels of less than 2mm in diameter
(Derderian et al, 1982).   This reduced bleeding in the area,
and thus makes ultrasonic instruments useful in highly vascular
organs such as the liver and spleen.   It has also been used
for tracheotomies, tonsillectomies, and in the lungs, bronchial
tubes, thoracic walls and eye (Derderian et al, 1982; Hodgson,
1979; Goliamina, 1974).   It is claimed that ultrasound has
advantages over cryosurgical techniques because the tip does
not stick to tissues, and the cut surfaces do not exhibit late
damage.   Ultrasound has an advantage over laser surgery in
that the operator has tactile feedback and tissue destruction
is less indiscriminate (Hodgson, 1979).

Ultrasonic saws may be used for cutting bone.   It is
thought to be easy to use, especially for performing accurate
osteotomies.   Bone healing appears to be initially slower
following ultrasonic cutting, but after six weeks appears to
be the same for both ultrasonic and conventional cutting techniques (Aro et al, 1981).

Ultrasonically driven tools are also used for tissue aspiration.   One common use is for the removal of cataracts from
the eye (phaco-emulsification).   The tip of the instrument
is a hollow tube.   This is inserted into a small perforation
in the eye.   The tip is vibrated thus breaking up the lens.
The fragments can then be sucked up through the tube (Kelman,
1967).   A similar technique can be used for debulking solid
tumours, for example in the rectum (Hodgson, 1979), and for
destroying renal calculi (Alken, 1982).

There is evidence from the published literature that ultrasound surgery may have considerable potential. However, there is a crying need for careful science and engineering to be performed in order that its full potential may be realized.

Ultrasonic scaling is now quite a widespread technique in dentistry (Ewen, 1966; Suppipat, 1974; Frost, 1977). These instruments operate by driving a small scraping tool in the shear mode at frequencies in the range 18-42 kHz. The tip is water cooled.

iii. Extracorporeal shockwave lithotripsy (ESWL)

One method of disintegrating renal calculi that is becoming more widespread is extracorporeal shockwave lithotripsy (ESWL) (Chaussy et al, 1984; Brendel and Enders, 1983). In this method, shock waves generated extracorporeally are focussed on the stone, with the intention of breaking it up. A spark discharge is generated at one focus of a rotationally symmetric semi-ellipsoid reflector. The patient is placed so that the stone is at the position of the second focus of the reflector. This is determined using X-ray imaging techniques. Short pulses ($\sim$ 1-2μs) are given to the stone until it has disintegrated. The pressure amplitude in one commercially available machine has been measured as 14 MPa at the focus. The focus is cigar shaped, pressures 80% of the peak being measured 5cm on either side of the focus on the long axis, and 1cm on either side in the perpendicular direction (Coleman and Saunders, private communication). There have been reports of skin bruising at the entry point of the shock wave, especially in female patients. It is worrying that very little work has been done on the effect of shock waves on normal tissues. This must be a high priority for research if these ESW lithotripters are to be used safely.

SUMMARY

Ultrasound is widely used for therapeutic applications, and its popularity seems to be increasing, especially in physical medicine. New work in this field should focus on providing an understanding of the way in which therapeutic benefit is derived, and thus in optimizing exposure conditions.

ACKNOWLEDGEMENTS

I should like to thank Dr. Mary Dyson for her help in preparing the lecture associated with this paper. I should also like to thank Dr. Coleman, St. Thomas' Hospital, for providing the technical information about the ESWL.

REFERENCES

Alken, P., 1982, Percutaneous ultrasonic destruction of renal calculi. Urologic Clinics of North America, 9:145.
Arslan, M., 1953, Treatment of Menière's syndrome by direct application of ultrasound waves to the vestibular system. Proc. 5th Int. Cong. Otorhinolaryngol. Amsterdam 429-436.
Borrelli, M.J., Bailey, K.I., Dunn, F., 1981, Early ultrasonic effects upon mammalian CNS structures (chemical synapses). J. Acoust. Soc. Am. 69:1514.

Brendel, W., Enders,G., 1983, Shock waves for gallstones:
    animal studies. <u>Lancet</u>, 1:1054.
Chaussy, C., Schüller, K., Schmiedt, E., Brandl, H., Jocham, D.,
    Liedl, B., 1984, Extracorporeal shock wave lithotripsy
    (ESWL) for treatment of urolithiasis. <u>Urology</u>, 23:59.
Coleman, D.J., Lizzi, F.L., El-Mofty, A.A.M., Driller, J.,
    Franzen, L.A., 1980, Ultrasonically accelerated resorp-
    tion of vitreous membranes. <u>Am. J. Ophthalm.</u> 89:490.
Coleman, D.J., Lizzi, F.L., Driller, J., Rosado, A.L., Chang,S.,
    Iwamoto, T., Rosenthal, D., 1985a, Therapeutic ultrasound
    in the treatment of glaucoma. I. Experimental model.
    <u>Ophthalmology</u>, 92:339.
Coleman, D.J., Lizzi, F.L., Driller, J., Rosado, A.L., Burgess,
    S.E.P., Torpey, J.H., Smith, M.E., Silverman, R.H.,
    Yablonski, M.E., Chang, S., Rondeau, M.J., 1985b, Thera-
    peutic ultrasound in the treatment of glaucoma. II.
    Clinical applications. <u>Ophthalmology</u>, 92:347.
Dunn, F., Lohnes, J.E., Fry, F.J., 1975, Frequency dependence
    of threshold ultrasonic dosages for irreversible struct-
    ural changes in mammalian brain. <u>J. Acoust. Soc. Am.</u>
    58:512.
Dyson, M., Brookes, M., 1983, Stimulation of bone repair by
    ultrasound, <u>in</u>: "Ultrasound '82", R.A. Lerski, P. Morley,
    eds.,Pergamon Press, Oxford.
Fallon, J.T., Stehbens, W.E., Eggleton, R.C., 1973, An ultra-
    structural study of the effect of ultrasound on arterial
    tissue. <u>J. Path.</u>, 3:275.
Frizzell, L.A., Linke, C.A., Carstensen, E.L., Fridd, C.W.,
    1977, Thresholds for focal ultrasonic lesions in rabbit
    kidney, liver and testicle. <u>IEEE Trans. Biomed. Eng.</u>,
    BME-24:393.
Frost, H.M., 1977, Heating under ultrasonic dental scaling
    conditions. Symp. on biological effects and characteri-
    zations of ultrasound sources. Hazzard, D.G. and
    Litz, M., eds. <u>DHEW(FDA)</u>78-8048:64.
Fry, F.J., 1978, Methods and Phenomena: Their applications
    in science and technology, <u>in</u>: "Ultrasound: its applica-
    tions in medicine and biology", F.J. Fry, ed. Elsevier
    Scientific Pub. Co., Amsterdam.
Fry, F.J., Kossoff, G., Eggleton, R.C., Dunn, F., 1970,
    Threshold ultrasonic dosages for structural changes in
    the mammalian brain. <u>J. Acoust. Soc. Am.</u> 48:1413.
ter Haar, G.R., Hand, J.W., 1981, Heating techniques in hyper-
    thermia. III. Ultrasound. <u>Brit. J. Radiol.</u> 54:459.
Johnson, R.L., Dunn, F., 1981, Ultrasonic hysteresis in
    biological media. <u>Radiat. Environ. Biophys.</u> 19:137.
Kossoff, G., Khan, A.E., 1966, Treatment of vertigo using the
    ultrasonic generator. <u>Arch. Otolaryngol.</u> 84:181.
Kossoff, G., Wadsworth, J.R., Dudley, P.F., 1967, The round
    window ultrasonic technique for the treatment of Menière's
    disease. <u>Arch. Otolaryngol.</u> 86:534.
Lee, A.J., Taberner, P.V., Halliwell, M., 1979, Severing the
    corpus callosum in rats using ultrasound: theoretical and
    experimental correlations. <u>J. Acoust. Soc. Am.</u> 66:1292.
Linke, C.A., Carstensen, E.L., Frizzell, L.A., Elbadawi, A.,
    Fridd, C.W., 1973, Localised tissue destruction by high
    intensity focused ultrasound. <u>Arch. Surg.</u> 107:887.
Lizzi, F.L., Coleman, D.J., Driller, J., Franzen, L.A., 1978,
    Experimental ultrasonically induced lesions in the retina,
    choroid and sclera. <u>Invest. Ophthalmol.</u> 17:350.

Pond, J.B., 1970, The role of heat in the production of ultra-sonic focal lesions.   J. Acoust.Soc. Am. 47:1607.

Warwick, R., Pond, J.B., 1968, Trackless lesions in nervous tissues produced by high intensity focused ultrasound (high frequency mechanical waves).   J. Anat. 102:387.

ULTRASONIC TISSUE CHARACTERIZATION[*]

Padmakar P. Lele and Gerard E. Sleefe

Laboratory for Medical Ultrasonics
Massachusetts Institute of Technology
Cambridge, MA. 02139

I. INTRODUCTION

For more than two decades, diagnostic ultrasound has been used as a non-ionizing means for imaging soft tissues and organs within the body[1]. Ultrasonic images, however, have not proved useful in unambiguously determining tissue pathology. Since the early 1970's, though, it has been recognized that normal tissues exhibit significantly different acoustic properties than ischemic, infarcted, structurally disorganized or other abnormal tissues[2,3]. As a result, the quantitative measurement of the acoustic properties of tissue has become a popular and important area of research.

The objective of this paper is to present an overview of the various acoustic parameters which have been investigated for tissue characterization and to summarize the methods used for their measurement. Both in-vitro and in-vivo measurement techniques will be presented. It will be seen that the transition from the in-vitro case to the in-vivo case is often non-trivial and requires sophisticated measurement techniques. These methods will be described in terms of their implementation and clinical usefulness. The practicality of these methods for future investigation into the ultrasonic characterization of tissues will be discussed.

---

[*]This work was supported partially by the U.S.P.H.S. through grant NCI-CA31303 and by the Fannie and John Hertz Foundation.

II. ACOUSTIC IMPEDANCE

The acoustic impedance, z, of a medium is defined as the product of its density, ρ, and its sound speed, c, viz.,

$$z = \rho c \qquad (2.1)$$

Although this section is entitled acoustic impedance, we also note that the individual components, ρ and c, can be used as tissue characterization parameters. It behooves us to treat these parameters together since the issues regarding their measurement are closely related.

There are two fundamental methods for in-vitro measurement of impedance. The first method entails individual measurement of ρ and c, where ρ is measured by any of a number of standard techniques. A comprehensive compilation of in-vitro data for density as well as several other parameters described in this paper has been published by Goss et al[4]. This paper also serves as an excellent bibliography for in-vitro measurement techniques. The sound speed, c is typically derived from a transit time measurement. If an acoustic pulse travels a distance x in a medium, then the transit time, t, for the pulse to propagate through that medium is

$$t = x/c \qquad (2.2)$$

The second fundamental approach to measuring z is from measurements of the reflection coefficient, R. Consider the parallel plane arrangement in Fig 1a. where a plane ultrasonic wave propagates in medium 1 and is normally incident upon an interface of acoustic impedance z_2. The ratio of the reflected amplitude to the incident amplitude of the acoustic wave is defined to be the reflection coefficient and is given by

$$R = \frac{z_2 - z_1}{z_2 + z_1} \qquad (2.3)$$

Hence the impedance of the unknown medium, z_2 can be determined from the ratio of the reflected amplitudes provided that the impedance of the reference medium, z_1 is known.

Acoustic impedance is considered to be a useful tissue characterization parameter since there are significant differences in this parameter among different tissue types. Table 1 lists some representative values of ρ and z for various tissue types, and Fig. 2 shows the differences which can exist in the reflection coefficient of normal and infarcted tissue. Note that these measurements were performed under in-vitro conditions.

The measurement of the acoustic impedance in-vivo is not a simple extension of the methods described above. In the first case, the sound speed can not be measured from transit times since tissue dimensions are not accurately known. In the second case, the ratio of reflected amplitudes does not yield the reflection coefficient as per Eq. 2.3 due to nonplanar interfaces (resulting in surface and internal scattering), and the loss of signal strength by attenuation with increasing depth. As a result, the determination of the acoustic impedance in-vivo requires alternative measurement schemes.

The methods used for mapping the acoustic impedance or sound speed of an inhomogeneous medium such as tissue, are generally referred to as inverse methods. In order to solve the inverse problem, the forward problem, which involves the specification of the wave equation for the medium, must

344

be defined. Due to the very complicated ordering and structure of tissues, especially _in-vivo_, various simplifying assumptions must be made in order to produce a mathematically tractable problem. In one investigation[7], for example, the medium is assumed to be composed of plane-parallel layers of homogeneous, non-attenuating tissue of varying-thickness. The inverse problem was solved for the determination of the impedance profile and was applied to various test media. The results were excellent for synthetic media, however, useful results have not been obtained for tissues _in-vivo_.

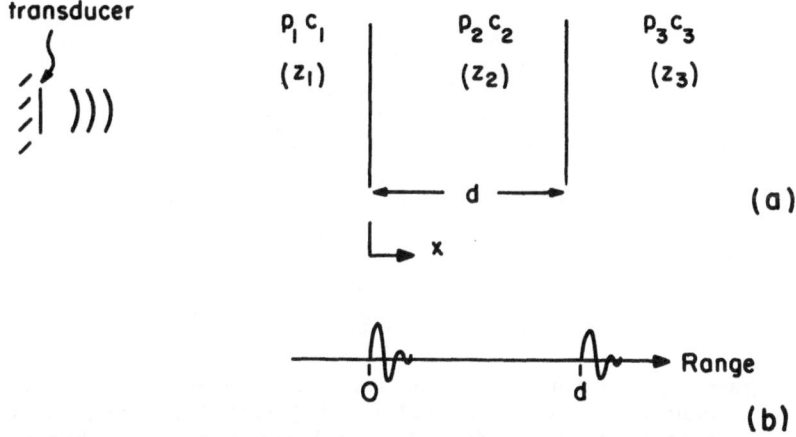

Figure 1: (a) Parallel-plane arrangement for describing reflection at an interface and wave propagation in homogeneous, attenuating media and (b) Typical reflected waveforms.

TABLE 1.

Representative Values of the Density (ρ) and Characteristic Acoustic Impedance (z) of some Biological Media. After Wells[5]

Material	ρ (g ml^{-1})	z (10^6 kg m^{-2} s^{-1})
Blood	1.06	1.62
Bone	1.38–1.81	3.75–7.38
Brain	1.03	1.55–1.66
Fat	0.92	1.35
Kidney	1.04	1.62
Liver	1.06	1.64–1.68
Lung	0.40	0.26
Muscle	1.07	1.65–1.74
Spleen	1.06	1.64–1.67
Water	1.00	1.52

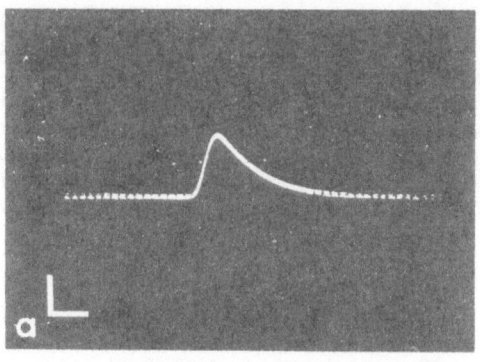

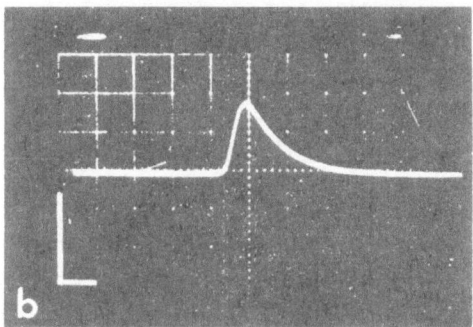

Figure 2. RF-rectified echo from front surface of excised
canine myocardium in saline: (a) normal myocardium, (b)
infarcted myocardium. Vertical bar = 5 volts; horizontal bar = 2 μs. Note that the amplitude of the echo
from the infarcted myocardium is 3.8 volts compared
with 7 volts for the normal myocardium. From Ref. 6.

With the advent of X-ray computed tomography (CT), there have been a
few efforts at using ultrasound CT for obtaining quantitative images[8]. A
detailed description of the theory of ultrasound CT is beyond the scope of
this paper and the reader is referred to Schueler et al[9]. The ideal objective of the ultrasound CT is to map a function of an acoustic parameter,
e.g. sound speed or attenuation. Unfortunately, the wavelengths of ultrasound used are much larger than those of X-ray CT resulting in considerable
diffraction and refraction effects. In essence, the ultrasound CT is an
inverse problem, which requires certain simplifying assumptions in order to
provide a reasonable solution. Although good quality images have been
obtained with ultrasound CT, these images lack the quantitative accuracy
required for tissue characterization.

Clearly, solution of the inverse problem for the determination of
the acoustic sound speed, density, or impedance, requires that the medium
be appropriately modelled. Although sophisticated models exist for the
interaction of ultrasound with tissues[10], there does not exist an appropriate formulation of the forward/inverse problem which yields useful results.
Hence, the determination of these parameters for tissue characterization
in-vivo remains a very complicated problem with a solution not foreseen in
the near future.

III. ACOUSTIC ATTENUATION

The measurement of acoustic attenuation (the loss of acoustic energy as it propagates through a medium) in tissues has certainly been the most promising and popular tissue characterization research area. This stems partly from the fact that the transition from the in-vitro case to the in-vivo case is relatively simple and partly due to evidence that the difference in acoustic attenuation in normal and diseased tissues is quite distinct[11]

The objective of all methods which use attenuation as a tissue characterization parameter is to measure its frequency dependence, which is typically linear with frequency. Thus it has become popular to characterize tissues by the slope of the attenuation coefficient versus frequency[12].

It would be worthwhile to discuss the in-vitro methods for attenuation measurement so that the in-vivo measurements can be more easily understood. Suppose that an ultrasonic beam is transmitted through the tissue and that a detector on the opposite side of the tissue receives the transmitted wave. The attenuation coefficient at a particular frequency is simply related by the ratio of the received energy in the attenuated wave to the energy in the unattenuated wave; the unattenuated wave measured using the same geometry, but with the tissue removed. This method for attenuation measurement, known as the through-transmission method, is unfortunately often inapplicable in clinical practice since the presence of air and bone prevents the complete transmission of sound through the body.

An alternative method for attenuation estimation is known as the pulse-echo method. In this case, the attenuation coefficient is simply related to the pulses reflected from the front and back tissue interfaces. Consider the parallel plane arrangement depicted in Fig 1. Here, a plane acoustic wave is emitted from a transducer into a homogeneous medium with sound speed c_1 and density ρ_1. Located at $x=0$ and $x=d$ are plane interfaces which are oriented perpendicular to the incident wave and bounded by an attenuating medium. Let the spectrum of the signal received at the transducer as a result of reflection from the first interface be $X(\omega)$. The signal spectrum from the back interface, $Y(\omega)$ is then given by

$$|Y(\omega)|=|X(\omega)| \ H(\omega) \tag{3.1}$$

where ω is the radian frequency. For acoustic propagation in homogeneous media,

$$H(\omega)=k \ e^{-\alpha(\omega)(0.23d)} \tag{3.2}$$

where $\alpha(\omega)$ is the frequency-dependent attenuation coefficient(dB/distance), and k is a constant which depends only on the densities and sound speeds of the three regions shown. It is seen from Eq. 3.1 and Eq. 3.2 that $\alpha(\omega)$ can be determined simply by taking the ratio between the back and front echo spectra. This is the method used for all in-vitro pulse-echo attenuation estimation schemes[13]. Fig 3. sequentially illustrates this approach to the in-vitro measurement of attenuation.

Now that some of the properties of signals reflected from homogeneous media, have been established, the nature of signals received from inhomogeneous media, e.g. in-vivo tissues can be discussed. Biological tissues in-vivo are well modelled as inhomogeneous media. Tissue boundaries are rough as opposed to planar and tend to distort impinging acoustic wavefronts. In addition, variations of the elastic constants within the tissue itself cause sound to be internally scattered. As a result, the signals received from such a medium exhibit random fluctuations as depicted in

Fig.4.   Hence, the determination of attenuation from such waveforms requires statistical methods which take into account the complex nature of these waveforms.

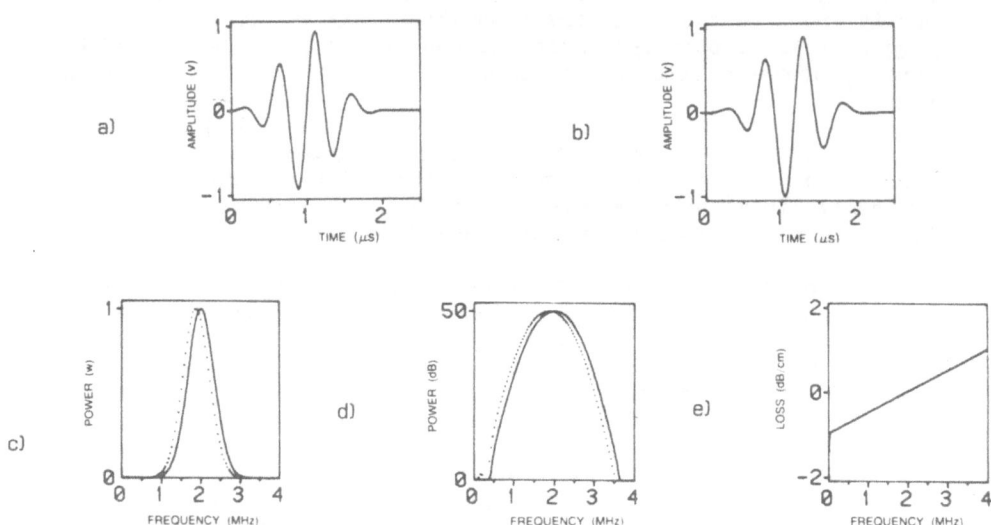

Figure 3.   Time and spectral waveforms of ideal reflections
            for d = 5 cm.   Amplitude normalized waveforms: (a)
            near-interface, (b) far-interface. Normalized spectra:
            (c) power spectra (near - solid, far - dotted) and (d)
            log power spectra (near - solid, far - dotted). (e)
            Attenuation coefficient is the log spectral difference
            divided by round-trip distance between interfaces (10
            cm). From Ref. 12.

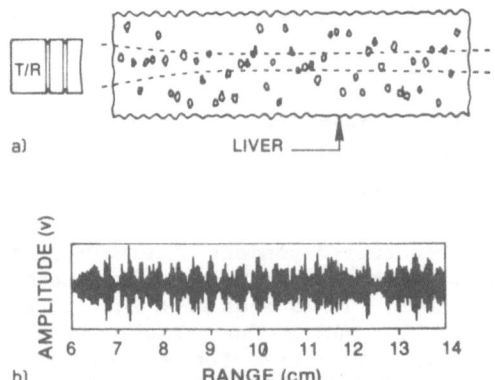

Figure 4.   Due to non-specular interfaces and randomly
            distributed scatterers, ultrasonic signals (A-scans)
            are random in nature. (a) The liver is shown permeated
            by a randomly distributed vascular system. (b) Typical
            A-scan. From Ref. 12.

The use of statistical methods for estimating the attenuation spectrum in tissue was pioneered by Kuc and Schwartz[14] in 1979. The tissue model used in their studies was based on the hypothesis that the tissue interfaces are not planer but are randomly "rough" in space. They further proposed that waves scattered from these random interfaces could be represented as the output of a linear space-invariant filter with an impulse response which depends on the statistical properties of the "roughness". By assuming a Gaussian impulse response with a short duration (such that attenuation is negligible), they arrived at an expression for the power spectrum of a signal reflected from the random interface. The received power spectrum, $Y(\omega)$ is given by

$$Y(\omega)=X(\omega)\ R(\omega) \tag{3.3}$$

where $X(\omega)$ represents the spectrum of the pulse incident on the reflector and $R(\omega)$ represents the distortion due to the spatial variations of the reflector.

Kuc and Schwartz further assumed that the shape of the pulse varies smoothly as it propagates through the medium. In other words, if $X_i(\omega)$ is the wave incident on the ith reflector and $X_j(\omega)$ is the signal incident on the jth reflector then

$$X_i(\omega)=X_j(\omega)e^{-0.23\ \alpha(\omega)\ d} \tag{3.4}$$

where d is the distance between the ith and jth reflectors. Note that Eq.3.4 is identical in form to that developed for the homogeneous case. Combining Eq. 3.3 and Eq. 3.4, the ratio of measured power spectrum of the signal reflected from the jth reflector to that of the ith reflector is

$$Y_j(\omega)/Y_i(\omega)=[R_j(\omega)/R_i(\omega)]\ e^{-0.23\ \alpha(\omega)\ d} \tag{3.5}$$

Hence, the problem of attenuation estimation was reduced to estimating the power spectrum from echoes at differing depths and taking the ratio (or logarithmic difference) between these power spectral estimates. We see from Eq. 3.5 that unless the tissue dependent parameters $R_j(\omega)/R_i(\omega)$ cancel, the attenuation estimate will be biased. Kuc and Schwartz proposed that averaging many independent attenuation estimates as per Eq. 3.5 will lead to unbiased, stable estimates. This is consistent with the assumption that the reflectors behave as zero mean independent stationary processes. The Kuc-Schwartz method for obtaining stable, unbiased spectral estimates is outlined below. The term "Periodogram" is simply the magnitude of the Fourier transform of a time-gated signal.

1. Compute periodogram of signal from reflector at depth x_1

2. Compute periodogram of signal from reflector at depth x_2

3. Perform log spectral difference between these two periodograms as illustrated in Fig 5.

4. Perform steps 1-3 for different reflectors within the tissue and average the log spectral differences.

Kuc[12] provides an excellent summary.

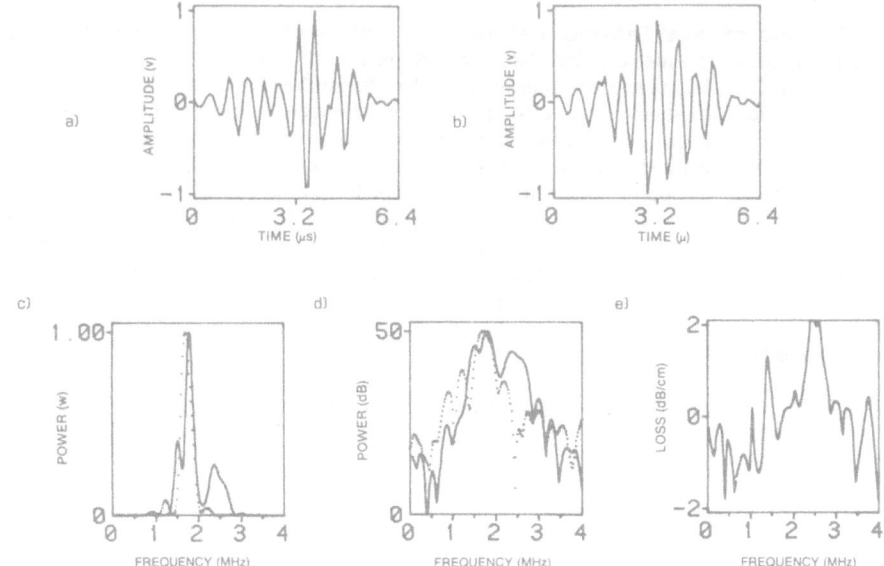

Figure 5. Time and spectral waveforms of actual windowed reflections from regions separated by 5 cm. Amplitude normalized windowed time waveforms: (a) near-region, (b) far-region. (c) Normalized periodograms (near-solid, far - dotted). (d) Normalized log periodograms (near - solid, far - dotted). (e) Attenuation coefficient is estimated from the log periodogram difference divided by round trip distance between regions (10 cm). From Ref. 12.

Since the work of Kuc and Schwartz was published, several variations on their method have been used. These methods all use the ratio of the power spectra at different depths, but utilize different techniques for eliminating the tissue dependent term R_j/R_i. These include spectral smoothing techniques[15] (which averages adjacent frequency bands to obtain estimate stability), combined spectral smoothing and statistical averaging[16], and short-time FFT techniques[17]. Leeman et al[18] provide an excellent summary of these methods.

There are four essential weaknesses to the above approaches:

    1. They assume that the signal is time stationary over short time periods. This may not be true for highly attenuating media.

    2. Because of the above assumption, they need to estimate the power spectrum of a short duration signal. It is well known that classical spectral estimators (e.g. periodogram) have poor performance for this class of signals[19].

    3. The distance d needs to be fairly large to obtain consistent estimates. This implies that the spatial statistics of the reflectors must be stationary throughout the entire medium.

    4. They are essentially one dimensional in nature.

Recently, evidence indicates that for both the _in-vitro_ and _in-vivo_ determination of attenuation, Eq. 3.2 and Eq. 3.4 are too stringent and it has become popular to require the weaker condition that

$$X_i(\omega) = H_j(\omega,d) \, X_j(\omega) \, e^{-0.23\alpha(\omega)d} \qquad (3.6)$$

where $H_j(\omega,d)$ is a complicated, non-stationary function known as the "diffraction correction"[20]. The diffraction correction is required in part due to the use of finite size piezo-electric receivers which average the ultrasonic field and can cause phase cancellation effects[21]. Phase cancellation effects cause the spectra of pulses arriving from drastically different ranges within tissue to be distorted. The diffraction correction has also been used heuristically to account for the non-stationary behavior of tissue as stated in weakness 3 above. Hence, all attenuation estimation schemes which use power spectral estimation techniques on pulses from drastically different depths require a calibration technique, which is complicated and theoretically questionable[18].

Based on the above discussions, it is not surprising that all currently proposed attenuation techniques have proved accurate only in characterizing profuse disease such as cirrhosis of the liver[22]. This is due to the requirement that a large number of estimates need be averaged, and that consistent estimates can only be achieved if the tissue statistics are stationary over long (many cms) acoustic path lengths.

IV. ACOUSTIC SCATTERING

Scattering is the process by which energy is redirected due to the presence of obstacles within the path of a travelling wave. At the wavelengths of ultrasound used in medical diagnosis, the ultrasound wave will undergo scattering as a result of rough interfaces and tissue inhomogeneities due to small variations in the medium's elastic constants. It is this process which gives rise to speckle and texture in ultrasound images of tissues. If changes in scattering characteristics could be correlated with specific tissue structure and pathologies, this property could become a valuable diagnostic aid.

Scattering is typically characterized by a quantity known as the scattering cross section. This is defined to be the ratio of total power scattered by the obstacle(s) to the incident wave intensity. Theoretical relationships for the scattering cross section in terms of the tissue pathology are mathematically involved and the reader is referred to an excellent review by Waag[23]. It is important to note, however, that the scattering cross section depends on the incident wave frequency, the size of the obstacle(s), the geometry of the obstacle(s) and the orientation of the obstacle(s) relative to the transmitting and receiving transducers. Hence, attempts have been made to study the frequency dependence and/or geometrical dependence of this parameter.

The angular dependence of scattering has been considered extensively in characterizing tissues by many investigators, for example Nicholas[24]. These methods are generally based on the hypothesis that the scatterers form a regular array, and that the inter-scatterer separation is relatively fixed, as shown in Fig. 6a. Ultrasound may then be used to determine the acoustical structure of tissue, on a scale corresponding to the wavelengths employed, in a fashion completely analogous to x-ray crystallography. Under the assumption of an ordered array of scatterers, there exists a relation known as Bragg's scattering condition which relates the insonating frequency and the geometry of the array;

$$n\lambda = 2d\,\sin(\theta) \tag{4.1}$$

where λ = ultrasonic wavelength
         n = integer
         d = distance between adjacent scatterers
         θ = angle from the horizontal to the scattered signal

This relation is derived by considering path length differences such that the scattered waves are exactly in phase, yielding maximum constructive interference, as indicated in Fig. 6a. The tissue parameter d may be determined by either fixing the frequency (and hence λ), and then varying the angle θ, or by fixing the angle θ and sweeping the frequency so that differences in path length vary over a number of wavelength. Theoretically, either technique should yield a succession of signal amplitude maxima or minima whose spacing is indicative of the target's internal structure. An example of a typical experimental arrangement for determining scatter as a function of source/receiver separation and typical results are illustrated in fig 6b and fig. 6c respectively. Methods for characterizing the geometry of the scattering region by fixing the scattering angle and sweep the frequency have been described by Fellingham and Somer[25]. Typical results are shown in Fig. 6d. Another method for inferring regular-geometry tissue structure is through the use of cepstrum analysis discussed by Lizzi et al[26].

Unfortunately, tissues do not generally exhibit the degree of regularity required by the Bragg condition, and consistent clinical results based on these methods have not been achieved. Work is currently on going in methods which do not require the Bragg condition[23]. These methods attempt to account for the random spatial distribution of scatterers within tissue. The success of these methods will depend on how well the scattering process in tissue is modelled. It should also be pointed out that a problem with scattering measurements is that in order to measure the frequency dependence of the scattering cross section of tissue, the frequency-dependent attenuation in the medium must be accounted for. It is thus true that only limited success has been achieved in estimating this dependence in-vivo due to uncertainties in the attenuation coefficient.

V. NON-LINEAR PARAMETER

All of the above methods are based on theories which utilize linear acoustics. Experimental evidence tends to indicate that there exist non-linear effects which can occur at higher acoustic intensities. One characterization of non-linear effects is referred to as the non-linear parameter B/A. This parameter is defined by:

$$B/A \approx 2\rho_0\, c_0\, \left. \frac{\partial c}{\partial P} \right|_s \tag{5.1}$$

where ρ_0 and c_0 are the density and sound speed at static pressure, P is the dynamic sound pressure, c is the local sound speed, and the bracketing subscripted by s implies at constant entropy.

Ichida et al[27] were perhaps the first to suggest the use of the B/A parameter as a tissue characterization parameter. It should be noted from the onset, that the acoustic intensities required to produce observable non-linear effects may be large enough to cause tissue damage. We therefore make the distinction that while the parameters described in previous sections were non-invasive, the measurement of B/A may be semi-invasive.

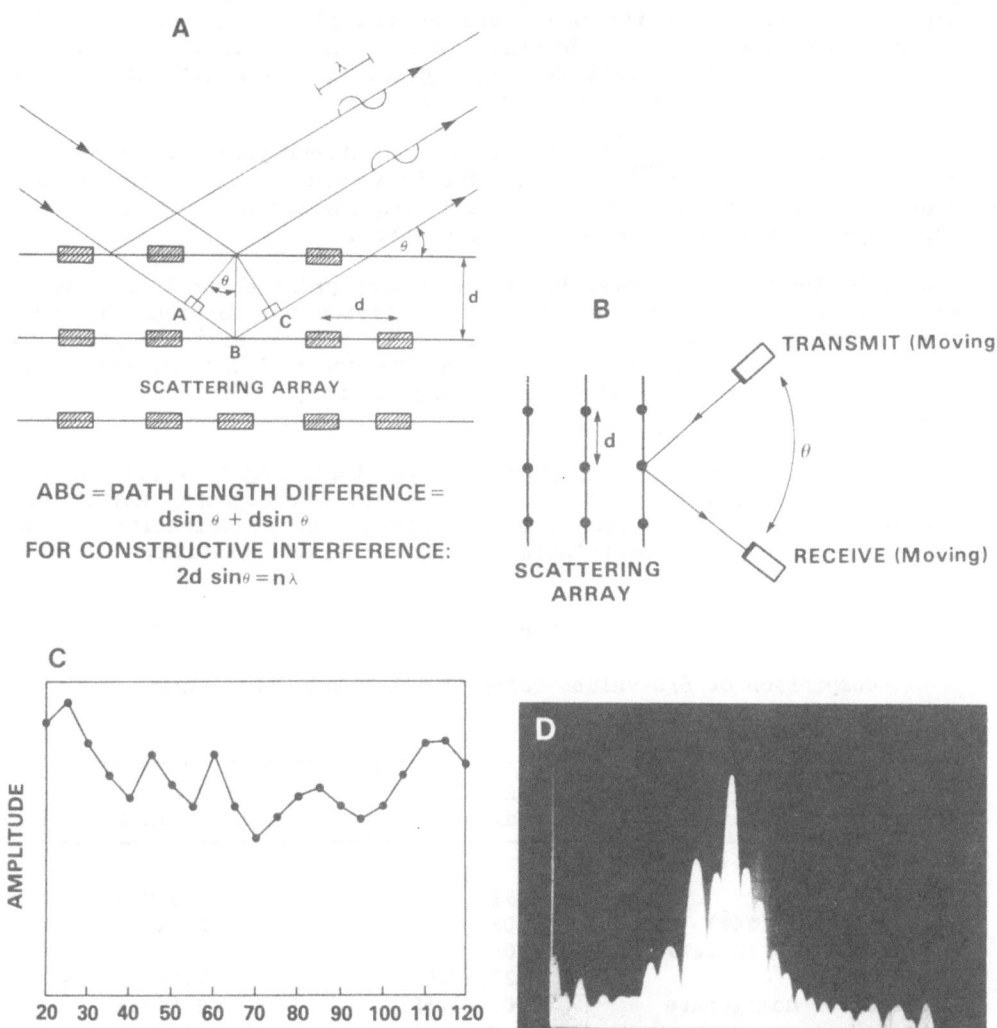

A

ABC = PATH LENGTH DIFFERENCE =
dsin θ + dsin θ
FOR CONSTRUCTIVE INTERFERENCE:
2d sinθ = nλ

SCATTERING ARRAY

B

TRANSMIT (Moving)

RECEIVE (Moving)

SCATTERING
ARRAY

C

AMPLITUDE

ANGLE 2θ

D

Figure 6. (a) Geometry for Bragg diffraction. (b) Double-
angle scanning method. (c) Double-angle scan at 2.25
MHz of fresh calf liver in degassed saline. Average of
5 runs, average periodicity equals 22 degrees of arc.
(d) Scattered frequency spectrum of cat liver. From
Ref. 11.

Several methods have been proposed for measuring the B/A parameter. One class of techniques, known as the finite amplitude methods, involve measuring the generation of a second harmonic component when the medium is insonated with a single frequency source[28]. The amplitude of the generated second harmonic depends not only on the amplitude of the fundamental and B/A parameter, but in addition, depends on the density, sound speed, and attenuation coefficient of the media and on the field properties of the transmitting and receiving transducers. Thus, quantitative measurement of B/A by this method holds promise for in-vitro measurements but not for in-vivo measurements due to uncertainty in the medium/system parameters.

Another method for measuring B/A is to use thermodynamic measurements and apply Eq. 5.1 directly[29]. Again, due to uncertainties in the parameters of the medium and the difficulty in making thermodynamic measurements in-vivo, results must be interpreted with caution.

The non-linearity parameter holds particular promise for tissue characterization since it is directly related to tissue composition. Results obtained from in-vitro experiments performed by Law et al[29] are given in Table 2. Although the results indicate a difference in B/A among different materials, the variation in the results may indicate that B/A is not a sensitive enough parameter.

Methods for measuring B/A in-vivo are just beginning to appear in the literature. Sato et al[30], for example, propose a tomography method for measurement of B/A. It is too soon to evaluate the practicality of the proposed methods and their usefulness in tissue characterization.

TABLE 2

Comparison of B/A values using thermodynamic and finite amplitude methods. From data in Ref. 29.

Material	B/A (Thermodynamic)	B/A (Finite amplitude)
Water	5.31	5.5±0.5
Dextran T150 (24%)	6.05	5.94
Dextran T2000 (26.4%)	6.03	6.2
Beef liver	7.23, 7.0	7.7±0.9
Beef liver homogenate	7.0, 6.53	6.8±0.4
Pig fat	10.9	11.0

VI. CONCLUSIONS

It has long been believed that ultrasound has the potential to non-invasively characterize tissue pathology. For more than a decade, investigators have attempted to obtain information regarding the structure and tissue type from quantitative measurements of acoustic parameters. The hope has been that these techniques would provide more information than is currently available from conventional ultrasound B-scans. To much disappointment, there currently does not exist a clinically consistent and reliable method for the non-invasive ultrasonic characterization of tissues.

The major technical difficulty in providing for a successful tissue characterization technique is clearly our lack of understanding of the interaction of ultrasound with in-vivo tissues. Models proposed for this purpose have either been too simple to produce useful results or too complex and thus mathematically formidable. In addition, attempts at tissue characterization tend to focus on only one parameter (e.g. impedance or attenuation) while it is obvious that the ultrasonic signals received from tissues in-vivo result from combined effects.

Among the parameters discussed in this paper, some appear much more likely to be successful than others. The measurement or mapping of acoustic impedance or sound speed of tissues in-vivo has been and will probably remain for sometime an unsolved problem. This is directly due to the fact that the measurement of these parameters requires the solution of a complex inverse problem. The measurement of attenuation, on the other hand holds considerable promise, since attenuation is a directly observable effect in tissues. Current methods of attenuation measurement can only provide very coarse (several cms) mapping of this parameter, and finer scale mapping will require a more thorough understanding of propagation of ultrasound in three dimensional inhomogeneous media. The solution to the scattering problem will also require this understanding, and the future success of scattering as a tissue characterization parameter is closely related to the success of attenuation estimation. Finally, new parameters, such as B/A, are beginning to appear as possible alternatives for tissue characterization. It is our hope and the hope of the entire medical community that perhaps someday, one or more of the parameters described in this paper will prove useful in the diagnosis of disease.

REFERENCES

1. G. B. Devey and P. N. T. Wells, Ultrasound in medical diagnosis, Sci. Amer. 238, No. 5, 98 (1978).
2. P. P. Lele and J. Namery, Detection of myocardial infarction by ultrasound, in: Proc. of the 25th Annual Conf. on Engng. in Med. and Biol. 14: 135 (1972).
3. N. Senapati, P. P. Lele and A. Woodin, A study of the scattering of submillimeter ultrasound from tissues and organs, in: 1972 I.E.E.E. Ultrasonics Symposium Proc., 72 CHO 708-8 SU, 446 (1972).
4. S. A. Goss, R. L. Johnston, and F. Dunn, Comprehensive compilation of empirical ultrasonic properties of mammalian tissues, J. Acous. Soc. Amer. 64, No. 2, 423 (1978).
5. P. N. T. Wells, "Biomedical Ultrasonics", Academic Press, London/ New York (1977).
6. P. P. Lele and J. Namery, A computer-based ultrasonic system for the detection and mapping of myocardial infarcts, in: Proc. of the San Diego Biomedical Symposium 13: 121 (1974).
7. J. P. Jones, Current problems in ultrasonic impediography, in: Proc. of 1st Conf. on Ultras. Tiss. Char., NBS Spec. Pub. No. 453, 253 (1975).
8. J. F. Greenleaf, S. A. Johnson and A. H. Lent, Measurement of spatial distribution of refractive index in tissues of ultrasonic computer assisted tomography, Ultrasound in Med. & Biol. 3: 327 (1978).
9. C. F. Schueler, H. Lee and G. Wade, Fundamentals of digital ultrasonic imaging, IEEE Trans. Son. and Ultrason., SU-31, No.4, 195 (1984).
10. J. C. Gore and S. Leeman, Ultrasonic backscattering from human tissue: a realistic model, Phys. Med. Biol. 22: No. 2, 317 (1977).

11. P. P. Lele and N. Senapati, The frequency spectra of energy backscattered and attenuated by normal and abnormal tissue, in: Recent Advances in Ultrasound in Biomedicine 1: 55, D.N. White ed., Research Studies Press, Forest Grove, Oregon (1977).

12. R. Kuc, Processing of diagnostic ultrasound signals, IEEE ASSP Magazine 1: No. 1, 19 (1984).

13. G. E. Sleefe and P. P. Lele, A non-invasive tissue characterization technique for use in hyperthermia studies, in: Hyperthermic Oncology 1984 1: 851, J. Overgaard, ed., Taylor & Francis, London and Philadelphia (1984).

14. R. Kuc and M. Schwartz, Estimating the acoustic attenuation coefficient slope for liver from reflected ultrasound signals, IEEE Trans. Sonics and Ultrason. SU-26: 353 (1979).

15. L. Hutchins and S. Leeman, Attenuation estimation by spectral smoothing, in: Ultrasonics International 1983, Z. Novak, ed., Guildford, England: IPC Science and Technology Press (1983).

16. L. Hutchins and S. Leeman, Pulse and impulse response in human tissues, in: Acoustical Imaging 12: 459, E. A. Ash and C. R. Hill, eds., Plenum Press, N.Y. (1982).

17. M. Fink, F. Hottier and J. F. Cardoso, Ultrasound signal processing for in vivo attenuation measurement: short time fourier analysis, in: Ultrasonic Imaging 5: 117 (1983).

18. S. Leeman, L. Ferrari, J. P. Jones and M. Fink, Perspectives on attenuation estimation from pulse-echo signals, IEEE Trans. Sonics Ultrason. SU-31: 352 (1984).

19. S. M. Kay and S. L. Marple, Spectrum analysis – a modern perspective, Proc. IEEE 69: No. 11, 1380 (1981).

20. M. Fink and F. Hottier, Short time fourier analysis and diffraction effect in biological tissue characterization, in: Acoustical Imaging 12: 493, E. A. Ash and C. R. Hill, eds., Plenum Press, N.Y. (1982).

21. P. W. Marcus and E. L. Cartensen, Problems with absorption measurements of inhomogeneous solids, J. Acoust. Soc. Amer. 58: 1334 (1976).

22. Program and abstracts for the Ninth Inter. Symp. Ultrasonic Imaging and Tissue Charact., June 3-6 1984 in: Ultrasonic Imaging 6: 201 (1984).

23. R. C. Waag, A review of tissue characterization from ultrasonic scattering, IEEE Trans. Biom. Engng. BME-31: No. 12, 884 (1984).

24. D. Nicholas, Orientation and frequency dependence of backscattered energy and its clinical application, in: Recent Advances in Ultrasound in Biomedicine 1, D. N. White, ed., Research Studies Press, Forest Grove, Oregon (1977).

25. L. L. Fellingham and F. G. Sommer, Ultrasonic characterization of tissue structure in the in vivo human liver and spleen, IEEE Trans. Sonics and Ultrason. SU-31: 418 (1984).

26. F. Lizzi, N. Feleppa and N. Jaremko, Liver-tissue characterization by digital spectrum and cepstrum analysis, Proc. 1981 Ultras. Symp. 575 (1981).

27. N. Ichida, T. Sato and M. Linzer, Imaging the non-linear ultrasonic parameter, Ultrasonic Imaging 5: 295 (1983).

28. R. T. Beyer, Parameter of non-linearity in fluids, J. Acoust. Soc. Amer. 32: 719 (1960).

29. W. K. Law, L. A. Frizzell, F. Dunn, Determination of the nonlinearity parameter B/A of biological media, Ultras. Med. Biol. 11: No. 2, 307 (1985).

30. T. Sato, A. Fukusima, N. Ichida, H. Ishikawa, H. M. Wa, Y. Igarashi, T. Shimura, and K. Murakami, Non-linear parameter tomography system using counterpropagating probe and pump waves, Ultras. Imaging 7: 49 (1985).

FUTURE TRENDS IN DIAGNOSTIC ULTRASOUND

Marvin C. Ziskin

Professor of Radiology and Medical Physics
Temple University Medical School
3400 N. Broad St.
Philadelphia, PA 19140

Ultrasound has become an essential diagnostic modality in medicine today and will undoubtedly continue to be so. The application of ultrasound has not been a one step process, but has actually evolved in increments over the past 25 to 30 years. The past evolution of diagnostic instruments is a guide for thinking about future trends.

The early A-mode techniques, although very popular in their time, have for the most part been discarded. The reason for this is that these one dimensional techniques have been superceded by two dimensional images in which localization and identification of anatomic landmarks can be performed much easier and with more confidence. Another important factor is that the two dimensional image provides a presentation to the sonologist that he can relate to his knowledge of anatomy much more closely than that of an A-mode scan. This is also true for two dimensional echocardiography in which numerical measurements in one dimension have been replaced by a two dimensional nonquantitative image. Nevertheless, this nonquantitative image provides the clinician with the desired diagnostic information in a very acceptable manner. The conclusions from these developments would imply that techniques will continually evolve toward producing a better image rather than merely a more quantitative measure of tissue properties.

Color has been added occasionally to the ultrasound image in various forms. Most early attempts have been a synthetic color coding of echo amplitudes as seen on the sonogram. This provides a very impressive esthetic image but one that is not really helpful diagnostically. In fact, an argument could be presented that this type of color addition does a good job of camouflaging anatomic structures and results in poorer diagnostic accuracy. However, there has been a meaningful use of color. That is when there is additional independent information to be added to the image. Primarily this is information coming from doppler techniques in which flow information is superimposed upon the anatomic structures. For example, rapid blood flow could be presented as a blue image and red could represent slower blood flow as may occur in veins. This use of color has been added to realtime imaging and has produced rather interesting demonstrations of various flow abnormalities such as patent ventricular septal defects.

Frequencies Utilized

The frequency chosen in diagnostic ultrasound is actually a compromise between penetration and resolution desired. The higher the frequency the less the penetration, but the greater the potental for increased resolution. The earliest frequency used in routine scanning was 2.25 MHz, but with increased sensitivity in instrumentation, the operating frequencies of choice have incremented up to 3.5 MHz for most routine examinations. For some of the more specialized examinations requiring higher resolution, particularly those close to the surface of the skin, frequencies as high as 10 and 15 mHz have been used. As future trends are concerned, it is not likely that ultrasonic frequencies will continue to increase and that frequencies as high as 20 to 25 mHz may actually be utilized in some very special imaging tasks.

There are also possibilities in which differing frequencies could be helpful in the same examination. Some ultrasound transducers have incorporated different frequency crystals on the probe. Different frequencies could also be utilized in reducing speckle in the image.

Acoustic Output Intensities

There appears to have have been a steady progression of increasing acoustic outputs in diagnostic instrumentation. Spatial peak, pulse-average intensities as high as 10,000 W/cm^2 have been reported. Spatial peak-temporal average intensities with dopplers have been measured as high as 1.5 W/cm^2, thus achieving therapeutic levels of ultrasound. There appears to be an increasing awareness of the output levels and increasing concern over the potential biological effects that might ensue. This is of course no accident, as evidenced by the amount of effort expended by the American Institute of Ultrasound in Medicine toward making these facts known. There now exists a delicate balance between the wish to minimize or limit the exposures to patients on one hand and on the other hand the avoidance of over restricting the development of the field to the point of stiffling advancement.

Contrast Agents

The use of contrast agents is not new. They were first introduced into diagnostic ultrasound by Gramiak in 1968. These have had considerable usefulness in cardiovascular ultrasonography. In some regions of the body natural contrast agents such as urine is found to be very valuable. That is, patients undergoing pelvic examination are instructed to drink considerable amounts of water to fill their bladder. This provides a natural highly transmitting body for better visualization of deeper structures. The inbibing of methyl cellulose has also been recommended as a contrast agent to visualize the stomach wall. Currently there is great interest in a new development of utilizing encapsulated gaseous microspheres as a contrast agent to be injected. This appears to be very promising but work remains to be performed.

Doppler Techniques

Interest in doppler ultrasound has increased markedly in recent years. A large part of this has been due to combining this modality with the cross sectional imaging of standard B-scans. This has resulted in the ability to visualize where the doppler signal is being obtained. Also possible is the ability to sample very small regions such as in specific arteries or veins. The combining of doppler with realtime B-scan is referred to as duplex scanning. It has become standard practice doppler. In addition, some manufacturers have added to this, continuous wave doppler for additional information and they refer to this as triplex imaging. The usefulness of dopplers for evaluating blood velocity and ultimately blood flow can be very valuable. One of the interesting newer techniques is evaluating blood flow to the fetus by measuring the blood flow in the umbilical vein. It is believed that this is an important advance in that it provides, in addition to morphological evaluation of fetal health, a physiological or functional evaluation.

Doppler has also been added to carotid artery scanning in realtime and has become effectively the modality of choice for screening in this procedure. Confidence in this imaging modality has increased in the estimation of surgeons and will no doubt continue to do so.

Tissue Characterization

The analysis of ultrasonic echoes returning from tissues has been used as a means by which tissue can be "finger printed". Certainly ultrasound interacts with tissue in a number of important ways and in turn is modified by the mechanical properties of the tissue through which it passes. By measuring such tissue properties as acoustic impedance, acoustic conduction velocity, ultrasonic absorption and the frequency dependency of these properties it may be possible to characterize and distinguish abnormal tissues from normal tissues. Most of the efforts in this area have been toward studies of liver. Although having some interesting results they have not achieved clinical utility at the present time. One area that has been successful for clincal use has been characterization of the tissues of the eye. This no doubt will continue to be of value. Instrumentation manufacturers are looking very seriously into those tissue characterization techniques that could be helpful clinically. No doubt several of these will become commerically available in the very near future.

FM Modulation

Echography is primarily concerned with the spatial location and amplitude of returning echoes from the body. However, one new approach is FM modulation or phase analysis of returning echoes. It is hoped that this approach will be less sensitive to resolution artifacts and specular reflection distortions in the sonogram. Imaging ultilizing this approach and also combining this with the standard B-mode type of display will be likely to appear soon.

Office Practice of Ultrasound

When ultrasound first became available, the instrumentation was awkward to use and required a great deal of sophistication, besides being expensive. Then centralized usage of ultrasound was the major way in which ultrasound was practiced in medical centers and hospitals. As instrumentation became more convenient, simple to use, and less expensive in many ways, instrumentation found its way into private physicians' offices, particularly in those of obstetricians. This trend has continued and is ever increasing. Manufacturers are now approaching general practitioners as a potential market for their instruments. There is no doubt that the employment of diagnostic units in private unit offices will increase.

The use of ultrasound in pregnancy is very well established as an indispensible diagnostic aide in clinical practice. Its use in routine screening, that is in examining women merely because of their being pregnant, is somewhat controversial at this time. Good arguments exist on both sides as to whether this should be performed. This ultimately should be a physician's judgement; however, economic concerns, namely reimbursement, may very well be the over riding driving force as to whether this is done or not.

As the use of ultrasound has increased in practice there has been an increase in a number of malpractice cases that have come to court in the United States. This, no doubt, will continue to increase as physicians are sued both for doing ultrasound with poor results and for not performing ultrasound when they should have.

An additional factor in the economics consideration for use of ultrasound lies in changes that are occurring in reimbursement procedures. We have now instituted a repayment scheme based upon diagnostic related groups (DRG). In this procedure a hospital is reimbursed a certain amount of money for a given diagnosis regardless of the resources or procedures that are performed on this patient in the hospital. The purpose of this is to encourage the hospital to reduce unnecessary utilization of resources. As applied to imaging, this will tend to increase the likelihood of performing ultrasound examinations when the ultrasound examination can provide the necessary diagnostic information. This is because ultrasound is typically considerabily less expensive than other imaging modality currently being used.

Computerization

The development of microprocessor technology resulting in more powerful units and yet much less expensive, has produced considerable benefit for ultrasound instrumentation. The incorporation of microprocessors into this instrumentation is now common place and an ever increasing number of tasks are being accomplished by them. For example, the properties of transducers and resulting sound beams can be adjusted for which producing the sonographic image. Multi element transducer arrays can be fired under microprocessor control and returning echoes processed and analysed in ingenious ways to maximize spatial resolution to permit the greatest possible anatomic detail visualization. Initially most multielement transducer arrays were fired in a sequential pattern. However, this seems to be changing such that the relative percentage fired as a phased array is ever increasing. In fact, many commercially available transducer arrays today have combined elements of both phased array and sequential firing in various porpotions. The phased arrays are tending to become smaller so that they are more easily handled, and thus internal anatomy is more easily interrogated with the ultrasound beam. The sector scan format of scanning has superseded the rectangular scan format of the old sequentially fired arrays.

System Design

There is a steady trend toward realtime imaging with small hand held devices with a sector format. These are in self contained units that are readily portable, and can be carried to the bedside or maintained in a office. The prices of these have remained constant or have actually decreased over the years. Relatively inexpensive units are available for physicians to use in their private offices.

At the same time, sophisticated large ultrasound instruments are continually being developed for major diagnostic facilities. These take advantage of the latest processing developments with computerized technology and the design to provide the maximum diagnostic quality in the images.

Fundamental Limitation for Ultrasonic Imaging

It is of interest to consider the question, how good can ultrasonic imaging become, or equivalently, what are the fundamental limitations on ultrasonic imaging. Are we presently close to that limit, or can we expect significant improvement in the future? To get a handle on approaching an answer to these questions, it is necessary to consider the three major goals of ultrasonic imaging: adequate temporal resolution, adequate spatial resolution, and adequate penetration (depth of view).

Adequate temporal resolution is required to visualize anatomic motion as it occurs. Realtime imaging requires a minimum of 15 frames per second. In order to see rapidly moving structures, such as the cardiac valves, higher frame rates are required. 30, and possibly 60 frames per second may be necessary.

Adequate spatial resolution is required for depicting fine anatomical detail in the ultrasound image. A major determinant of this is the number of independent scan lines in an image. Each scan line is initiated by an ultrasonic pulse as it leaves the transducer, and the scan line displays all returning echoes up to the time of the successive pulse emission. As many as 400 scan lines per image may be necessary for high quality images.

Penetration or depth of view is the third important consideration in imaging. The depth of view is proportional to the time interval between pulses. Whereas some diagnostic procedures, such as ophthalmic or thyroid imaging, may require a depth of view of only 3 or 4 centimeters, some diagnostic procedures will require a depth of field of over 20 centimeters. It takes 13 microseconds for a sound pulse to leave the transducer, reflect off of an object one centimeter into the body, and then return. Thus, the depth of view (in cm) is equal to the pulse interval divided by 13 microseconds. Alternatively, penetration can be expressed as one half the speed of sound divided by the pulse repetition frequency.

The above three desirable quantities can be related in a equation. That is:

$$\text{FRAME RATE X NUMBER OF LINES X PENETRATION} = 77{,}000$$

This is the fundamental limitation for imaging. The product of the three goals is a constant. If you wish to improve on any one of these, one or both of the other aims will have to be diminished. The constant equals one half the sonic speed in soft tissue expressed in centimeters per second, and thus the limiting factor for diagnostic imaging is in fact the speed of sound. We are at this limit at the current state of the art. In order to produce any significant improvment in imaging over the future, we will need to either encode pulses, utilize multiple transducers, or employ some other clever scheme to circumvent this theoretical limitation.

Summary

Predicting future trends is certainly a difficult task. These have been my personal thoughts and may or may not have any correlation with ultimate reality. However, I trust that the above may provide some idea as to what may be expected in the near future.

PANEL DISCUSSION ON MECHANISMS AND BIOLOGICAL EFFECTS

Nyborg, W. L. (Chairman), Carstensen, E., Giese, K.,
ter Haar, G., Lele, P. and Williams, A. R.

To guide the discussion, a series of proposals, or statements, (controversial to a varying extent) were presented by
the chairman and displayed for panelists and audience to
examine. It was explained that these represented or resembled
ideas that had been advanced at one time or another by one or
more individuals. For each of the proposals, one of the
panelists was asked to give a brief initial assessment, after
which the topic was opened to discussion by other members of
the panel, and the audience.

Proposal 1: "All cellular changes produced by
ultrasound in vitro are caused by cavitation."

Dr. Williams was asked to give the initial response to this
proposal. He expressed general agreement with it, based on
his recollection of reports in the literature, dealing with
cellular effects produced in vitro. When there are positive
findings, and the mechanisms have been successfully identified, they usually involve microstreaming stresses generated
by cavitation bubbles. Exceptions would be experiments where
vibrating wires or other special methods are used to generate
microstreaming by noncavitational means.

Dr. Repacholi asked, "If this is true, why do in vitro
experiments?" There is little evidence that ultrasound
affects mammalian tissue via cavitational mechanisms. Hence
results obtained in vitro would seem to have little relevance
to clinical situations.

Dr. Williams agreed that this consideration does cause
difficulty in extrapolating from in vitro experiments to in
vivo situations. However, there is a growing body of evidence
that cavitation-related activity might occur in vivo. Dr.
Lele gave his support to the use of well-planned in vitro
experiments. Any effect observed in vitro may occur in vivo,
though to a different extent.

Dr. Williams added that cells are often affected indirectly, in that cavitation destroys some cells, thus releasing

enzymes or other factors which produce changes in remaining cells. It is good experimental practice to test for this possibility: when ultrasound is found to produce some kind of change in a cell suspension, add a small quantity of homogenized cells to a control suspension and observe whether a similar change occurs.

> Proposal 2: 'Intensity' has no value for characterizing near-field features of medical devices".

Dr. Giese began the discussion by reviewing experimental methods available for measuring acoustic quantities. The methods involve the use of radiation-force devices, optical arrangements, thermocouples, thermistors or hydrophones. Of these, only the latter, which measure acoustic pressure rather than intensity, offer the spatial and temporal resolution required for characterizing the complex fields encountered in medical applications of ultrasound. Hence "pressure" is preferred over "intensity" because of measurement considerations.

In addition, pressure is preferred over intensity because of its greater relevance to physical mechanisms for producing biological effects. For example, at a point in the near field of a transducer the local rate of heat production (Q) typically bears little relation to the local value of intensity. Instead, for an important class of media, Q is proportional to the square of the local acoustic pressure. (For this to be true, however, the medium must be such that the shear viscosity coefficient, also called the imaginary part of the shear modulus, is of negligible importance).

Dr. Carstensen pointed out that in therapeutic applications, the tissue exposed to ultrasound lies in the near field. He asked, "Would you recommend that physical therapists speak in terms of pressure from now on? Would use of 'intensity' lead to significant error?" Dr. Giese replied that since heating is involved he believes a description of the pressure distribution would be a correct step. Use of intensity instead of pressure can lead to errors up to a factor of two (for Q, the local rate of heat production) in small regions, but would be less for averages over larger regions. Dr. Williams observed that in accepted practice the transducer is continually moved during a therapeutic application. Since this causes additional averaging, he suggested that the above-mentioned errors would be minimal.

> Proposal 3: "Temperature elevation is the primary cause of significant effects produced by ultrasound in living mammals."

Dr. Lele initiated the discussion by stating that he would support a revised statement, as follows: "Temperature elevation is the primary cause of any significant biological effects produced by current diagnostic-ultrasound techniques in organized or nonfluid tissues in living mammals." He went on to say that in fluid tissues there can be other mechanisms, and that at higher intensities cavitation occurs, even in solid tissues. Whether at these higher levels the temperature elevation is accompanied by shear stresses and acoustic streaming in intercellular spaces is at present not known.

Also it is not known what biological significance these latter phenomena may have, in themselves.

Questions were raised from the audience about the applicability of these ideas when the ultrasound is delivered in repeated short pulses, as in diagnostic ultrasound. Dr. Lele replied that this topic would be treated further in his lectures.

Dr. Ziskin observed that no hazard presented by pulse-echo ultrasound has yet been identified clinically. In spite of over 25 years of continued and extensive clinical usage, there has been no known instance of an adverse effect caused by the use of ultrasound in diagnosis.

> Proposal 4 "For diagnostic ultrasound, nonlinear waveform distortion is important in water, but not in mammalian tissue."

Dr. Carstensen gave the initial assessment of this statement. He remarked that, like most of the five proposals considered by the panel, it is neither completely true nor completely false. In respect to Proposal 4, if one allows for some exceptions, it is a reasonable statement. Most applications of ultrasound can be handled very nicely with linear theory. This includes the analysis of important biological effects caused by heating. On the other hand there is convincing evidence from the work of Starritt et al (1985) that harmonics are generated under some circumstances during the propagation of diagnostic ultrasound through (human calf) tissue. It is not clear how important this is for diagnostic procedures.

Dr. Ziskin remarked that it may be very important in diagnostic techniques to be aware of distortion produced by nonlinearity, in the analysis of returning echoes. He and Dr. Carstensen agreed that awareness of saturation phenomena may influence manufacturing practice. For example, manufacturers may find that little is gained by generating pulses of extremely high intensity.

> Proposal 5: "Nonthermal mechanisms are always involved in effects produced by therapeutic-level ultrasound on mammalian tissues (even when the primary mechanism is thermal).

Dr. ter Haar, who made the initial response to this proposal, expressed support for it. She stated her thesis that at therapeutic levels temperature rise is unavoidable, but that as the temperature gets high, so does the cavitational and noncavitational-nonthermal activity. She illustrated possibilities by describing an example where heat and cavitation act together. In experiments on bubble growth induced by therapeutic ultrasound in the leg of a guinea pig, more bubbles appeared when the ambient temperature was 43 $^{\circ}$C than under otherwise comparable conditions when the temperature was 37 $^{\circ}$C. (She also reported recent findings that bubble growth occurs in a gel when it is exposed to diagnostic pulsed ultrasound instead of therapeutic ultrasound.)

Dr. Lele found it to be "totally obvious" from the work

cited, and from previous work, that temperature enhances cavitation. (He has also found that cavitation enhances heating). The question is not whether nonthermal activities occur in non-fluid tissues but whether they are biologically significant at therapeutic levels.

Dr. ter Haar believed it would be difficult to distinguish between damage from nonthermal and thermal causes when the two exist together. Dr. Lele disagreed; he considered it possible to distinguish regions of uniformly coagulated materials produced by heat from highly localized regions of disrupted materials produced by cavitation. Dr. Carstensen referred to earlier work of Pond (1970) in which the lesion produced by focused ultrasound was shown to appear very similar to a lesion produced by heat from a small heated wire. Dr. ter Haar replied that the apparent similarity does not rule out cavitation events occurring in the midst of the lesion; these would not be seen since the tissue there is completely coagulated.

Dr. Ziskin suggested that judicious use of pulsed regimes would help in distinguishing thermal from nonthermal mechanisms. Dr. ter Haar agreed that this would be possible in future work.

In further comments, Dr. Mazzeo pointed out the importance of knowing thresholds for cavitation effects. Dr. Mariutti suggested that it would be useful to compare findings on nonthermal phenomena for ultrasound with those for other radiations. Dr. Williams stressed the importance of research collaborations which include expertise in both biology and physics.

REFERENCES

Pond, J. B., 1970. The role of heat in the production of ultrasonic focal lesions, J. Acoust. Soc. Am. 47:1607.

Starritt, H. C., Perkins, M. A., Duck, F. A. and Humphrey, V. F., 1985. Evidence for ultrasonic finite-amplitude distortion in muscle using medical equipment, J. Acoust. Soc. Am. 77: 302-306.

INDEX